This book is dedicated to:

Barb and Murray

Who have been brave enough to stand up
for what they wanted in their personal lives

And to all the other individuals
With developmental disabilities
who have charted our pathway to
understanding

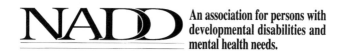

Acknowledgements

Firstly, we are grateful for the opportunity to develop this book. In saying that, Barbara Vyrostko, Executive Director of the Welland District Association for Community Living deserves particular recognition, as her support and flexibility made it all possible. She trusted us to take a chance with the conference, then had the confidence for us to continue the journey toward the completion of this book.

Our thanks to the group leaders who kindly volunteered their time and expertise and to all participants who attended the conference, we were encouraged by your presence and valuable suggestions.

In addition, we acknowledge the exceptional contributions of the chapter authors. Your masterful skills captured the essence of both a clinical and human viewpoint.

A special debt of gratitude to Dick Sobsey, at the University of Alberta, for his many years of invaluable research that greatly influenced the pathway of several chapters.

David DiGaetano, thank you for your amazing computer knowledge. Your patience with us was admirable.

We also thank everyone else who believed in this project from the initial meetings to the final stages. You encouraged us through the uncharted waters in the hope of making a difference in the sexual lives of people who have developmental disabilities.

Thank You

Ethical Dilemmas: Sexuality and Developmental Disability

D. Griffiths, D. Richards, P. Fedoroff, & S. Watson (Editors)

Page

Foreword

Jason's Story

Jason is a kind-hearted, soft-spoken, twenty-seven year old man who has a moderate degree of developmental disability.

Jason and his family have always been strong in their religious faith. His mother and father devoted their parenting years to supporting Jason. Supporting Jason, however, became increasingly difficult as they aged.

Three years ago, Jason moved into a residence operated by an agency that supports individuals with developmental disabilities. There were six men and five women living in this home.

This agency had a sexuality policy which placed sanctions against any sexual behaviour other than masturbation. Jason's family were initially in agreement with this policy, given their religious background.

This policy had been approved ten years previously by the Board of Directors of this agency. Statements in the policy arose from concern regarding the prevention of pregnancies and transmission of sexually transmitted diseases, family disapproval of sexual relationships, community perceptions, and concern regarding consent issues (includes religious beliefs that could not condone sexual relationships outside of marriage). Front-line staff received training regarding this policy and were expected to follow its guidelines regardless of their own personal value system.

While living at this residence, Jason developed a friendship with Sarah, a 24 year old woman who also resided at the group home. They began spending time together. Jason and Sarah would go for walks, play card games, eat meals together, go to the movies, and frequently just sit and talk. Staff supported this friendship and encouraged their daily interactions. This relationship became intimate over the next year, and Jason and Sarah began to have a sexual relationship without staff awareness. To prevent getting "caught", they became not only cautious, but also very secretive.

However, on one occasion, a staff person discovered Jason and Sarah having sexual intercourse in Sarah's bedroom. The staff were appalled, despite their previous beliefs that this was a healthy relationship. Consequently, Sarah was sent to live in another group home and Jason was told he had to attend sex education classes as well as being supervised on a one-to-one basis at the group home.

Approximately one year later, Jason became interested in a woman named Paula, who attended the same workplace as Jason. The two had lunch and breaks together. Several months later, staff walked into the shipping and receiving area and discovered Jason and Paula engaged in heavy petting. Paula was sent to another workplace against her desire to stay. Jason was told he would be attending social skills training. One-to-one supervision was now extended to the workplace.

Jason disliked being supervised and would often wander off when staff would become distracted. Approximately twenty elopements were recorded in one month. On one of these occasions, Jason was found in the bathroom at the workplace having sexual intercourse with Cathy, a female who also worked at the same place as Jason. This woman had limited verbal skills and it was believed she was more cognitively impaired than Jason. Her ability to provide informed consent in this sexual relationship was therefore questioned.

A police investigation was initiated. They questioned both Jason and Cathy, but found it difficult to confirm that non-consensual sexual contact had occurred.

Cathy's parents wanted the legal matter against Jason dropped, but were threatening action against the agency for failing to adhere to its sexual policy and provide adequate supervision.

Jason was referred to a psychiatrist for an evaluation to investigate the possibility of "hypersexuality" and "rape tendencies". Staff requested the doctor prescribe Depo-Provera to decrease "inappropriate" sexual arousal displayed by Jason.

What happened to the kind hearted, soft-spoken man named Jason? Anything? Did the system fail him? Was Jason expressing himself inappropriately? Was Jason ever given opportunity to express himself appropriately? Was there a victim in this case? Who was it? Are staff obligated to follow a policy statement, if it violates the rights of individuals regardless of disability or ability? Can people with developmental disabilities have sexual relationships that are satisfying and fulfilling? Is this possible when the people who are involved in their lives struggle with ethical dilemmas surrounding the topic of sexuality? Are there answers to these questions? For Jason and people who have experienced similar problems, we hope so.

Preface

Sexuality and Developmental Disabilities: Rights for Sexual Health

Eli Coleman

Like anyone else, individuals with developmental disabilities are sexual beings. They have sexual feelings, attitudes, and engage in sexual behaviour. Similarly, they are entitled to the same rights for basic and fundamental sexual health.

Before one can define sexual health, one needs to define sexuality. There have been many attempts to do so. At the Program in Human Sexuality at the University of Minnesota, the following definition has been used for the past 30 years:

"Sexuality is, in the broadest sense, the psychic energy which finds physical and emotional expression in the desire for contact, warmth, tenderness, and love."

The World Health Organization has defined sexuality in a similar way:

"Sexuality is an integral part of the personality of everyone: man, woman, and child. It is a basic need and an aspect of being human that cannot be separated from other aspects of human life" (World Health Organization, 1975).

The WHO goes on to say:

"Sexuality is not synonymous with sexual intercourse, it is not about whether we have orgasms or not, and it is not the sum total of our erotic lives. These may be part of our sexuality, but equally they may not be. Sexuality is so much more: it is in the energy that motivates us to find love, contact, feel warmth, and intimacy; it is expressed in the way we feel, move, touch and are touched; it is about being sensual as well as sexual. Sexuality influences thoughts, feelings, actions, and interactions and thereby our mental and physical health" (World Health Organization, 1975).

Defining Sexual Health

The World Health Organization (1975) defined sexual health as containing three components. The definition includes the following: (i) a capacity to enjoy and control sexual and re-productive behaviour in accordance with a social and personal ethic, (ii) freedom from fear, shame, guilt, false beliefs, and other psychological factors inhibiting sexual response and impairing sexual relationship, and (iii) freedom from organic dis-orders, diseases, and deficiencies that interfere with sexual and reproductive functions.

In my own definition, I try to incorporate many of the same components with some elaboration. Sexual health is certainly more than freedom from diseases and disorders. It involves the capacity to derive pleasure from sexual activity and inti-mate relationships. It is non-exploitative, respectful of self and others. Ultimately, it is rewarding and joyous. It depends upon an individual's well being and their sense of self-esteem. And, it requires trust, honesty and communication between partners (Coleman, 1997).

In all the attempts to define sexual health, there is recognition that these definitions are bound by cultural norms and behaviours. It is difficult to say that there is a universal definition of sexual health. However, these definitions give some parameters of which the sexual health of an individual, relationship or community could be judged. And, I believe that this definition would be applicable to most people with developmental disabilities.

Promoting Sexual Health among Individuals with Developmental Disabilities

We need to advocate for sexual health as a basic human right—especially for those who are sexually disenfranchised. At the conclusion of the 13th World Congress of Sexology, the Valencia Declaration on Sexual Rights (adopted in Valencia, Spain on June 19, 1997) was presented (Borras Valls & Perez Conchillo, 1997).

As President of the World Association for Sexology, I formed a commission at this conference to study this document and to gain input and support from its various member societies around the world. The purpose was to adopt a consensus declaration during the 14th World Congress of Sexology in 1999 in Hong Kong. This commission completed its work, and a new Declaration of Sexual Rights was adopted unanimously by the General Assembly on August 26, 1999. The preamble of the declaration states:

"Sexuality is an integral part of the personality of every human being. Its full development depends upon the satisfaction of basic human needs such as the desire for contact, intimacy, emotional expression, pleasure, tenderness and love. Sexuality is constructed through the interaction between the individual and social structures. Full development of sexuality is essential for individual, interpersonal, and societal well being. Sexual rights are universal human rights based on the inherent freedom, dignity, and equality of all human beings. Since health is a fundamental human right, so must sexual health be a basic human right. In order to assure that human beings and societies develop healthy sexuality, the following sexual rights must be recognized, promoted, respected, and defended by all societies through all means. Sexual health is the result of an environment that recognizes, respects, and exercises these sexual rights." (World Association for Sexology, 1999)

The rights of persons with developmental disabilities is covered specifically in the fourth point of the declaration, The right to sexual equity. This refers to freedom from all forms of discrimination regardless of sex, gender, sexual orientation, age, race, social class, religion, or physical and emotional disability. This implies that persons with developmental disabilities should have the same rights to the remaining sexual rights including the right to comprehensive sexuality education, sexual activity, form relationships, marry, and reproduce (balanced with right of offspring and society). As with all rights, they come with responsibilities. One of the most important responsibilities is to respect the rights of others.

Our challenge as professionals working with persons with developmental disabilities is clear: *We have the responsibility to provide persons who have a developmental disability with their rights to sexual health. This is our responsibility and our duty.*

References

Borras-Valls, J.J. & Perez-Conchilllo, M. (Eds.) (1997). *Sexuality and human rights.* Valencia, Spain: Instituto de Sexologia y Psicoterapia.

Coleman, E. (1997). Promoting sexual health: The challenges of the present and future. In J.J. Borrás-Valls & M. Pérez-Conchillo (Eds). *Sexuality and human rights* (pp. 25-35). Valencia, Spain: Instituto de Sexología y Psicoterapia.

World Association for Sexology. (1999). *Declaration of sexual rights.* Author.

World Health Organization. (1975). *Education and treatment in human sexuality: The training of health professionals.* Technical Report Series Nr. 572. Geneva, Switzerland: Author.

Introduction

Dorothy M. Griffiths, Debbie Richards, Paul Fedoroff, and
Shelley L. Watson

Professionals who work in systems that support individuals
who have developmental disabilities, are constantly faced with
ongoing ethical dilemmas in regards to issues of sexuality.
What is common practice? Would it be fair to say you would
prefer others to make the final decision? Do you struggle with
balancing the rights of individuals with parental or societal expectations? What would be considered ethically correct? In
1998, a conference was planned to address these questions and
develop a consensus among participants regarding ethical
practice in the area of sexuality.

Ethics is a "common" word in many professions. Physicians
and psychologists must meet the ethical standards set for the
well-being of each patient. Research-oriented clinicians are
guided by ethics committees to ensure individual rights are not
being violated. Social workers are governed by a code of
ethics that guides the treatment of people in different social
environments. Scientists have to consider the Bio-ethics of
their research and the effects it may have on humans. Ethics
are recognized in many professions, yet when it comes to what
is ethical regarding sexuality and persons who have a
developmental disability, there are no set standards or
practices. Basically, each case is treated differently, depending
on who is in the position to make decisions. Occasionally, a
person with a disability may be assertive enough to stand up

and address what they want. However, this is rare.

At the turn of the last century, clinicians were confronted with a growing awareness that sexual behaviour was ubiquitous and could not be ignored. By the end of the century, major changes had occurred. Masturbation was accepted as "normal", female sexuality had become a topic outside of pathology journals, homosexuality was no longer listed as a psychiatric disease, pornography had become a major industry, birth control was now a primary school topic, syphilis was curable, and AIDS was controllable. Times had changed for the "average citizen".

But what happened to the needs and concerns of citizens with developmental disabilities? This is the question the editors of these volumes asked themselves in 1998. The literature was largely silent, yet front-line workers kept posing questions. "We have a client who masturbates. Is it OK? We think two of our clients are gay; What do we do? Should we censor mail? Is it okay to provide condoms? Is it okay not to?; One of our clients is HIV positive. Who do we tell? What do we do?"

Recognizing it was no longer acceptable to do nothing or to rely on limited personal or professional experience, we decided to ask the experts. At this point in time, the experts are the people involved in the practice of clinical, medical, legal, and family support to persons with developmental disabilities.

Rather than re-inventing the wheel, the editors turned to the rich literature and experience of the field of continuing education. Continuing education (CE) has dealt with related issues of assessing problems, measuring them, and developing interventions in ways that are client-oriented to produce demonstrable results. The process we adapted was as follows:

Needs Assessment

A questionnaire was distributed to approximately 100 people who were affiliated with agencies that served individuals who have a developmental disability in the province of Ontario, Canada. Participants were asked what types of "ethical issues involving sexuality and individuals who have a developmental disability keep them awake at night". They were instructed to list 3 issues or case examples that are representative of the ethical issues they face in their day to day work.

In response to our inquiry, 50 respondents identified ethical issues which had been encountered while addressing the issue of sexuality in the lives of people with developmental disabilities. These responses were reviewed and categorized into themes and sub-themes. Questions were then developed that reflected each of these themes.

The following case scenario is illustrative of the outcome of the process:

A 19 year-old female with a mild disability is referred to an obstetrician-gynecologist requesting a tubal ligation. She is the daughter of two prominent members of a local church. A year ago, she was involved with a young man who talked her into engaging in sexually intimate behaviour with him. She refers to the incident as "sexual abuse". Her parents responded to the incident by punishing the young woman and saying that she "should set a better example for the young people in the church". The ob-gyn refers the girl for counselling because he is reluctant to do the procedure despite the girl's well-rehearsed "consent". In the interim, the girl is prescribed Depo-Provera. She is obliged to personally purchase this medication while on a limited budget and experiences side effects.

This case raises many issues with regards to the sexuality of individuals who have a developmental disability. Specifically, issues of *Birth Control and Sterilization* and issues regarding *Guardianship (informed consent)* were identified. Questions were then created for the discussion groups based on these issues.

For the Birth Control and Sterilization discussion group, the following question was posed:

Following the case of Eve (Supreme Court of Canada decision), are sterilization procedures (e.g. tubal ligations) ever viable options? If so, when? Who gives consent for these procedures?

For the Guardianship discussion group, the following question was posed:

Does a guardian have the right to impose medical procedures (hormone therapy or arousal reduction drugs, sterilization, tubal ligation, birth control) on the individual without the individual's fully informed consent?

The questionnaire data served as the basis for selected topics for the sessions. For those themes that were repeated in the information collected, two sessions were created with a slightly different perspective than the other.

The editors sent letters to the agencies inviting them to send representatives to attend a two-day conference to discuss the issues they had identified. The CE literature refers to this as "recruitment". Conference attendees were asked to sign up for two of the sessions that most interested them. Consumers, parents, front line staff, police, administrators, medical doctors, psychiatrists, psychologists, social workers, teachers, religious sector, therapists, nurses and mental health professionals were invited. "Experts" were selected to lead small group sessions dealing with the issues identified by the conference attendees. All the "experts" were professionals prominent in a field related to the topic of interest. For example, a police detective currently working in a sexual assault unit was selected to lead the session on reporting sexual assault. A medical doctor who specialized in obstetrics and gynecology led the session on "birth control and sterilization". A Crown Attorney, who was well versed in the legalities of consent agreed to be a group leader. Another lawyer specializing in advocacy for vulnerable people became the "guardianship" group leader. However, the editors made it clear that the true "experts" were those dealing with the issues first hand.

Small consensus sessions were held for each topic. The consensus group comprised of 10 – 20 participants along with the group leader and leader's assistant who documented information from the sessions. The questions created from the themes of the original questionnaire were the topics of discussion with the main objective to create consensus.

Following the completion of the consensus group sessions, a

poster board session was held in which all conference participants could review each group's deliberations and add comments. Group members were available to clarify the sometimes intense and complex discussions.

At the conclusion of the conference, each group leader (in
most cases the identified expert in the field) was asked to
summarize the literature, present a representative case, discuss
the ethical issues, and present the group consensus about what
should be done. The result is the text of these volumes.

Conclusion

The following chapters are a compilation of consensus perspectives on ethical issues involving the sexuality of people
with developmental disabilities. The editors would like to
make several caveats clear:

- The opinions expressed are "North American"-centric. A
  common theme expressed by conference participants was
  the need to individualize care to the person and the community in which the person resides. The opinions and
  practices must be tempered by the cultural and legal needs
  of the community in which policies are enacted.
- A recurrent theme expressed by the chapter authors was
  the dearth of peer-reviewed papers on the topics at hand.
  While recognizing this limitation, the editors of these volumes hold that to do nothing or say nothing is itself a decision. While evidence-based findings are important, ethical
  decisions often rely on the considered opinions of people
  who must make decisions today.
- Ethics is by definition, a field of study in which decisions
  are not simply "right or wrong", but rather outcomes of a

review of two or more options that have merit. The editors have intentionally included chapters with divergent opinions to highlight areas where well-intentioned "experts" disagree and to encourage further investigation and debate about what is best for the people who will be affected by the decisions we make, namely the community, the agencies, the caregivers, the professional "experts", the families, and most importantly, the many people with a developmental disability who daily entrust their lives to our care.

- People with a developmental disability were present but under represented in the conference deliberations. The editors acknowledge this as a serious flaw and strongly encourage readers to bear this in mind.

Having said this, the purpose of these deliberations was to deal with the ethical concerns of health care providers. Like it or not, decisions on all topics covered in these volumes are made every day. The editors hope that this text will provide a springboard for future studies, surveys, and consultations designed to improve the lives of a population which has been left behind by the advances in our knowledge of healthy human sexuality.

Chapter 1

Sexual Rights and Individuals who have a Developmental Disability

Shelley L. Watson, Thomas Venema, William Molloy, and Meg Reich

"All human beings are born free and equal in dignity and rights" (United Nations, 1998).

"Sexual Health is a basic and fundamental human right. Human Sexuality is the origin of the deepest bond between human beings and essential to the well being of individuals, couples, families, and society. Therefore the respect for sexual rights should be promoted through all means" (Instituto de Sexologia Y Psicoterapia Espill, 1997).

To deny a person's sexuality is to deny part of his or her personhood. To deny that an individual who has a developmental disability is a sexual being is thus to treat him or her as less than a full person. This is clearly an ethical issue.

Introduction

Individuals who have developmental disabilities have the same basic legal, civil, and human rights as other citizens. Sexuality and fertility concerns are natural experiences for persons who have disabilities. However, the violation of human rights is nowhere more evident for individuals who have developmental disabilities than in the area of sexuality. Sexuality is often denied for individuals who have a developmental disability. This is a direct violation of human rights.

Until the 1960's, denial and suppression were the means of dealing with the sexuality of individuals who have developmental disabilities (Kempton & Kahn, 1991). The Eugenics movement of 1880-1940 led to forced mass sterilization and the segregation of members of our society who had developmental disabilities. The civil rights movement and the "sexual revolution" were among the catalysts for change as was the move toward normalization and deinstitutionalization of people who have developmental disabilities. In the last 30 years, professionals and caregivers have begun to work together to find ways to help individuals who have developmental disabilities to understand their sexuality and to engage in appropriate self-affirming sexual behaviours (Kempton & Kahn, 1991).

Despite much progress in expanding public policy at all levels, the fundamental rights of people who have developmental disabilities have yet to be fully acknowledged or secured (Medlar, 1998). Much of society remains ignorant about the capabilities and rights of people who have developmental disabilities. They have not been given the respect to which they are entitled as citizens nor have most received the support they need to enable them to exercise their rights (Medlar, 1998).

When it comes to sexuality, personal issues can become public and contentious. When couples or individuals explore their sexuality, staff and family members often become involved, leading to conflict. Difficulties arise when staff and family members demonstrate negative attitudes and have little tolerance for discussions on sexual matters, often denying these individuals their human rights. Individuals who have developmental disabilities face many barriers including a lack of privacy, the inability to find partners, and restrictive institutional policies or rules. Society has not been comfortable addressing sexual and reproductive rights and this is even more true when dealing with an individual who has a developmental disability. Many people harbour feelings of ambivalence, confusion, and discomfort in relation to the sexuality of individuals who have a developmental disability (Szollos & McCabe, 1995).

The sexual rights of individuals who have a developmental disability are recently receiving more attention and recognition. Service providers, professionals, and caregivers must deal with these rights and the desires of the individual. This acknowledgment of rights is required so that the individual may experience the fulfillment of their own sexual desires and/or the joys of intimate relationships (Stavis, 1991).

Current normalization trends are towards provision of education and natural opportunities for individuals who have developmental disabilities to experience their sexuality. However, the rights of these individuals to their own sexuality has become an emotionally discussed topic among professionals and lay people because of concerns about unwanted pregnancies, sexually transmitted diseases (STDs), and sexual exploitation. The key ethical issue is the acceptance of the human rights of personal inviolability and self-determination. It has been argued that in discussing ethical aspects of the sexuality of individuals who have developmental disabilities, consistent standards should be upheld by applying principles fundamental to modern ethics (Held, 1993).

Tim is a 28 year old adult male, labelled as moderately delayed. He lives at home. He has been referred for individual counselling by his parents at the suggestion of a local agency. His parents described the presenting issue to the therapist as "self-esteem / depression". He has no criminal record, nor has he ever been known to be "inappropriate" with any other individual on a physical level. He has been "discovered" to be masturbating two times per day in his room. His parents express strong concern that he is "potentially dangerous". According to his parents, because he has an intellectual disability, his capacity to contain his sexual interests may not be within his own control and he therefore *"might* molest a young niece or nephew". They want him placed on a libido-lowering medication as soon as possible. The family is requesting the family doctor to medically "neutralize" his sexuality. They have informed the therapist that they will go to another specialist if this doctor fails to comply with their wishes. The family is sincerely convinced that their objective is to *protect* both their son and potential extended family victims. The therapist is not of the opinion that Tim, as a 28 year old adult, is in fact a sexual risk to anyone. The therapist also believes that with ongoing education, he will be able to control his sexuality. Individual assessment of Tim through eight sessions of psychotherapy plus Tim's life-history of "appropriate" behaviour have provided sufficient evidence for the therapist to conclude that Tim is not the "risk" his parents fear he may be.

It is the therapist's belief that Tim presents "normal" sexual feelings that the parents are attempting to violate based on their own beliefs. When confronted by the therapist with this differing perspective, the parents indicate that:

a) they intend to terminate therapy for their adult son, and
b) it is not the therapist's right to interfere with their family's business by contacting Tim's doctor with his concerns.

Tim has a positive, emotional bond with his parents. One conversation between the therapist and Tim regarding the situation results in Tim indicating that he believes he should trust his parents' directives. He does, however, give permission to the therapist to share his opinions with the family doctor. The family doctor listens to the family's concerns. He has known the family for years and believes the parents have honest concern. He knows the parents are Tim's guardians and trusts their intentions to be in Tim's best interests. He endorses the parental decision without private discussion with Tim (although a "family talk" did occur at the office).

Case Study
Literature Review

Before sexuality rights can be discussed, it must first be noted that sexuality is more than simply sexual behaviour. It encompasses one's feelings of femininity or masculinity, sense of worth and desirability, and ability to give or receive affection, love, and caring in personal relationships (Medlar, 1998). All individuals are sexual and express their sexuality in different ways throughout the life cycle. Acquired physical and mental impairments may alter one's sexual drives, but they do not eliminate basic sexual drives or human needs for affection, intimacy, and need for a healthy and positive self-concept (Medlar, 1998).

"Masturbation is normal" (Edwards, 1976, p. 36). This statement in Edwards' 1976 book, *Sara and Allen: The right to choose,* caused sizable dispute. It is difficult to know whether the controversy was because of the discussion of masturbation itself or to the fact that Edwards' book was addressing sexuality in people who have developmental disabilities. By taking the stance that masturbation is healthy sexual behaviour and more importantly that people with developmental disabilities are sexual beings, Edwards advanced the cause of sexuality and education for people who have developmental disabilities (Hingsburger, 1994). However, while considerable progress has been made, much of society still has difficulties acknowledging the sexuality of people who have developmental disabilities.

In 1997, the World Congress of Sexology held a conference, where Sexual Rights were specifically addressed. This conference resulted in a document entitled the Valencia Declaration

The right to freedom, which excludes all forms of sexual coercion, exploitation and abuse at any time and situations in life. The struggle against violence is a social priority.

The right to autonomy, integrity, and safety of the body encompasses control and enjoyment of our own bodies free from torture, mutilation, and violence of any sort.

The right to sexual equity refers to the freedom from all forms of discrimination, paying due respect to sexual diversity, regardless of sex, gender, age, race, social class, religion, and sexual orientation.

The right to sexual health includes availability to all sufficient resources for the development of research and necessary knowledge. HIV/AIDS and STDs require more resources for research, diagnosis and treatment.

The right to wide, objective, and factual information on human sexuality in order to allow decision-making regarding sexual life.

The right to a comprehensive sexuality education from birth and throughout the life cycle. All social institutions should be involved in this process.

The right to associate freely means the possibility to marry or not, to divorce, and to establish other types of sexual associations.

The right to make free and responsible choices regarding reproductive life. The number and spacing of children and the access to means of fertility regulation. All children should be desired and loved.

> **The right to privacy** implies the capability of making autonomous decisions about sexual life within a context of personal and social ethics. Rational and satisfactory experience of sexuality is a requirement for human development.
>
> (Instituto de Sexologia Y Psicoterapia Espill, 1997)

on Sexual Rights. This document outlined a list of sexual rights for all individuals. These rights included:
The following literature review will analyze the World Congress of Sexology declarations as they relate to people with developmental disabilities.

The right to freedom

Regardless of age, individuals who have a developmental disability appear to be more vulnerable to abuse than nondisabled individuals (Goldman, 1994). In a survey of 85 women with a disability, 70% indicated that they had been violated sexually (Goldman, 1994). In a comparative study of the patterns of sexual abuse in three countries, Sobsey (1992) also found that the setting or placement of individuals influences their vulnerability. Individuals who reside in institutional settings are at greater risk for abuse than individuals in other settings.

There are a number of factors that render individuals who have a developmental disability particularly vulnerable to sexual abuse. There are many false assumptions that many people make about abuse and disabilities: The following are examples:

- No one would take advantage of an individual who has a disability;
- Any form of sexual contact is enjoyed by individuals who have disabilities as they are more stimulated sexually than other people;
- Individuals who have disabilities have impaired sexuality (Carmody, 1991).

The right to autonomy, integrity, and safety of the body

Historically, individuals who have a developmental disability have been involuntarily sterilized and denied the right to sexual expression (Sobsey, 1994). However, not everyone has considered these actions to be abuse; some of them have been permitted and even condoned by law. For example, the sterilization programs in the United States and Nazi Germany were permitted by law (Kempton & Kahn, 1991; Sobsey, 1995; Wolfensberger, 1981). The Eugenics movement provided the rationale for these actions.

Eugenics is defined as "the science that deals with the improvement (by control of human mating) of the hereditary qualities of a race or breed" (Sobsey, 1994, p. 119). Increased urbanization in the late 19th century brought about greater visibility for people who had disabilities, together with the idea that not all individuals are created equal after all. Mentally "defective" persons were seen as ultimately criminal as well as sexually promiscuous (Kempton & Kahn, 1991). It was also believed that these individuals reproduced more quickly than the rest of the population and would therefore overwhelm civilization if their sexuality were not controlled. Developmental disabilities came to be viewed as one of civilization's most serious problems. Poorly designed "research", such as the infamous studies of the Jukes and the Kallikaks (see Goddard, 1912), linked mental deficiency to heredity criminal behaviour. Selective breeding or eugenics thus became the proposed solution to society's problems. Involuntary castration, hysterectomies, and/or oophorectomies were recommended and thousands were performed (Kempton & Kahn, 1991).

Although the earliest sterilization practices were punitive in intent, the laws that followed were regarded as protection for society, children, and individuals who had a developmental disability. Between 1907 and 1957, about 60,000 individuals were sterilized without their consent and many, without their knowledge (Kempton & Kahn, 1991; Sobsey, 1995). However, by 1935 research studies showed that many patients who had genetic developmental disabilities were infertile and/or incapable of sexual intercourse. In addition, less than one-fifth of those sterilized were known to have been sexually active in the first place (Kempton & Kahn, 1991).

According to Sobsey (1994), the eugenics movement in the United States had three major components. Starting in the late 1800's, restrictive marriage and reproduction laws were passed that prohibited marriage or sexual intercourse involving any woman of a reproductive age who had a developmental disability or epilepsy . Many of these laws remain in effect today. Compulsory sterilization soon followed due to the failure of the aforementioned marriage and reproduction laws. Finally, institutionalization with strict sexual segregation was implemented when sterilization programs failed (Sobsey, 1994). Each of these attempts were intended to eliminate developmental disabilities by controlling human reproduction (Sobsey, 1994).

Not all individuals in the field of disabilities can agree on what constitutes abuse. Some believe that sterilization is an appropriate medical intervention to avoid the problems of menstrual management and adjusting to sexual development for young women who have a developmental disability (Conway, 1994). According to Held (1993), a frequently used argument in favour of compulsory sterilization of individuals who have a developmental disability has been the right of a child to be born free of a genetic defect or any other serious health problem. However, this is an indefensible position since every pregnancy has a risk of a congenital defect and children of people with developmental disabilities do not necessarily inherit "defective" genes. In addition, this argument is based on the incorrect notion of a genetic cause of all developmental disabilities (Held, 1993). A large proportion of developmental disabilities are due to non-genetic causes such as fetal alcohol syndrome, malnutrition, and child maltreatment (Griffiths, 1999; Percy & Brown, 1999). Involuntary sterilization in order to control reproduction is therefore a direct violation of human rights.

Held (1993) believes that "[t]he principle of equality requires that sterilization should be available as a method of contraception to mentally disabled persons of all ability levels to the same extent as to the general population" (p. 257). He argues there is no reason to assume that individuals who do not have a developmental disability would not accept sterilization as a method of choice for contraception if they were incapable of coping with the emotional or physical stress of pregnancy. But, it is the performance of such operations without the consent or knowledge of the individual that is the violation of rights (Rioux, 1990). "Whenever the concerns of the society are placed above the rights of the individuals, this results in the long run in a suspension of human rights" (Held, 1993, p. 258).

The right to sexual equity

The right of the individual who has a developmental disability to their own sexuality results directly from the principles of universalizability and equality. It is therefore not a matter of the generosity of individuals who do not have disabilities to grant this right to individuals who have developmental disabilities. In essence, this means that all forms of sexuality that are compatible with human dignity are acceptable (Held, 1993).

According to the United Nations' Declaration of Human Rights (1999), the individual who has a developmental disability has "to the maximum degree of feasibility, the same rights as other human beings". All persons are sexual, and are endowed with dignity and self-worth, regardless of race, sex, disability, sexual orientation, or medical condition (SIECUS, as cited in Medlar, 1998). We cannot artificially separate sexuality from the spectrum of life for anyone (Cole & Cole, 1993).

Individuals who have developmental disabilities are often the object of many stereotypes and misconceptions regarding their sexuality. It is often contended that sexual activity is "inappropriate" for people who have disabilities (Corbett, Shurberg Klein, & Luna Bregante, 1989). Some believe they cannot "handle" a sexual relationship or that individuals who have a developmental disability need "helpers" not lovers. Women who have disabilities are considered to be too fragile for sexual activity. Another common perception is that an individual who has a developmental disability should be grateful if they find someone who wants a "cripple" (Corbett et al.,

1989). If they are "granted" a relationship, and if this is a disabled/nondisabled partnership, the nondisabled partner is the one to define when the relationship begins and ends. Sexual activity may be allowable for a married individual who has a developmental disability, but it is often assumed that an individual who is not married is also (or should be) celibate (Corbett et al., 1989).

Another assumption is that all individuals who have a developmental disability are heterosexual (Corbett et al., 1989). However, ten percent or less of the population in North America has a homosexual orientation, including those who have a developmental disability (Cole & Cole, 1993). Hingsburger (1993) has discussed the problems faced by homosexual individuals who have a developmental disability, whom he refers to as "a minority within a minority" (p. 19).

Coleman and Murphy (1980) conducted a survey of care providers within a facility for individuals who have a developmental disability. The researchers found that staff who approved highly of sex education (75%) and masturbation (73%) were less approving of heterosexual petting (42%) and intercourse (32%) and least approving of homosexual behaviour (23%). Adams, Tallon, and Alcorn (1982) conducted a similar study, with community-based staff and college students. The researchers found that community-based staff were no more liberal in their attitudes than were those who worked within institutions and facilities.

Griffiths, Quinsey, and Hingsburger (1989) however found different results in practice when they conducted therapeutic interviews. These researchers found that homosexual behaviour is more likely to be tolerated than heterosexual behaviour.

They suggest two explanations for this finding. First, because heterosexual behaviour has the potential consequence of pregnancy, it needs to be more actively discouraged than homosexual behaviour. Second, because of the predominantly same-sex residential services for individuals who have a developmental disability, homosexual behaviour is more prevalent (Monat-Haller, 1992). Kempton and Kahn (1991) support the second explanation in their finding that homosexual activity in institutions has been "practically universal, representing not such innate orientation or arrested development, but simply environmental conditioning or lack of alternative means for sexual expression" (pp. 96-97).

Notwithstanding, much has changed since these studies. Hingsburger (1993) conducted a similar study to those of Coleman and Murphy (1980) and Adams et al. (1982). Hingsburger (1993) found that a much smaller percentage indicated high approval of homosexual behaviour for individuals who have a developmental disability. In a sample of 231 individuals, 98% of the participants approved of sex education, 97% approved of masturbation, 80% approved of heterosexual petting, 70% of heterosexual intercourse, but only 30% approved of homosexual behaviour. Hingsburger (1993) reported anecdotally that individuals who were previously able to engage in homosexual behaviour, although covertly, are now reporting that their behaviour is being curtailed and even punished. These findings therefore suggest that staff members still disapprove of homosexuality, but now this disapproval is being mirrored in practice.

Conclusion: Individuals who have developmental disabilities are human beings and therefore have the same rights as other human beings. This includes the right to express their sexuality.

The right to sexual health; The right to wide, objective, and factual information on human sexuality; The right to a comprehensive sexuality education

Although there is limited information available on the sexual attitudes of individuals who have developmental disabilities, the data that are available indicate that they are poorly informed and hold largely negative attitudes toward the expression of their sexuality (McCabe, 1999; McCabe & Cummins, 1996; McCabe & Schreck, 1992; Szollos & McCabe, 1995). Civil rights, that are the rallying points of those who are oppressed, include the right to reproductive information that is comprehensive and accurate (Cole & Cole, 1993). Individuals who have and do not have disabilities have the same rights to information, to services, and to health service providers with adequate knowledge, sensitivity, and experience in the areas of sexual development. Self-empowerment issues, life skills, parenting, and medical concerns are common to everyone, but these issues may need special attention in individuals who have disabilities (Cole & Cole, 1993). However, if individuals who have a developmental disability are not made aware of their own sexual feelings and their rights to choose or not choose sexual partners, the possibility of sexual exploitation increases. A lack of sex education and opportunities to develop a sexual identity result in confusion and uncertainty about what is acceptable behaviour by the individual and from other people (Carmody, 1991; Sobsey, 1994; Sobsey & Varnhagen, 1991).

In a study conducted by Szollos and McCabe (1995), it was found that the sexual knowledge of individuals who have developmental disabilities is often partial, inaccurate, and inconsistent. These researchers also found several misconceptions such as the belief that sexual intercourse is intended to hurt the female, that women can give birth without being pregnant, that masturbation causes harm, that men have menstrual periods, and that in heterosexual intercourse the penis generally goes into the woman's anus. A lack of education increases the risk of sexual exploitation. This conclusion is supported by Sobsey and Varnhagen's (1991) findings that the biggest risk factor for abuse was the victim having inadequate knowledge about appropriate sexual behaviours and/or having poor judgment.

Information about sexuality has generally been withheld to prevent interest in sexual activity due to negative attitudes toward the sexuality of individuals who have a developmental disability (McCabe, 1999; Szollos & McCabe, 1994). However, people with developmental disabilities need not only general information about sex but also specific information on individual disabilities and sexuality. There should also be an opportunity for discussion to explore feelings about being different and specific information about more than just the anatomy and physiology of sex and its adverse consequences. Specific discussion is also needed about the unique problems that people with developmental disabilities may have (e.g., concommitant physical disabilities, medication side effects). It would also be beneficial to have documentation of cases showing that adults with disabilities can have fulfilling sexual lives (Corbett et al., 1989).

Conclusion: All individuals have a right to proper education, training, rehabilitation, and guidance about sexuality, particularly those who also have a developmental disability.

The right to associate freely

There is limited information in the literature about marriage and individuals who have a developmental disability. This may be due in part to the fact that these individuals are often denied the right to marry. Couples who both have developmental disabilities often report that they are not taken seriously by people who do not have disabilities (Corbett et al., 1989). They are frequently told that they "look cute" together, but it is assumed that the relationship is nonsexual and has no potential for commitment and/or marriage. Kempton and Kahn (1991) report that individuals who have developmental disabilities are receiving more support for marriage, but it is often a difficult battle.

Although individuals who have developmental disabilities are now receiving more help and support from their support providers and families, there are still a number of states in the United States that have laws prohibiting marriage for individuals who have developmental disabilities (Kempton & Kahn, 1991). They are often regarded to be incompetent or unable to sustain a long-term relationship. However, this notion has been challenged (Held, 1993). To determine "marital incompetency" one would have to ask for the degree of intelligence necessary to qualify for having a meaningful sexual relationship and for a definition of the specific characteristics of "meaningful" (Held, 1993). As well, to set higher standards in respect to compatibility and stability for long-term relationships of individuals who have a developmental disability as compared to individuals who are nondisabled is an ethical violation of human rights.

Some studies have indicated that individuals who have a developmental disability and who marry have the same statistical chance of success (50%) as the general population. In fact, some unpublished studies have found that their marriages without children have a better chance of success than the non-disabled population. Kempton and Kahn (1991) believe that this is often because sexual fulfillment is not the main aspect of their marriage.

Conclusion: Individuals who have a developmental disability have the same right to marriage as nondisabled individuals. To deny this right is to deny basic human rights.

The right to make free and responsible choices

The right to bear children is a fundamental human right that is most often denied to individuals who have a developmental disability. It is often thought that these individuals cannot be parents, or if they do have children, that their children will be "short changed" (Corbett et al., 1989). Silence from the health care community concerning disability, sexuality, and reproductive issues relays the stronger message of rejection and repression and gives the impression that parenting is not to be considered by individuals who have a developmental disability (Cole & Cole, 1993; Schultz & Adams, 1987).

The contention that a child has a right to satisfactorily functioning parents is understandably shared by many (Schultz & Adams, 1987). However, as discussed by Rioux (1990), individuals who do not have developmental disabilities are not expected to prove that they know how to care for a child before they are permitted to reproduce. There is no requirement that females who do not have disabilities understand the process of delivery nor demonstrate their maternal instincts. However, parents who have developmental disabilities often undergo much scrutiny regarding their ability to raise their child free from harm or neglect (Griffiths, 1999). This will be discussed further in Chapter 8 on *Parents who have Developmental Disabilities*.

As discussed in the section on *the right to safety of the body,* a frequent argument in the discussion about compulsory sterilization is based on the notion of the right of a child to be born free of a genetic defect or any other serious health problem. However, as stated by Held (1993), there are logical and ethical problems with this position. Every pregnancy presents a risk of congenital defects, so it is fair to say that genetic risks are an integral part of being human. However, mental disability is often not genetic in nature and the recurrence risk is low in most cases (Held, 1993). Even if a person who has a developmental disability is disabled due to a genetic condition, it is not always passed on (Griffiths, 1999). Recessive genes must be paired with similar recessive genes and if a dominant gene was the cause of the disability, the chance of passing the disability to the fetus is only 50% (Griffiths, 1999; Percy, Lewkowicz, & Brown, 1999). Even in cases in which genetic disabilities have a high probability of transmission, the ethical questions raised need to be developed on a case by case basis with full participation by the individuals affected. In ethical societies, sterilization is not imposed on individuals found to be at a high risk for transmitting a serious genetic disease if they are of normal intelligence (Held, 1993).

Conclusion: The principle of routine or involuntary sterilization of individuals with developmental disabilities for the purpose of preventing procreation is a direct violation of human rights.

The right to privacy

In the course of normal development, children demonstrate independence and curiosity, including curiosity about themselves and their genitals. The child who has a developmental disability may be more closely observed or supervised by family or caregivers and therefore less able to be spontaneous and private with sexual curiosity than a typically developing child. This lack of privacy can affect a child's perception of his or her body, its function, and personal boundaries regarding appropriate or inappropriate touch (Cole & Cole, 1993).

Parents or staff need to respect privacy (Hingsburger, 1994). This includes never assisting someone to dress or toilet with the door open, never discussing highly private issues with others present, and knocking and receiving permission to enter the room. According to the Valencia Declaration on Sexual Rights (Instituto de Sexologia y Psicoterapia Espill, 1997), the right to privacy also implies the capability to make autonomous decisions about sexual life within a context of personal and social ethics.

Personal relationships are another area where the privacy of individuals must be respected. When an individual who has a developmental disability enters a sexual relationship or begins to express his or her sexuality, it often triggers much discussion among care-takers about competency or consent. Whether the individual lives with his or her family or in a residential setting, staff and/or family often enter into long discussions about the sexual activities of that individual (often without including the individual!). Conahan, Robinson, and Miller

(1993) present a case where an individual's mother began legal action to terminate a presumed homosexual relationship. This began a plethora of tests and procedures to determine if the individual was in fact engaging in homosexual behaviour or was in fact homosexual. The matter came to trial and the individual's right to express his sexuality was discussed. This 30-year-old man was not permitted to engage in a sexual relationship. It is an example of how individuals who have a developmental disability are still treated as children whose decisions must be sanctioned by adults who "know better" (Conahan et al., 1993, p. 317). Again it shows how people with developmental disabilities are vulnerable to having their human rights violated. In this case: the right to privacy, and the right to make autonomous decisions about sexual life.

Masturbation is a key area where lack of privacy causes problems. Historically, attitudes toward masturbation, even in private, have ranged from tolerance to ridicule, to harsh punishment. Sex educators profess that masturbation is a healthy form of sexual expression for both males and females (Hingsburger, 1994). Privacy for this activity in the typical institutional setting was hard to find; in some places, even the bathroom stall lacked doors (Kempton & Kahn, 1991). Despite growing acceptance of masturbation for individuals who have a developmental disability, there is little information that suggest proactive approaches to teaching about this and other forms of sexual behaviour (Hingsburger, 1994). Consequently, staff and parents often respond to behaviours as they occur, usually through punishment.

Conclusion: Individuals with developmental disabilities have the same rights to personal privacy and autonomy as individuals who do not have a disability.

Conference Deliberations

In respecting the rights of an individual, there are often several competing influences. Specifically, the way the rights of the 1) *individual* interact with the rights/mandate of 2) *guardians* (family or assigned), the 3) *agency policies,* the 4) individual *staff* interpretations of rights, and 5) basic *societal values/ rights/ guidelines.*

An added variable for agencies (and therefore clients) might often be the subjective and changing interpretation of agency policy by the board of directors. It was discussed that a clear delineation of the boundaries of these varied interest groups must be established for any agency to function ethically and without confusion or conflict.

Concerns were also raised about the ability of individuals who have developmental disabilities to discern their own value systems. While this is an issue for any person, it poses a major challenge for people with developmental disabilities, particularly those in institutional settings.

In addressing the broad topic of human rights as it pertains to individuals who have developmental disabilities, the group concurred on several basic issues. These included education; advocacy; communication; rights vs. responsibility; inherent human rights vs. agency values; and due process.

Education

It is paramount that any person considering admission to an

agency be clearly informed of exactly what rights he or she will have in the context of agency functioning. This must be done in a way that respects the cognitive abilities of the individual. Agency policy should respect human rights including sexual rights.

It is acknowledged, however, that agencies may differ in their interpretation of how best to protect human rights (e.g., a religious based agency vs. a state-run agency). Our group agreed that all agencies should be mandated to clearly define its policies regarding all aspects of sexuality including education, privacy, reporting, contraception, and respect for sexual behaviours including masturbation, same-sex activities, pornography, and established relationships.

A person should be given assistance to understand agency rights and rules. It was agreed that the person's peer group might be helpful in communicating policies and procedures. This is especially true at the point of "intake". The family and guardians should also be educated.

For education to be effective, it must also be ongoing and geared to the specific needs of the individual. Finally, ongoing education of staff and agency management is also mandatory.

Advocacy

Basically the role of an advocate is to "plead on behalf of another". Concerns were raised that advocates of persons with developmental disabilities need to be particularly sensitive to the danger of imposing their own views about sexuality on the process of representation.

The consensus group also felt that a distinction must be made between a) *advocating* and *assisting* and b) *infantalizing*. The latter involves treating the person like a child by over-compensating and doing too much, thereby infringing on the person's capacity to learn, grow, and change. For example, if, out of love, parents persist in "helping" an individual who has a disability to tie his or her shoes, in actuality, they are depriving a person from learning, through frustration, to master the task.

Inherent rights

Discussion often went back to basic inherent rights - equal to all human beings and subject to societal values. Although each agency is individualized in terms of policies, several parties in the discussion presented the notion that if inherent right is truly present, maybe agencies do not need a "rights policy". Further discussion produced the statement: "*The law has been formulated, therefore boards, families, and guardians should not have the power to over-ride the law of inherent human rights*". Of course, discussion also produced the reality that many individuals who have developmental disabilities do not have the capacity to understand or indicate their right to choose or may have never been granted this opportunity.

Individual rights relative to the rights of others

Discussion explored the concept of "freedom to sexualize does not mean that all parties in the living milieu will choose or believe in the same expression and/or interaction of sexual expression". There must always be a context or a sense of limitation. For example, because a person feels comfortable with masturbation or copulation does not mean that they have the right to violate others' privacy or molest other unwilling persons.

Due process

All participants in discussion concurred that there must be an

- to ensure that justice occurs, an appeal committee must have some unbiased participants. How can this occur in an agency, when we all automatically bring our value base and biases into any discussion, such as staff, board members, and therapists? It was suggested that a minimum of 1/3 of any appeals committee be composed of individuals who are unrelated to agency peers, but aware of human rights.
- that peers who have disabilities must be involved in any appeals process and their input be treated equally
- that this committee also deal with ongoing staff ethical dilemmas
- that persons who have developmental disabilities have ongoing education about their rights and be encouraged to voice their own opinions.

appeals process to deal with disputes about agency sex policies. The group had several recommendations:

The group also agreed that policy cannot be a substitute for human rights. Policy is intended to serve as a guideline for interpretation for staff and clients. Instead of a policy on sexuality, because human rights are already a given, a statement on sexuality may be more appropriate.

Balance between rights and responsibilities

Education will always be needed in the area of social behaviour and social boundaries, such as what will be interpreted as acceptable or unacceptable behaviour. A warning was issued to all front-line staff by a front-line staff member to be aware of one's own values and how they influence judgments. Personal values affect vision of when and if rights may be violated.

Summary

The State of the Art

Despite much progress in expanding public policy at all levels, the fundamental rights of people who have developmental disabilities have not yet been fully acknowledged or secured. Much of society remains ignorant about the capabilities and rights of people who have developmental disabilities. Persons with developmental disabilities have not been given the respect which they are entitled as citizens, nor have most received the support they need to enable them to exercise their rights.

There are a range of attitudes and values in the area of human relations and sexuality. Many parents and care staff deny sexual expression to the individual who has a developmental disability by overreacting to displays of bodily curiosity, avoiding discussions of sexual topics due to fear of arousal and uncontrollable sexual impulses, and historically have frequently implemented female sterilization (Szollos & McCabe, 1995).

Attitudes are influenced by concern for the protection of individuals who have a developmental disability from exploitation.

However, this concern needs to be balanced with the person's right to live a full and "normal" life, including the right to sexual expression (Carmody, 1991). Caregivers and support workers to individuals who have a developmental disability must deal with these rights and must address the desires of these individuals to experience the fulfillment of their own sexual desires or the joys of intimate relationships. This can also include marriage and children (Stavis, 1991).

Clinical and Agency Implications

As the discussion of human sexual rights develops, the responsibilities of stakeholders to ensure ethical implementation will increase. As stated in the literature review, according to the Valencia Declaration on Sexual Rights, the right to sexual health is a basic human right and should be promoted in all aspects of the individual's life. This includes the right to freedom; autonomy; the right to sexual equity; the right to sexual health; the right to sex education; the right to associate freely; the right to make free and responsible choices; and the right to privacy.

According to Sobsey and Doe (1991), one of the agency's primary responsibilities is to provide a safe environment for the individual. As more is known regarding the patterns of sexual offenses and abuse, agency responsibility must be addressed. For example, if an agency fails to screen employees for history of abuse, should the agency be held responsible for future abuse committed by that person while in their employ? If an agency clusters known offenders with vulnerable individuals without providing adequate safeguards against assaults, is the agency responsible for the abuse that results? (Sobsey & Doe, 1991). Courts are considering such questions across North America and agencies are increasingly being held responsible.

No agency or institution can be expected to provide an absolutely risk-free environment, but every agency must provide at least the same level of safety available within the community. Due to the increased risks that are being currently experienced by individuals who have developmental disabilities, prevention strategies must be recognized and implemented (Sobsey & Doe, 1991).

Kempton (cited in Kempton & Kahn, 1991) lists the sexual rights that should be ensured by all agencies for their clients. They believe all persons with developmental disabilities have the following rights within agencies:

- to receive training in sexual behaviour that will open more doors for social contact with people in the community
- to have access to all the knowledge about sexuality they can comprehend
- to enjoy loving and being loved by either sex, including sexual fulfillment
- to express sexual impulses in the same forms that are acceptable to others
- to marry and have a voice in whether or not to have children
- to have supportive services, as they are needed and feasible (Kempton & Kahn, 1991).

It is also imperative that every institution or agency that supports individuals who have developmental disabilities, put in writing a policy committing them to the sexual rights of their clients, accompanied by the accepted procedures to implement it (Kempton & Kahn, 1991).

Final Consensus Statement

According to Held (1993), "[t]he key ethical issue is the acceptance of the human rights of personal inviolability, self-determination in marrying and founding a family and voluntary procreation of mentally disabled persons in respect to prevailing parent-family and parent-citizen models" (p. 255). Sexuality and fertility concerns are natural experiences for individuals who have developmental disabilities. These cannot be artificially separated from the spectrum of life for anyone (Cole & Cole, 1993). "Sexuality is a fundamental need of (men and women). It is an integral part of being human and part of one's personality" (Held, 1993, p. 255).

As stated in the Canadian Human Rights Act, "Every individual should have an equal opportunity with other individuals to make for himself or herself the life that he or she is able and wishes to have, consistent with his or her duties and obligations as a member of society, without being hindered in or prevented from doing so by discriminatory practices based on race, national or ethnic origin, colour, religion, age, sex, marital status, family status, *disability*, or conviction for an offense for which a pardon has been granted". Agencies must therefore respect the human rights of all individuals they support. This includes the respect for sexual rights.

References

Adams, G. L., Tallon, R. J., & Alcorn, D. A. (1982). Attitudes toward the sexuality of mentally retarded and nonretarded person. *Education and Training of the Mentally*

Retarded, 17(4), 307-312.

Carmody, M. (1991). Invisible victims: Sexual assault of people with an intellectual disability. *Australia and New Zealand Journal of Developmental Disabilities, 17(2),* 229-236.

Cole, S. S. & Cole, T. M. (1993). Sexuality, disability, and reproductive issues through the lifespan. *Sexuality & Disability, 11(3),* 189-204.

Coleman, E. M. & Murphy, W. D. (1980). A survey of sexual attitudes and sex education programs among facilities for the mentally retarded. *Applied Research in Mental Retardation, 1,* 269-276.

Conahan, F., Robinson, T., & Miller, B. (1993). A case study relating to the sexual expression of a man with developmental disability. *Sexuality and Disability, 11(4),* 309-319.

Conway, R. N. F. (1994). Abuse and intellectual disability: A potential link or an inescapable reality. *Australia and New Zealand Journal of Developmental Disabilities,* 19(3), 165-171.

Corbett, K., Shurberg Klein, S., & Luna Bregante, J. (1989). The role of sexuality and sex equity in the education of disabled women. *Peabody Journal of Education,* 198-212.

Edwards, J. P. (1976). *Sara and Allen: The right to choose.* Portland, OR: Ednick Communications.

Goddard, H. (1912). *The Kallikak family: A study in the heredity of feeblemindedness.* New York: McMillan.

Goldman, R. L. (1994). Children and youth with intellectual disabilities: Targets for sexual abuse. *International Journal of Disability, Development and Education, 41(2),* 89-102.

Griffiths, D. (1999). Sexuality and people with developmental disabilities: Mythconceptions and facts. In I. Brown & M. Percy (Eds.), *Developmental disabilities in Ontario* (pp.

443-451). Toronto, ON: Front Porch Publishing.

Griffiths, D., Quinsey, V. L., & Hingsburger, D. (1989). *Changing inappropriate sexual behavior: A community-based approach for persons with developmental disabilities*. Baltimore, MD: Paul H. Brookes.

Held. K. R. (1993). Ethical aspects of sexuality of persons with mental retardation. In M. Nager (Ed.), *Perspectives on disability: Text and readings on disability* (2nd edition), pp. 255-260. Palo Alto, CA: Health Markets Research.

Hingsburger, D. (1993). Staff attitudes, homosexuality, and developmental disability: A minority within a minority. *The Canadian Journal of Human Sexuality, 2(1),* 19-21.

Hingsburger, D. (1994). Masturbation: A consultation for those who support individuals with developmental disabilities. *Canadian Journal of Human Sexuality, 3(3),* 278-282.

Instituto de Sexologia Y Psicoterapia Espill (1997). *Valencia declaration on sexual rights.* Valencia, Spain: Author.

Kempton, W. & Kahn, W. (1991). Sexuality and people with intellectual disabilities: A historical perspective. *Sexuality & Disability, 9(2),* 93-111.

McCabe, M. P. (1999). Sexual knowledge, experience, and feelings among people with disability. *Sexuality and Disability, 17(2)*, 157-170.

McCabe, M. P. & Cummins, R. A. (1996). The sexual knowledge, experience, feelings, and needs of people with mild intellectual disability. *Education and Training in Mental Retardation and Developmental Disabilities, 31(1),* 13-21.

McCabe, M. P. & Schreck, A. (1992). Before sex education: An evaluation of the sexual knowledge, experience, feelings, and needs of people with mild intellectual disabilities. *Australia and New Zealand Journal of Developmental Disabilities, 18(2),* 75-82.

Medlar, T. (1998). The manual of policies and procedures of the SHIP sexuality education program. *Sexuality & Disability, 16(1)*, 21-42.

Monat-Haller, R. K. (1992). *Understanding and expressing sexuality: Responsible choices for individuals with developmental disabilities.* Baltimore, MD: Paul H. Brookes Publishing Company.

Percy, M. & Brown, I. (1999). Causes and contributing factors, and approached to intervention. In I. Brown & M. Percy (Eds.*), Developmental disabilities in Ontario* (pp. 223-251). Toronto, ON: Front Porch Publishing.

Percy, M., Lewkowicz, S., & Brown, I. (1999). An introduction to genetics and development. In I. Brown & M. Percy (Eds.), *Developmental disabilities in Ontario* (pp. 199-222). Toronto, ON: Front Porch Publishing.

Rioux, M. H. (1990). Sterilization and mental handicap: A rights issue. *Journal of Leisurability, 17(3), 3-11.*

Schultz, J. B. & Adams, D. U. (1987). Family life education needs of mentally disabled adolescents. *Adolescence, XXII (85)*, 221-230.

Sobsey, D. (1994). *Violence and abuse in the lives of people with disabilities: The end of silent acceptance?* Baltimore, MA: Paul H. Brookes Publishing Co.

Sobsey, D. & Doe, T. (1991). Patterns of sexual abuse and assault. *Sexuality and Disability, 9(3), 243-259.*

Sobsey, D. & Varnhagen, C. (1991). Sexual abuse, assault, and exploitation of Canadians with disabilities. In C. Bagley & R.J. Thomlinson (Eds.), *Child sexual abuse: Critical perspectives on prevention, intervention, and treatment* (pp. 203-216). Toronto: Wall & Emerson.

Sobsey, D. (1995). Enough is enough: There is no excuse for a hundred years of violence against years of violence against people with disabilities. In D. Sobsey, D. Wells, R.

Lucardie, & S. Mansell. (Eds.), *Violence and disability: An annotated bibliography* (pp. ix-xvii). Baltimore, MD: Paul H. Brookes Publishing.

Stavis, P. (1991). Sexual expression and protection for persons with mental disability. *Sexuality and Disability, 9(2),* 131-141.

Szollos, A. A. & McCabe, M. P. (1995). The sexuality of people with mild intellectual disability: Perceptions of clients and caregivers. *Australia and New Zealand Journal of Developmental Disabilities, 20(3),* 205-222.

United Nations (1998). *Universal declaration of human rights.* New York: Author.

Wolfensberger, W. (1981). The extermination of handicapped people in World War II Germany. *Mental Retardation, 19,* 1-7.

Chapter 2

Sexual Policies in Agencies Supporting Persons who have Developmental Disabilities: Ethical and Organizational Issues

Frances Owen, Dorothy M. Griffiths, and Kimberly Arbus-Nevestuk

Introduction

Issues related to sexuality are among the most emotionally loaded and potentially complex facing agency leaders. It is difficult for administrators, professionals, consumers and the community at large to address issues of sexuality from a neutral viewpoint. For this reason, there may be a tendency to avoid addressing the issue directly and, instead, to deal with issues as they arise. However, in the absence of clear, values-based guidance, consumers and staff are left to struggle alone with emotionally complex and, potentially, legally and ethically risky issues. A clear policy statement related to the agency's values, vision and mission, supported by clear procedures, can provide much needed guidance for staff and consumers.

Case Examples

Case 1: A situation that occurs all too frequently is inappropriate sexual contact between care staff and consumers. Such a situation was faced by Tom Welch (fictitious person). Tom had lived in the Pine Street group home for five years when he met Ted Snyder (fictitious person), a direct care staff counselor who had worked in another group home for two years before transferring to Pine Street. Tom needed hand-over-hand guidance for personal care of all kinds. He had tardive dyskinesia and his tremors became worse when he was anxious and especially when he was transferred to a new caregiver, so he needed considerable help when Ted first took responsibility for his care. Tom's diagnosis was moderate developmental handicap and bipolar disorder. His symptoms were quite well controlled with medication.

Tom and Ted got along quite well at first. Ted went out of his way to insure that Tom had everything he needed. Tom appreciated this extra attention. He had a history of difficulty making friends and often felt lonely so Ted's attention was a ray of sunshine for him. Tom began to look forward to Ted's shifts and made it clear to Ted that he appreciated his kindness. However, as Tom's emotional dependence on Ted increased, so did Ted's sexual demands. It started with Ted spending a little longer than needed in assisting Tom with his personal care. Gradually Ted demanded more access to sexual touching of Tom and he pushed Tom to touch him. Initially, Tom tolerated the inappropriate behaviour because he trusted his "friend" Ted who told him he was just insuring that Tom was cared for properly. However, he became increasingly uncomfortable as Ted's advances progressed and his demands became more intrusive. When he tried to protest, Ted threatened him, saying he would tell Association management that it was Tom who had initiated the inappropriate behaviour.

The outcome of this situation for both Tom and Ted depends on a combination of factors, not the least of which is the mechanism that the agency responsible for Tom's group home has in place to support people who are being victimized. The remedies available to Tom would be very different depending on which of the following organizations ran his group home.

Consider first the situation faced by Tom in a community service that does not have a clear sexuality policy. Whitefield Association for Disabled Citizens (fictitious organization) employs two hundred part time and full time staff to support its ten residential programs. The Association has grown rapidly over the past ten years as local institutions have been reducing their populations and, in some cases, closing their doors. While the Association's management has been delighted with the organization's growth and has been philosophically supportive of the move to community living for persons with developmental disabilities, at a corporate level there has been little time to focus on issues beyond basic program development and financial survival concerns. The Board of Directors of the Association has been generally supportive of the increase in services but its members have been feeling quite overwhelmed by the service delivery pressures the organization is facing.

The organization has, traditionally, been quite conservative in its approach to service delivery. Its approach to sexuality has been to ignore the issue officially, a strategy that the members of the Association's Board of Directors feel has been successful since there have never been any complaints from consumers, their families or the community. The feeling among management and Board members has been that sexuality is dangerous for persons who have developmental disabilities and, as such, it is a topic best left unspoken within their programs.

The danger with this culture is that there is no guidance provided for consumers or staff, leaving them to fend for themselves. What is even more dangerous in this scenario is that, since it is clear that the culture of the organization does not value and, in fact actively suppresses discussion of sexuality, inappropriate behaviour related to sexuality is never discussed. This is potentially fertile ground for the development of inappropriate relationships between caregivers and consumers, or victimization by one consumer of another. In the absence of a clear policy and procedural guidelines, staff and consumer training, and staff supervision regarding the maintenance of appropriate professional boundaries, consumers have no idea to whom they may turn for help when they are victimized. By the same token, there are no guidelines for healthy and appropriate sexual self expression.

Case 2: Contrast this scenario with the situation in the Redfield Association for Disabled Services (fictitious organization). Redfield has faced growth at a rate similar to that at the Whitefield Association. However, for the past ten years, Redfield has had a consistent commitment to staff training in a variety of program areas, including sexuality. While the organization's Board of

Directors initially was quite hesitant about articulating a sexuality policy and, in fact, some members resigned over the issue, the Association's management and Executive Committee recognized the importance of addressing this difficult issue. They realized that, without a clear policy and attendant implementation guidelines, staff and consumers would be left to deal with difficult issues without guidance.

Redfield initiated the process of policy development recognizing that the task would not be accomplished quickly or easily. A consultant was hired to interview consumers, both individually and in groups, regarding their perception of the issues that should be included in the organization's policy and guidelines. This consultant, who had experience in establishing sexuality policies and procedures in community organizations, was also available for consultation on an ongoing basis throughout the process.

All staff members completed an anonymous survey regarding their perception of the elements that must be included in the policy to insure that it would be clear, appropriate, culturally responsive and practical. Staff consensus building groups were held at every level of the organization to develop the themes that arose from the questionnaires. A committee comprised of consumers, front line counselors and management staff reviewed the results of the surveys and consensus groups, and developed a draft policy which was circulated for comment to all consumers, staff, managers, Board members and professionals from related constituencies including counseling agencies and government departments that worked with the Association. The final policy and procedures were developed based on the feedback received on the draft.

The Redfield Association did not consider that its job was complete once the policy had been adopted by the Board of Directors. The Association's managers recognized that policy and procedures without a practical implementation plan were hollow. To insure that these documents were useful to both consumers and staff, the Association's management undertook an extensive training plan with everyone associated with the organization from consumers to Board members, part time staff to maintenance personnel. In addition to the initial training, the policy and procedures were reviewed with all staff and consumers on an annual basis.

It is not difficult to guess which of these Associations would be better prepared to respond in an appropriate and professional manner when faced with an issue such as Tom's. In the absence of a clear reporting mechanism and in an organizational culture that discouraged discussion of issues related to sexuality, it is likely that Tom would delay reporting the situation if he lived in a group home operated by the Whitefield Association. He would not know who he could trust, especially in the face of Ted's threats. He might be afraid that he would be forced to leave his home. Once the situation was brought to light, Tom, staff members and managers in the Whitefield Association would be faced with two concurrent problems: the issue itself and the need to devise a strategy for dealing with it. However, if Tom was fortunate enough to be associated with the Redfield Association he would know how to report the problem with Ted and what to expect as a response from staff and management of the Association. While the situation would be traumatic for Tom, and challenging for his direct care staff and managers, the existence of clear procedures would allow them all to focus on Tom's needs rather than using their energy to develop new procedures. Ideally, the Redfield Association policies would allow staff to identify Ted's vulnerabilities before he ever acted on them.

While the development of policies and procedures concerning sexuality is difficult, a failure to address the issue does not prevent the occurrence of problems. It is more likely that organizational avoidance of the issue creates fertile ground for abuse.

Literature Review

Rights and Freedoms

The task of clarifying organizational values concerning sexuality can be very challenging. It includes an examination of what constitutes a good society and how to translate this vision into reality (Prilletensky, 1997). As with policies in other areas of the agency's functioning, sexuality policies must be based on the organization's vision and mission statements, both of which reflect the organization's values. In all cases, the process is guided by the rights of persons who have developmental disabilities. These rights are enshrined in documents including the United Nations Declaration on the Rights of Disabled Persons (1975), which "states that all people with disabilities have an inherent right to respect for their human dignity, as well as a right to protection from all degrading treatment, discrimination, and abuse" (Sobsey, 1994, p. 2). In Canada, section 15 of the Charter of Rights and Freedoms specifies that, "Every individual is equal before and under the law and has the right to equal protection and equal benefit of the law without discrimination and, in particular, without discrimination based on race, national or ethnic origin, colour, religion, sex, age or mental or physical disability" (Government of Canada, 1982, p. 15).

The Americans with Disabilities Act (ADA) provides similar protection. The preamble to the ADA cites the historic segregation and isolation of persons with disabilities in all areas of their lives, including "...employment housing, public accommodations, education, transportation, communication, recreation, institutionalization, health services, voting, and access to public services" (Americans with Disabilities Act of 1990, p. 3). The stated purpose of the ADA is "...to provide a clear and comprehensive national mandate for the elimination of discrimination against individuals with disabilities" (Americans with Disabilities Act of 1990, p. 3) with clear standards and a national mechanism for enforcing them. This reflects the Constitutional rights that protect people who have developmental disabilities just as they protect all other American citizens. These rights include the right to privacy, the right to marry, and the right to have children (Rowe & Savage, 1987). Nevertheless, despite the growth in public awareness of the need to protect the fundamental rights of persons who have disabilities, there is no specific legislation that guarantees their rights to sexual self expression in particular. The interpretation within an agency of what is appropriate sexual behaviour is influenced by the larger environment, not directed by legislation.

From the perspective of strategy, agencies attempting to

develop policies and procedures should start with an environmental analysis that examines relevant pressures, both internal and external to the organization (Certo, Sales, & Owen, 1998). These include consumer perspectives, community values and tolerance, and professional ethical guidelines. These must all be viewed with a sensitivity to issues of cultural and religious diversity. In the case of setting sexuality policies, community values and standards of behaviour have tended to make a major impact. Naturally, the agency's mission and objectives, including those related to sexuality, must be developed in response to these local pressures. To support the policy, strategic controls in the form of standards of practice, clear job descriptions, appropriate training and supervision, must also be in place.

Because of the variation in tolerance and behavioural expectations from community to community, it is difficult to imagine that there would ever be one universally accepted policy concerning sexuality. However, some published policies are available as models to assist organizations that are grappling with this issue. The Arc's (a national organization on mental retardation) national policy on sexuality articulates the organization's position that "The Arc recognizes and affirms that individuals with mental retardation are people with sexual feelings, needs and identities, and believes that sexuality should always be seen in the total context of human relationships" (The Arc , 1997, p. 13). Specific policies and procedures are necessary to translate this belief into action for persons who have developmental disabilities. One such policy is the Intimate Sexuality in Long Term Care Facilities: Policy for Institutions Draft (Essex County Consensus Group on Sexuality in Institutions, 1998), which provides definitions of key terms, such as intimacy and sexuality, and delineates the roles of the staff and of the institution. It also provides examples illustrating the strategies that could be applied in accordance with the policy guidelines. These are potentially useful training tools for staff being introduced to decision making in this complex area.

The Sexuality Rights Protection Policy of the Colorado Developmental Disabilities Planning Council is another example of a policy that has been designed to "guide the community and empower persons with disabilities in Colorado to ensure that their inherent sexual rights and basic human needs are affirmed, defended, promoted, and respected" (Colorado Developmental Disabilities Planning Council, 1992, abstract). This document was developed in response to a request to the Colorado Developmental Disabilities Council made by Speaking for Ourselves, a self-advocacy group concerned about the need to address sexuality issues. The result was a series of focus groups and a retreat from which the policy was developed. This policy asserts the rights of all persons to privacy, to sexual self expression, to access service and community resources. It also clarifies the responsibilities of agencies and the need for ongoing staff training (Colorado Developmental Disabilities Planning Council, 1992).

Training For Staff

The distance between policy development and policy implementation can be bridged by coherent procedures and ongoing staff training and consultation. Consumers and staff should be trained in the organization's policy regarding sexuality and, especially, in the procedures for reporting inappropriate sexual conduct. Suggestions for training specifically for consumers will be addressed in the next chapter.

With regard to staff training, there are several key areas of training that are needed in order to support the implementation of an agency's sexuality policies and procedures. The first is the issue of professional self awareness and, especially, awareness of the issue of countertransference in work with consumers. Staff self awareness is key to the maintenance of appropriate professional boundaries. This is often especially challenging for staff who work in residential programs where there is a high level of personal care provided for consumers. Staff must be mindful of the possibility of their relationship with consumers being colored by their own needs. This countertransference "...occurs when a counselor's own needs or unresolved personal conflicts become entangled in the therapeutic relationship" (Corey , 1996, p. 39). Corey emphasizes that unrecognized countertransference "blurs" the ability of counselors to maintain their professional objectivity. For this reason, supervision should include discussions of the counselors' personal reactions to their consumers. Transparency in the counselling relationship is one of the keys to maintenance of professional boundaries and avoidance of ethical violations. While sexuality is by no means the only area in which staff-consumer relationships can become confused, it is certainly one of the most serious.

Self awareness and countertransference

Organizations sometimes choose to avoid an open discussion of the topic of sexuality because of the feelings that the topic promotes in each individual. The intimate nature of the topic can make it difficult to maintain an objective per-

spective. This personalization of the topic can present a serious problem at an administrative and, more importantly, at
a clinical level. For this reason, Anderson (1992), in a discussion of preparation of health care professionals to address
sexuality issues in persons who have physical disabilities,
stresses the need for professionals to become aware of their
own attitudes toward sexuality before undertaking to assess
issues related to their consumers. Staff who may be experiencing personal sexual or more general relationship difficulties may be less able than others to provide appropriate
training for consumers. Even more importantly, there is the
danger that staff struggling with their own issues may be at
greater risk of boundary violations with consumers. Awareness of the limits of one's fitness to practice in a given area
is one of the foundations of professional practice in many
professions (Orr, 1997). Sensitization of staff to the impact
of their own personal issues on their ability to provide guidance for consumers and to maintain appropriate professional
boundaries should be a cornerstone of any discussion of
sexuality policy and procedures. It is unlikely that all members of an organization will be equally suited to developing
sexuality policies and procedures, or to providing training
programs for consumers on the topic, but every member of
an organization must be prepared to carry out the policy and
part of that process includes keeping personal needs in the
proper perspective.

One of the most difficult aspects of professional sexual misconduct is the reluctance of professionals to seek consultation when they feel tempted to cross professional boundaries. Celenza (1998) stresses that the inherent tension in a
therapist-patient relationship should be a topic for open discussion among professionals. A similar argument can be

made for the need for an open dialogue among professionals working in the field of developmental disabilities. The taboo associated with the temptation to violate professional boundaries should be replaced by an acknowledgement of the need for clear, supportive and ongoing supervision to help people to maintain these boundaries rather than leaving individual professionals to struggle with countertransference alone and confused. It has also been suggested that the use of supervision is one of the factors that helps professionals to manage countertransference in a positive and proactive manner. Other management factors include reflecting on the therapeutic interaction with consumers and insuring that one's personal needs are met outside the work setting (Hayes et al., 1988).

Decision Making

No policy statement or set of procedures can possibly cover all the situations that consumers and staff may face in the course of their work together. Therefore, a cornerstone of any training program related to policy implementation must be the development of skills in ethical decision making. Family therapist and counselor educator Michele Burhard Thomas (1992) has outlined a ten step process in making ethical decisions.

Thomas (1992) suggests that practitioners begin with a clear definition of the problem situation they are facing. This includes asking fundamental questions: who is involved, what happened, when did it happen, where did it happen, and how did it happen?

The next step is to consult codes of ethics, standards of practice, relevant legislation and agency policies that pertain to the situation. This is the point where ethical decision making breaks down if policies and procedures have not been spelled out in advance of a difficult situation. At this stage of the decision making process, if the staff member has no prescribed guidelines to consult, he/she is functionally cast adrift.

The third, fourth, fifth and sixth steps focus on action alternatives. The staff member is encouraged to determine the range of viable and ethical choices and to evaluate each in terms of its impact on the consumer, its appropriateness given the responsibilities of the staff member and the likely consequences of each alternative.

In steps seven and eight, the staff member chooses the alternative that appears to be the most responsible based on the analysis performed in the previous steps, and then consults his/her supervisor or obtains consultation from informed peers or a formal consultant to insure that the decision is appropriate. As discussed above, the consultation process is critical given the challenges of decision making in the context of an intense caregiving relationship. In serious situations, consultation with a supervisor is always advisable. This insures that the decision is professionally responsible and that it is congruent with organizational policy. In addition, support from a supervisor can insure organizational support for the decision. Making an appropriate ethical decision can be personally uncomfortable, especially if it means the individual must take a position that may set him/ her apart from a group. However, appropriate supervision can help the staff member to keep a clear focus on the welfare of the consumer (Fly, van Bark, Weinman, Kitchener &

Lang, 1997).

In the last two steps, nine and ten, Thomas recommends the implementation of the decision and careful documentation of the process used in reaching it. The latter step is vital to insure that the process is open to scrutiny by supervisors, consumers and advocates.

Organizational culture and supervision

The existence of a clear organizational policy regarding sexual issues, and staff training in its implementation, provides objective guidance for staff, opens the issue to general discussion and leaves no room for serious ambiguity which could provide the opportunity for staff to rationalize an inappropriate relationship. However, policies should not consist of a list of rigid rules and regulations. Instead, they should clarify the values of the community and the values to which all levels of the organization subscribe and which are reflected not only in the policy and its attendant procedures, but in the culture of the organization itself. Sexuality policies should not be window dressing. They should be rooted in the heart of the organization and reflected in the actions of all its members.

Organizational culture "provides a sense of identity for its members. The more clearly an organization's shared perceptions and values are defined, the more strongly people can associate themselves with their organization's mission, and feel a vital part of it." Organizational culture also encourages commitment to a mission, and strengthens standards of behaviour (Greenberg, Baron, Sales, & Owen, 1996, p. 498). It is created through the influence of founders, through interaction with the external environment and through contact among groups within the organization. The latter point is of particular importance to trainers attempting to communicate sexuality policies. Since different work groups may have different points of view on the issue, it is important that training events encourage a high level of intergroup interaction in order to promote a shared understanding of the policy. Training of subgroups in isolation could result in intergroup confusion about policy application (Greenberg, Baron, Sales, & Owen, 1996; Dekker & Barling, 1998). This could prove to be especially difficult for consumers who may, as a result of this fragmented training, be given very different messages by staff who have been trained in different groups. Instead, to insure that the policy reflects the values of the organization and becomes embedded in the organization's culture, all levels of the organization must "buy into" one policy and live by it.

Included in the notion of living by the policy is the consistent and equitable application of sanctions against people who violate its principles. In a study of sexual harassment in the workplace, Dekker and Barling (1998) found that the existence of a sexual harassment policy was not the major factor in preventing sexual harassment. Instead, it was the perception staff had of the content of the policy and its enforcement that predicted the incidence of harassment. Generalizing from this experience, it would be advisable for organizations to include clear sanctions for policy violation. Training in the procedures to be used in the investigation of alleged violations should be provided for both consumers and staff.

Attitudes And Values Of Personal Dignity

Policies, even when carefully thought out and congruent with organizational values and vision, are at best hollow and at worst false when not internalized by all those associated with the organization. The process of establishing policies must involve all those associated with the organization including consumers, staff, managers, volunteers and community constituencies that have a vested interest in the work of the organization. The process of values clarification (Huber, 1994) offers a mechanism to guide both personal reflection and organizational discussion of the process of valuing. It includes three processes: choosing, prizing and acting on beliefs. The process challenges staff to examine the source of the inspiration for their beliefs, to evaluate these beliefs, to examine their willingness to share their beliefs with others and to consider the consistency with which they act on their beliefs. This process is not static. With the evolution of individuals and organizations there is the danger that beliefs once held dear and used to guide the life of an organization can fall into disuse. For this reason, it is critically important that value systems be reviewed on a regular basis and that they be used to guide all decisions, from policy to program development and implementation.

Conference Deliberations

In discussion with conference participants there was support for the utility of clearly established policies and procedures. The reasons the participants gave for establishing such policies included the need for consistency, the need for the delineation of clear rights and responsibilities of both staff and consumers, the need for direction to guide the nature of interpersonal contact and the need to insure professional safety and security. It appears that, in the absence of clearly articulated policies, the sometimes conflicting feelings and views of staff tend to become de facto policy.

In discussing the process of organizational planning, the participants at the conference expressed concern that policies and procedures provide clear but not restrictive guidance. Participants stressed the need to avoid a "cook book" approach and recommended, instead, an approach that supports informed decision making.

As the conference participants emphasized, sets of rules and regulations may be useful as guidelines but training in ethical decision making is key to insuring that appropriate boundaries are maintained. Participants at the conference emphasized the need for training to focus on decision making models that staff members can use when faced with concerns about when and how to intervene in sexual matters in an appropriate and sensitive manner. To be both effective and respectful, staff training must parallel the training provided for consumers.

Rather than existing as a set of rules, conference participants emphasized that policies should clarify the values of the community and the organization. These must be values to which all levels of the organization subscribe and which are reflected not only in the policy and its attendant procedures, but in the culture of the organization itself. Participants expressed concern that policies and procedures may not be supported by agency administration. They also emphasized the need for policies to be comprehensive in the sense of discussing expectations concerning all manners of sexual behaviour.

Participants discussed the fact that residential services are a place where consumers must feel at home. It is important that policies concerning intimate behaviour such as sexuality be developed with consumers and not imposed by others. Policies should specify a philosophy that guides the teaching of responsible sexuality which reflects the need for mutual respect of staff and consumers in the home.

Summary

State of the Art

The state of the art of policy development varies from organizations that do not address the issue directly and formally to those, such as the ones described above, that have engaged in lengthy and in depth policy development and training processes. Cultural, religious, legislative, legal and social factors all impact on an agency's willingness to undertake the challenging process of sexuality policy development. For this reason, there is considerable controversy regarding whether sexuality policies should exist and, if they should, what freedoms they should enshrine and what limitations they should describe. It is unlikely that one policy will be adopted by all organizations that provide services for persons with developmental disabilities. In fact, such a notion flies in the face of the need for policies to reflect local values and standards. However, the consensus of the conference deliberations and the trends in the professional literature emphasize the need for organizations to develop a clear statement of policy and procedures to guide both staff and consumers.

Clinical Implications

Sexuality policies are far more than intellectual exercises perpetrated by managers and Board members. Sexuality policies reflect the clinical commitment that the organization makes to its consumers in a very important area of their lives. In the absence of clear policy statements and procedural guidelines there are two major clinical dangers. The first is that consumers will be treated in an inconsistent manner by staff. Some staff may tolerate or even encourage certain behaviours that other staff may punish, leaving consumers frustrated and confused. An even more serious consequence of this lack of policy guidance is the possibility that sexual abusers can take advantage of the procedural vacuum to justify their actions. Consider the example of Ted and Tom. Ted would be much freer to manipulate the situation in an association that had not articulated a sexuality policy and in which there were no clear procedures for Tom to use to obtain help. Furthermore, it is possible that some abusers could rationalize the lack of a clear policy as tacit approval of their actions.

Agency Implications

From an agency perspective, organizations that have not developed a clear sexuality policy may leave themselves open to the kinds of clinical problems described above. They could be criticized for failing to provide appropriate protection for consumers or guidance for staff who will, inevitably, face issues related to sexuality in their work with residential consumers.

Nevertheless, as described above, the process of establishing policy, procedures and training programs is far from simple and will require significant evaluation of the organization's values and its commitment to consumers and staff.

What Should Be Done Now

The clear message in the literature and in the deliberations of conference participants was the need for agencies to develop clear sexuality policies with implementation procedures and training to support these procedures. Agencies should begin the process of establishing policies by articulating an agency statement of values and vision. This process should be undertaken with full participation of all key stakeholders, especially consumers. In addition to training on the specific policies and procedures, agencies should insure that staff have training in systematic ethical decision making processes including strategies for problem assessment, familiarization with codes of ethics and appropriate use of supervision. Staff should also receive training and supervision in issues related to countertransference including regular open discussion of the complex relationship that develops between a caregiver and consumer in long term care settings. Staff training should be conducted with all staff together or, in larger organizations, with ample opportunity for information sharing across departments, to insure consistent understanding of policies and their enforcement at all levels of the organization.

Since sexuality policies are a reflection of the agency's and the community's values, organizations should engage in an ongoing process of values clarification.

Final Consensus Statement

The avoidance of difficult issues does not make them go away. The consensus of the conference discussion and the literature is that every organization that provides services for persons who have developmental disabilities should develop a policy and procedures regarding sexual behaviour. These documents should be supported by training for staff and consumers, and should be reviewed on a regular basis to insure that they remain relevant and practical.

References

Americans with Disabilities Act of 1990, Available at: gopher://wiretap.spies.com/00/Gov/disable.act

Anderson, L. (1992). Physical disability & sexuality, *The Canadian Journal of Human Sexuality, 1,*177-185.

Celenza, A. (1998) Precursors to therapist sexual misconduct preliminary findings. *Psychoanalytic Psychology, 15,* 378-395.

Certo, S. C., Sales, C. A. & Owen, F. A. (1998). *Modern management in Canada.* Scarborough, Ontario: Prentice Hall Canada Inc.

Colorado Developmental Disabilities Planning Council (1992). *Sexuality rights protection policy.* Denver, CO: Author.

Corey G. (1996). *Theory and practice of counseling and psychotherapy (Fifth Edition).* Pacific Grove, CA: Brooks/Cole Publishing Company.

Dekker, I. & Barling, J. (1998). Personal and organizational predictors of workplace sexual harassment of women by men. *Journal of Occupational Health Psychology, 3,* 7-18.

Essex County Consensus Group on Sexuality in Institutions (April, 1998). *Intimate sexuality in long term care facilities: Policy for institutions: Draft* Unpublished manuscript.

Fly, B. J., van Bark, W. P., Weinman, L., Kitchener, K. S. & Lang, P. R. (1997). Ethical transgressions of psychology graduate students critical incidents with implications for training. *Professional Psychology, 28,* 492-495.

Government of Canada (1982). *The charter of rights and freedoms: A guide for Canadians.* Minister of Supply and Services Canada.

Greenberg, J., Baron, R. A., Sales, C. A. & Owen, F. A. (1996). *Behaviour in organizations (Canadian Edition).* Scarborough, Ontario: Prentice Hall Canada Inc.

Hayes, J. A., McCracken, J. E., McClanahan, M. K., Hill, C. E., Harp, J. S. & Carozzoni, P. (1998). Therapist perspectives on countertransference qualitative data in search of a theory. *Journal of Counseling Psychology, 45,* 468-482.

Huber, C. H. (1994). *Ethical, legal and professional issues in the practice of marriage and family therapy (Second Edition).* Upper Saddle River, NJ: Prentice-Hall, Inc .

Orr, P. (1997). Psychology impaired? *Professional Psychology: Research and Practice, 28,* 293-296.

Prilletensky, I. (1997). Values, assumptions, and practices assessing the moral implications of psychological discourse and action. *American Psychologist, 52,* 517-535.

Rowe, W. S. & Savage, S. (1987). *Sexuality and the developmentally handicapped.* Lewiston, NY: Edwin Mellen Press.

Sobsey, D. (1994). *Violence and abuse in the lives of people with disabilities.* Baltimore: Paul H. Brookes Publishing Co.

The Arc. (1997). *Sexuality and policy procedures manual.* Arlington, TX: The Arc of the United States.

Thomas, M. B. (1992). *Introduction to marital and family therapy,* New York: Macmillan Publishing Company.

Resources

Job Accommodation Network: http://janweb.icdi.wvu.edu/links

The ARC *Sexuality Policy and Procedures Manual.* Arlington, Texas.

American Association on Mental Retardation (AAMR) Guidelines to Professional Conduct:
http://www.aamr.org/Policies/guidelines.html

American Association on Mental Retardation (AAMR) Fact Sheet: Human Rights:
http://www.aamr.org/Policies/faqhumanrights.html

Chapter 3

Sexual Policies in Agencies Supporting Persons who have Developmental Disabilities: Practical and Implementation Issues

Dorothy M. Griffiths, Frances Owen, Louis Lindenbaum, and Kimberly Arbus-Nevestuk

Introduction

In recent years, there has been growing recognition of the sexuality of persons with developmental disabilities and an increased interest in sociosexual education and advocacy for the sexual rights of persons with developmental disabilities. This represents a significant shift from historical perspectives.

Historically, persons with developmental disabilities were regarded as sexually innocent in need of protection, sexually dangerous or promiscuous in need of sanctioning. Until the 1970's the prevailing sexual policies in North America were largely based on the Eugenics practices adopted at the beginning of the 20th century. Restrictive measures included controlled marriage, sterilization, and segregation through institutionalization (Scheerenburger, 1982). In the 1950's segregation of men from women and both from society was still standard practice. In the past three decades there has been a significant attitude shift largely heralded by the normalization and desinstitutionalization movement (Whitehouse and McCabe, 1997).

There has been a growing awareness of the need for agencies

to develop sociosexual policies to ensure that the sexuality and reproductive rights of persons with developmental disabilities is respected. However, many agencies still fail to provide opportunity for the persons they support to experience meaningful social and intimate relationships. A positive sexuality policy would represent a significant policy change for most North American agencies (Stiggall Muccigrosso, 1991).

Sexual Policy: To be or not to be?

There are five basic arguments that have been presented against the development of sexual policy: fear of probibition, protection from exploitation, liability, individuality, and board/ community perception.

One of the primary arguments against development of sexuality policy provided by some service providers is the concern that policies could be too restrictive and prohibitive. Staff and administrators have resisted policy development because Boards of Directors or government agencies might impose prohibitions based on ignorance, bias, fear for the safety and protection of the consumer, or protection from liability. Restrictive policies have indeed been written that prohibit all sexual contact between persons with developmental disabilities who are served by an agency. In addition, there is concern that individuals who fail to meet the prohibitive standards of abstinence may be excluded from service or punished for their behaviour.

A second concern raised has been protection from abuse and exploitation. Service providers have questioned whether allowing sexual activity will result in increased sexual abuse or exploitation. Sexual abuse is commonly defined as unwanted or forced sexual contact. Sexual policy should set out standards for reducing sexual abuse of this nature. However, in 1993 Health and Welfare Canada concluded that for persons with disabilities, the "denial of sexuality, denial of sexual information/education and forced abortion or sterilization" is also sexual abuse (Roeher Institute, 1994, p.12). Thus policy must also include issues of education, information, and self-determination.

A third concern has been that written sexual policies will create liability for an agency should a problem arise. This view has been disputed. "Polices exist whether they are expressed or implied. The absence of a formal written policy only ensures that informal policy will be developed and implemented in an inconsistent manner based on personal bias of individual workers." (Rowe & Savage, 1988, p. 148). Without written policy and procedures, each staff responds to a sexual situation in their own way. Without formal policies, the messages people with disabilities hear about what is sexually appropriate and inappropriate are inconsistent. The same sexual behaviour may be ignored, encouraged, or even punished by different staff from the same agency. This inconsistency was noted by Deisher (1973) who demonstrated that staff shared very different beliefs about what should and should not be permitted. Consequently, consumers of an agency may be afforded divergent, conflicting and inconsistent messages that are counterproductive to an atmosphere of responsible sexual behaviour.

Fourth, the argument has been posed that it is best to deal with sexual issues on an individual basis, rather than by universally written sexual policies. As with the arguments reviewed above, while the spirit of this argument appears person-centred, unless power is handed to the people governed by the policy, the result is the haphazard imposition of values by stakeholders whose lives are simplified by "just saying no".

Lastly, agencies have expressed concern regarding what parents, board members, or the community might think if policies were made explicit (Shore, 1978). If policies are written they are more likely to become known. Policies need to be developed in an inclusive atmosphere of education to ensure that interested parties are aware that the policy is to promote a responsible and healthy attitude toward sexuality and to reduce potential for abuse.

While debate continues over whether to have or not to have sexual policies, the reality is that agency staff are being confronted on a daily basis with situations that require an immediate response. In some cases people have been punished, ridiculed and abused. In other cases, sexual behaviour of a criminal nature has been ignored. It appears that client rights are more at risk and agency risks are more apparent without written policies than with them. Policies and procedures, that are unwritten or left to the individual staff to determine, may actually be of greater risk to the civil liberties of the clients and may leave the agency open to greater risks. In some areas, failure to have policies and to respond appropriately to sexual situations has resulted in law suits against the host agencies. Thus sexual policies may reduce the legal liability of agencies rather than increase it.

Should we have sexual policies and procedures in our agencies that support persons with developmental disabilities?

Yes. Staff members are required to respond to situations that are delicate and controversial. It is unthinkable that they are doing so without guidance and direction from their agency. It is also discomforting to think that such important client behaviours and rights are being determined by an individual care provider.

The authors argue that agencies may be asking the wrong question. The question is not whether there should be policies but what the policy should say. Are policies a list of sexual behaviours that people can and cannot do? No, that would be redundant.   There are already laws that govern socially accepted sexual behaviour.   These laws can (and should be) applicable to persons with developmental disabilities.

So what are agency policies about then?

The purpose of any agency policy is to provide consistent direction for staff and to delineate agency responsibilities. The same should hold true for sexual policies. A sexual policy is not really about the sexual behaviours of the consumers, but about beliefs, principles and programs that the agency offers with regard to the sexuality of persons with developmental disabilities, together with guidelines for staff about how to implement those beliefs and programs.

Case Examples

These six examples point to the need for policies and procedures in the following areas: consumer training, staff training, access to clinical and medical services, abuse prevention and reporting, and relationship development. Each of these will be explored in the literature review that follows:

Case 1: *Sara is a 25 year old woman living in a local association supporting persons with developmental disabilities. The staff were aware that Sara was sexually active and so she was prescribed birth control pills. Sara now felt safe to have sexual relations. She did not get pregnant but did acquire an STD. Sara thought she was safe. Is the agency liable for not teaching her that "the pill" did not protect her from disease?*

Case 2: *John Smith began to work as an instructor at a vocational program six months ago. One day he found two male clients engaging in oral sex in the washroom of the workshop. John was extremely upset. He felt these men were engaging in an immoral and illegal act. He physically hauled them out of the bathroom with their pants down and put them in separate rooms to wait while he called the police. Was this response appropriate? Is John at risk for legal or employment sanctions? Is the agency liable because they had no policy or guidelines for John to follow? What is the agency's responsibility to the two men who have been treated in this way? Would the response be the same if it had been a male and female client? or two female clients?*

Case 3: *Peter is 27 years old. He was out for a walk and began to talk to some children in a park. He picked up one of the children and put her on his lap. When he did this, he grabbed her between the legs to lift her up. The mother came running and accused him of sexually interfering with her daughter. The police were called by someone who heard the commotion but charges were* *not laid because the woman would not give a statement. The staff in Peter's group home are unsure if his touch was sexual. They decided to restrict his access to the community as a precaution. Are the staff infringing on his rights? What if they do nothing? Should he be assessed? What happens if he has a sexual interest in children? Do staff have an obligation to inform the police of what occurred?*

Case 4: Ralph has been prescribed seizure medication. As a result, he developed inhibited orgasm (inability to sexually climax). Ralph does not understand that this is the cause of his sexual dysfunction. Ralph is often seen touching himself in public and in his room. The staff approach is tell him to stop. One day he was found using a vacuum cleaner to masturbate and was seriously injured. Who is responsible for this situation?

Case 5: Paula lives in a small residential program. A male staff has been seen by other staff going into Paula's room in the evening and closing the door. This has occurred nightly for more than a week. Paula confided a secret to one of the female staff members that she was in love with the male staff and was going to get married. Paula showed the staff member a "cheap" ring that the male staff member had given to her. What should the female staff member do? Staff may be concerned about getting the male staff in trouble. She does not feel she really knows what went on. Who should she tell? What will the other staff think of her if she tells? But what about Paula, is she being sexually exploited or is it ok because she is consenting?

> *Case 6: Steven and Grace want to have sex. The agency says only married clients can have sex. Now Steven and Grace say they want to get married. Is the agency policy ethical? Is the agency obliged to investigate the motive for marriage?. Does the couple understand what marriage is? If they get married how can they take care of themselves? What will her parents say and could they try to stop it? What about children?*

Literature Review

The following literature review provides policy implications in several areas: training for consumers, training for agency staff, counselling and therapy services, access to medical services, sexual risk reduction, as well as sexual and relationship development.

Training for Consumers

Individuals who receive full care service from an agency require training to develop appropriate sociosexual knowledge and to learn responsibility with regard to their sexuality. Sociosexual education has been defined as follows:

A formal training program designed to provide the learner with an opportunity to develop an understanding of the physical, mental, emotional, social, economic, psychological and moral ethical aspects of human development and interpersonal relationships. The purpose of this training is to help the learner develop responsible personal behaviour and so should be geared toward the comprehension level of the participants (Polk Center, PA., 1998, p. 7).

Sexuality Education

Persons with developmental disabilities should have the right to sexual pleasure, to develop meaningful and loving relationships and have access to information about their sexuality (Strong, 1989). Although the field generally recognizes the importance of sociosexual education for persons with developmental disabilities, most agencies do not provide ongoing access to sociosexual training for the persons they support. Often people are sent for sociosexual training only after they have engaged in a sexually inappropriate behaviour or are becoming overtly sexual (Griffiths, 1999). The goal of sociosexual education is to teach responsibility for one's sexual feelings and desires, *not* to eliminate sexual interest and responses (Griffiths, 1999). Sociosexual education should be provided proactively as a routine part of habilitation training, and incorporated into personal planning goals, just as we do transit training, self-care, and other typical life experiences.

Agencies undertaking sociosexual education should carefully select their curriculum. A wealth of training materials that have been developed to teach persons with developmental disabilities. However, there is little empirically-based research regarding the effectiveness of these training materials. Whitehouse and McCabe (1997) argue that most sexuality programs have been developed from the perspective of the professionals and their beliefs about what is important. Few studies (Lunsky & Konstantareas, 1998; McCabe & Cummins, 1996; McCabe & Schreck, 1992) have taken the perspective of the person with a disability and most fail to recognize that men and women may have different needs.

Agencies need to examine curriculum resources to ensure (a)

they provide the range of important topics, and (b) the method of instruction is appropriate for the experience and learning needs of the pupils.

An example of one of the most widely used commercially-available sociosexual education programs is the Life Horizons I and II program by Winifred Kempton (1988). This program is very comprehensive and includes hundreds of slides to aid in instruction. Winnifred Kempton, one of the founding sex educators for persons with developmental disabilities, identi-fied eleven goals for sexuality education: provision of accurate information, to learn about their bodies, to avoid potential ex-ploitation, to teach social skills, to find the best sexual expres-sion relative to personal abilities and needs, to provide access to social programs and the social skills to benefit from them, to enjoy the company of both sexes, to teach responsibility, to help with birth control, to provide insight into marriage and parenthood, to communicate about sexuality without guilt, and to clarify attitudes (Kempton, 1993). She suggests that socio-sexual education should include male and female anatomy, human reproduction, birth control and sexual health, including safer sex practices. However, she also recommends that train-ing should include the moral, social and legal aspects of sexu-ality, male and female sociosexual behaviour, dating, parent-ing, marriage, prevention/coping with abuse, building self-esteem, and establishing relationships.

Relationship Training

All sexually active people, (including persons with develop-mental disabilities) need to develop relationship skills (Foxx, McMorrow, Storey, & Rogers, 1984) and learn to exercise choice in the development of those relationships (Ames &

Samowitz, 1995). One of the most widely used relationship training programs is Circles, designed by Walker-Hirsch and Champagne (1986). This approach uses a visual cue of colored concentric circles to teach about different types of social relationships and the social behaviour that should accompany each type of relationship. The approach is very appealing to people with developmental disabilities in that it provides practical guidelines about whom it is appropriate to interact with and how. Despite its popularity and appeal, there is no validation of its effectiveness in the literature (Whitehouse and McCabe, 1997).

Valenti-Hein, Yarnold, and Muser (1994) developed a dating skills program to teach individuals with developmental disabilities sociosexual skills. Although they were able to demonstrate an increase in dating knowledge, they found that the anxiety about dating mediated the ability of the participants to apply the new learned information.

Responsibility Training

An accepted part of sociosexual education involves teaching that sexual expression comes with responsibilities (Kempton, 1978). Page (1991) suggested that persons with developmental disabilities must be taught to understand personal limitations and abilities, learn the requirements of specific situations, be able to select and carry out appropriate responses to each situation, and additionally, must have the skills to self-monitor the responses. Thus, although the sexuality of a person with developmental disabilities is acknowledged, sexual expression is governed by responsibility to oneself and one's partner(s). The goal of sociosexual education is not only to provide knowledge, but an understanding and ability to act responsibly on this knowledge.

There are different areas of responsibility that need to be taught: personal, legal, medically-related, abuse prevention, and parent training, for those parents who are developmentally disabled. In the following sections each will be discussed.

(i) Personal Responsibility

Being sexual comes with personal responsibilities. Persons with developmental disabilities need to be taught that they have the right to decide who, how and when another will be allowed to touch their body. Sociosexual education should provide the means to help persons with developmental disabilities explore their own feelings and develop their personal values and morality.

(ii) Legal Responsibility

Persons with developmental disabilities should learn the standards and values of society, including legal standards. Many persons with developmental disabilities have been sheltered from knowledge about what is considered appropriate by social standards, or they have experienced a very different set of standards. Ignorance of legal responsibility can create a vulnerability that could increase the potential for a person to inadvertently breach a legal or social standard, and/or result in learning social interactions that are considered inappropriate by social standards.

(iii) Medically-related Responsibility

In the past, the emphasis of teaching individuals with develop-mental disabilities about medical responsibility regarding sexuality was solely on prevention of pregnancy, with a secon-dary emphasis on disease prevention. Since the discovery of AIDS/HIV, the importance of medical responsibility and sexu-ality has become paramount. Safer sex practices must therefore be a mandatory component to any sociosexual education pro-gram. However, the objective of training is not to frighten peo-ple out of having sex, as some programs have attempted, but to educate and promote responsible sex.

Could an agency be accused of neglect if it fails to provide sociosexual education that teaches individuals about these risks and when and how to prevent the risk of disease? The increasing medical risks and responsibilities of sexuality place a greater onus on agencies to provide effective sex education. Thus, it is not only important to teach the subject of sexuality but also to provide outcome measures of training to ensure that knowledge was acquired, skills were learned, and the person was able to implement the learned strategies when needed. Thus improved knowledge (pre to post measures), mainte-nance over time, and generalization to the *real* world must be demonstrated in order to claim programmatic success. Agen-cies that operate sexuality education programs must be able to demonstrate effectiveness, or they cannot assert that they have actually provided training that will change behaviour.

Sexual Risk Reduction Training

It has been estimated that people who have developmental dis-abilities are one and one half times more likely to experience abuse than people who do not have a disability (Sobsey &

Varnhagen, 1991). Kempton (1993) suggests that persons with developmental disabilities may be more likely to be abused because they lack "awareness of what is really happening to them" and the "knowledge, ability or opportunity to report effectively or to appropriate authorities" (p. 201).

A correlation study conducted by Hard (cited in Roeher Institute, 1988) revealed that among a sample of females who had never been afforded sex education, all had been sexually abused. In comparison only 12% of a sample of females who had sex education had experienced abuse. Similar data for the males demonstrated a difference in abuse rates from 38% when there was no education to 20% with education. Although this study is only correlational, and therefore causality cannot be assumed, it does point to the potentially positive influence of sex education on the reduction of risk for abuse.

An increasing number of training materials have become available to teach persons with developmental disabilities to identify, resist, and report unwanted sexual advances. For example, Life Facts 2: Sexual Abuse Prevention (Stanfield & Cowardin, 1992); Life Horizons #1 Set 7: Sexual Abuse (Kempton, 1988); Circles 2: Stop Abuse (Walker-Hirsch & Champagne, 1986). Some of the content areas include personal safety skills, individual rights, assertiveness and self-esteem, communication, social skills, sex education, and self-defense (Sobsey & Doe, 1990). To date, the impact of abuse prevention programs is, with rare exception, unknown (Sobsey, 1994). Most of the programs have been developed on intuitive rather than empirical foundations (Roeher Institute, 1988). While some programs report improvement in consumer knowledge of appropriate and inappropriate sociosexual interactions (Lee & Tang, 1998), few programs have systematically evaluated the impact of training on the actual behaviours of the consumers. Researchers who have evaluated the social validity of the protection skills using generalization probes have shown discouraging results (Lumley, Miltenberger, Long, Rapp, & Roberts, 1998). A recent encouraging exception to these findings is the work of Miltenberger et al. (1999) who found better generalization when training was embedded in the natural environment.

It appears that sociosexual education may produce some benefit to sexual abuse risk for persons with developmental disabilities. However, as will be discussed later in this chapter, consumer education is only one part of a comprehensive intervention plan to reduce the risk of sexual abuse within agencies.

Parent Training
(Parents who have a Developmental Disability)

Although many persons with developmental disabilities may not choose and/or be physically able to become natural parents, there is a small percentage of individuals for whom having and raising children is both possible and desired by the person. This topic is covered extensively in Chapter 7, Parents with Intellectual Disabilities: Impediments and Supports by Maurice Feldman. From time to time agencies may be faced with the opportunity to support a parent with a developmental disability. Special parent education and support resources have been successfully developed to assist a parent with developmental disabilities to learn the skills of parenting.

The above literature review would support the following recommendations:

Recommendation 1:

Sociosexual policy should ensure that persons with developmental disabilities be afforded the opportunity to take part in Sociosexual Education, that includes Relationship and Dating Skills, Responsibility Training, and Sexual-Risk Reduction Training. These programs should be offered on an ongoing or regular basis for all service recipients, and the effectiveness of the programs should be evaluated for each individual relative to knowledge, skill and ability to transfer the skill from the classroom to the real world.

Training for Agency Staff

Implementing policy is closely tied to staff training. No policy, regardless of how well it is written, will be effective unless the staff have the attitudes, knowledge and skills to put the policy into practice. See Chapter 2 on Sexual Policies in Agencies Supporting Persons who have Developmental Disabilities: Ethical and Organizational Issues.

Training on Agency Policy

In an unpublished study, "front-line" staff and managers in community agencies were asked to answer a number of questions about their agency's sexual policy and how they would handle various on-the-job sexual scenarios (Griffiths, Haslam, & Richards, 1994). The authors found that 28% of the front-line staff did not know there was a sexual policy for their agency. Only 21% of the front-line staff had been informed about or trained in sex education issues for consumers, although 67% of the managers had been trained. Moreover, there was a vast difference in the perspectives between and among front-line staff and managers on to how to respond to various sociosexual situations.

Staff, particularly front-line staff, require (i) training in the sexual policy and procedures of the agency, (ii) education regarding the nature of the sociosexual training that is being provided for consumers, (iii) direct instruction on how to implement the policy with particular training in how to respond to various scenarios regarding sexual behaviour, both appropriate and inappropriate, and (iv) training in abuse awareness, prevention and response procedures. The latter two topics will be explored more fully below.

Procedures for Responding to Sociosexual Situations (appropriate and inappropriate)

Agencies need to develop policies to ensure that staff are consistently and objectively responding to sociosexual situations (Howe, 1993). There should be very clear guidelines to provide staff direction on how to manage sexual situations. The policies should deal with a variety of potential examples and potential responses. A decision model is often useful in providing staff training for these complex areas. This model looks at several variables and generates various potential response paths. Let's take as example, a couple who is engaging in sociosexual behaviour. The first consideration would be to determine if the couple is age-appropriate and consenting. If not, the immediate response is to intervene and protect the non-consenting or age-inappropriate partner. Next it would be important to assure if the couple engaged in the behaviour in an appropriate place or time. If not, the staff should point out that this location is a public place and suggest a more suitable location.

As part of the decision model, it is important that staff determine if there is a need to provide or access follow-up for the
incident. For example, a staff may encounter a consumer masturbating in a public area. The immediate response is for the
staff to say, "that is not appropriate to do here, that is something you should do in your bedroom". However, the staff
should ascertain if this was a singular event or a pattern. They
should also ascertain whether or not the exposure was inten-
tional and whether anyone who observed it was adversely affected. If it is a pattern, then the reasons for the public masturbation need to be investigated and an appropriate intervention
plan developed.

The flowchart, Figure A, depicts how a policy, such as ARC's
Sexuality Policy (1998) on Masturbation might look when
translated into a decision-model.

Abuse Prevention and Reporting Procedures

Agency staff need to be aware that most sexual exploitation
and abuse of persons with developmental disabilities occurs
within the person's natural environments and that the offender
generally gains access to the victim through the disability service. Sobsey and Varnhagen (1991) report that most sexual
abuse occurs in services for persons with disabilities and that
in 43.7% of the cases, the perpetrators had an established relationship with the victim because of the victim's developmental
disability. Offenders include caregivers or staff (37%) or other
people with disabilities (6.7%).

Policy Direction: A person may engage in masturbation in private

If masturbation occurs in private and does not infringe on the rights of others, then staff shall not interrupt.

If masturbation is public or infringes on the rights of others, interrupt in a non-punitive way and redirect to a private

If the person expresses frustration with ability to masturbate or is causing harm to self, consult with physician.

The supervisor will discuss privacy in a manner appropriate to the person's level of understanding.

If there is no medical reason found, consult the Clinical Services Unit to determine if there is a need for follow-up.

Incidents of public masturbation in residence will be documented in the daily log; incidents outside of residence will be documented as incident report.

If masturbation continues to occur in public, consult with Clinical Services.

Figure A– ARC's Sexuality Policy (1998)

Recommendation 2:

Policy should commit to the provision of training for all agency staff in the sexual policy and procedures of the agency. Additionally, it is important that staff be aware of the areas of sociosexual knowledge and attitudes consistent with that provided for consumers. Specific instruction is needed to ensure that the staff have direction for implementing the policy and procedures for both appropriate and inappropriate sexual behaviours, and abuse prevention and response procedures.

Staff training in this area should cover at least:

- ✓ General abuse statistics and nature of abuse situations,
- ✓ Sensitization to attitudes that disempower persons with disabilities and increase the vulnerability of abuse,
- ✓ Training in appropriate client-staff social behaviors (i.e. touch, respect for privacy),
- ✓ Training in respectful provision of personal care,
- ✓ Training with regard to response to known or suspected abuse or allegations of abuse, including reporting, and
- ✓ Strategies for dealing with and reporting inappropriate sociosexual contact between a client and themselves.

Counselling and Therapy Services

Educational services are not always enough. Some individuals may require access to clinical services to assist with relationship or couple issues, abuse counselling following victimization, or assessment and treatment for inappropriate or deviant sexual behavior. Agencies should commit in policy to seek appropriate therapeutic services as needed, and specify guidelines for when this may appear warranted.

Sexual Counselling

Couples may require specific counselling to assist them through difficult periods or in planning for a change in their relationship, such as cohabitation, marriage, parenting, or divorce. Counselling issues often include pre-marital counselling, financial responsibilities, housing, employment, relationship development, family planning, sexual relations, communication, emotional responsibilities, roles, and commitment.

Victim Counselling

Persons with developmental disabilities are more often sexually victimized, and the victimization is often repeated and committed by multiple perpetrators (Sobsey, 1994). Yet, counselling or therapeutic support services are not often provided. When they are, they often are minimal. Agencies typically fail to adapt services to the needs of the person with disabilities (Sobsey, 1994).

Ryan (1994) reported 51 cases, who met the DSM III-R criteria for Post Traumatic Stress Disorder (PTSD), in which the identified problem was violent or disruptive behaviour on the part of the victim. Each case included a history of a traumatic event and symptoms lasting more than one month involving persistent re-experience of the event, avoidance of stimuli associated with the event, and hyperarousal. Ryan recommended a six point protocol for treatment that includes judicious use of medication for psychiatric symptoms, treatment of associated medical problems, minimization of iatrogenic complications, psychotherapy, control of triggering events, and education and support of staff.

"Sexual abuse treatment goals include alleviating guilt, regaining the ability to trust, treating depression, helping victims express anger, teaching about sexuality and interpersonal relationships, teaching self-protection techniques, teaching an affective vocabulary to label feelings, teaching sexual preference and sexual abuse issues when appropriate, and treating secondary behavioral characteristics" (Mansell, Sobsey, & Calder, 1992, p. 410).

As with any sexual counselling it is important to take a sexual history and to be mindful of possible psychological and physical factors and their interaction (Sandowski, 1993). Often a thorough medical evaluation is also required. Sandowski (1993) suggests that other areas that need to be addressed when counselling persons with disabilities are self-image, adjustment, physical concerns, and intimate relationships.

In recent years, the field has responded to the needs of sexual offence victims who have a developmental disability by developing sexual assault support groups (i.e., Fresco, Philbin & Peters, 1993) and psychotherapy programs (Razza & Tomasulo, 1996). A sexual counselling method called **PLISSIT** (Annon, 1976) suggests that intervention should be based on the following principles:

✓ Provide *Permission* for the individual to discuss sexual issues in a nonthreatening manner.
✓ Give *Limited Information* that may be lacking or misun-
  derstood.
✓ Give *Specific Sugggestions* to assist the individual or couple in their sexual needs.
✓ Provide *Intensive Therapy* for those who require this.

Annon (1976) suggests that sexual counselling can be provided by different levels of service providers. However, specific suggestions require persons with appropriate training and
intensive therapy such as by trained sexual therapists or counselors.

Sexual counselling often occurs through generic services;
however, clients with disabilities often have concerns and
needs that require special attention (Sandowski, 1993).
Szymanski and Tanguay (1980) suggest that treatment for persons with developmental disabilities is unavailable because of
the lack of experience, training, and confidence of professionals in working with persons with special needs. Therefore, intensive therapy is often difficult to access because of a lack of
trained relationship, marital counsellors and/or sexual therapists with interest in working with persons with special needs.

Assessment and Treatment of Inappropriate Sexual Behaviour

Persons with developmental disabilities generally commit less
serious sexual offence behaviour than nondisabled persons, but
are more likely to commit non-contact behaviours such as public masturbation, exhibitionism and voyeurism (Gilby, Wolf,
& Goldberg, 1989). However, it is often these inappropriate

behaviours that result in persons with developmental disabilities being categorized the same as contact sex offenders (e.g., rapists), thereby excluding them from programs or the community, and subjecting them to very restrictive and intrusive management and control practices.

In 1991, Hingsburger, Griffiths, and Quinsey differentiated between 'deviance' and 'counterfeit deviance' in persons with developmental disabilities. "Sexual misbehaviour" by some persons with developmental disabilities can be differentially influenced by atypical experiences, environments, or learning. These influences include a lack of privacy, modeling, inappropriate partner selection or courtship skills, lack of sexual knowledge or moral training, maladaptive learning histories, and medical or medication reactions.

The implications of the Hingsburger et al. (1991) model for agency policy are very clear. If a person with a developmental disability is demonstrating a sexually inappropriate behaviour it behooves the agency to conduct an appropriate evaluation to determine the cause of the behaviour and to then treat the cause. In the majority of cases, intervention requires some socio-environmental change accompanied by an educational program to teach functional alternative social skills, dating or relationship skills, or sociosexual knowledge. Without this type of assessment, persons with developmental disabilities are vulnerable to being treated using restrictive or coersive measures that will not solve the cause of the problem, and may be inappropriate, ineffective, and a violation of the persons freedoms and rights.

Persons with developmental disabilities develop sexual offending behaviour for the same reasons as nondisabled persons:

- psychological factors such as a lack of attachment bonds, childhood sexual trauma, deficit in empathy skills, and a lack of prosocial inhibition ,
- biomedical factors involving neurological/biomedical abnormalities, mental illness, and medical influences, and
- socio-environmental factors (Griffiths, in press).

Treatment of Sexually Deviant Behaviour

A small percentage of persons with developmental disabilities develop more complex and challenging sexual behaviours, such as deviant sexual expressions. It is imperative that the agency access appropriate professional resources to assess the nature of the problem for the individual and make recommendations for medical, psychiatric, socio-environmental, and psychological services.

In the past two decades there has been considerable knowledge gained with regard to the assessment and treatment of persons with developmental disabilities who commit sexual offending behaviour. Agencies serving persons with developmental disabilities have successfully provided community-based and institutionally-based interventions to treat these behaviours (Griffiths, Quinsey, & Hingsburger, 1989; Haaven, Little & Petre-Miller, 1990; Ward et al., 1992).

A corollary to the treatment of persons in the program who have sexually invasive or predatory behaviour, is the obligation to save from harm persons within the program who might be vulnerable to such advances. As such, the obligation to treat is often closely tied to the obligation to protect.

Recommendation 3:

Agencies should commit in policy to access appropriate clinical treatment for persons within their programs who require couple/relationship counselling, victim counselling, or intervention for sexually inappropriate or deviant behaviour.

Access to Medical Services

Medical Information

Persons with developmental disabilities may have many questions about their sexuality, but lack access to resource persons who can provide reliable answers. Staff or family members may not know the answer, may not agree that the person has the right to know the answer, or may decide that the information requested should be given in a biased or uniformed way. One of the important aspects of a policy is the provision of accurate, informed, and unbiased information to the individual upon which important medical issues can be decided (e.g., birth control, sexually transmitted disease, sexual dysfunction and medication).

Birth Control

Whether oral contraceptives, depo-provera, condoms or even sterilization, persons with developmental disabilities should be afforded an opportunity to gain information regarding options for birth control, should they choose to be sexually active and not get pregnant. In Canada prior to 1986, guardians were providing consent to sterilize their children as a precaution to pregnancy. However, the Supreme Court of Canada ruled on the case of Eve that it was illegal to perform non-therapeutic sterilization without the person's consent (Rioux & Yarmol, 1987).

Kramer Monat-Haller (1992) suggests that when explaining contraception, it is important to be as explicit as possible. She suggests showing different forms of birth control and explaining the reproductive anatomy and physiology using drawings. Additionally, she suggests that the shared responsibility of both partners should be discussed. Often Planned Parenting or Public Health Centres are very helpful in providing this type of education and helping a couple decide on the most appropriate type of birth control for them.

Sexually Transmitted Disease

Persons with developmental disabilities may require medical education and/or treatment regarding sexually transmitted diseases. Scotti, Speaks, Masia, Boggess and Drabman, (1996) argues that persons with developmental disabilities are not receiving the full educational benefits of media messages on HIV/AIDS, other than condom use and avoidance of contact with blood. Their findings suggest that training produces improved knowledge but things were uncertain that training would lead to behaviour change (i.e., increased condom use).

In this day and age it is irresponsible for any sexual education program to *not* address such vital and life-saving information as safer sex practices. However, knowledge-training should also be linked to skills-training and support for use these skills (Scotti et al., 1996). Moreover, persons with developmental disabilities need to know the symptoms of sexually transmitted diseases and how to access appropriate medical attention if needed.

Sexual Dysfunction

Persons with developmental disabilities may experience sexual idiosyncracies related to their syndrome. The following examples are provided by Rowe and Savage (1988):

✓ Persons with Down Syndrome may experience slower growth rates. Females may experience delayed or irregular periods. Both male and female fertility may be questionable.

✓ Persons with Turner's Syndrome do not experience puberty, are sterile, and do not fully develop physically. Hormonal therapy may aid in the ability to have sexual relations, however sterility remains.

✓ Persons with Klinefelter's Syndrome experience delays in their secondary sexual characteristics, pubic hair is often distributed as a female and testes are small. Sexual drive may be diminished, however males can achieve erection and ejaculation. They are sterile and often experience gender identity problems .

✓ Persons with Prader-Willi Syndrome are often interested in sexual intimacy; they may, however, be unable to be actively involved because of their incomplete sexual development. Males have delay in secondary sexual characteristics and underdeveloped male genitalia. Females have delayed or sporadic menstruation and incomplete secondary sexual development.

In the cases described above, medical and counselling services, in addition to adaptation of educational programs, need to be available.

Access to medical professionals regarding sexual dysfunction is perhaps one of the most neglected areas. If a person with a developmental disability is unable to be sexually active or achieve sexual satisfaction, there is generally no action taken unless the individual is engaging in an inappropriate behaviour. Sexual dysfunction can affect a person in many ways including desire, excitement, orgasm or resolution and may involve pain (APA, 1994). Some of the challenges are lifelong and generalized, whereas others are acquired or situational. The causes may be psychological, medical, substance use, or combined factors.

Medication

Many persons with developmental disabilities are prescribed medication for a variety of medical and behavioural/ psychiatric reasons. Often medications can have side effects on sexual desire or performance. In our example at the beginning of this chapter, Ralph had been receiving seizure medication that rendered him unable to masturbate to orgasm. Often persons with disabilities are not informed of the side-effects of the medication. In Ralph's case, the physician did not think it was important to tell Ralph because he was "developmentally disabled" and assumed to be nonsexual. Persons with developmental disabilities should be afforded the same opportunity to be informed of the major side-effects of medication as are other medical care consumers.

There is however a second issue of sexuality and medication that should be addressed in policy. Medications are often used to manage sexual behaviour and desire. In *rare* cases of dangerous sexual behaviour, such medications may be considered by the consumer to assist in self-management or relapse pre-

vention. However, such extreme measures would only be considered with the person's informed consent and only in combination with other habilitative and rehabilitative treatments (See
Chapter 4).

Recommendation 4:

***Policy should commit to the provision of accurate, informed
and unbiased information to the individual regarding areas
such as birth control, sexually transmitted disease, sexual
dysfunction.***

Sexual Risk Reduction

Persons with developmental disabilities are more vulnerable to
sexual abuse than nondisabled persons and the abuse typically
occurs within known and often care-giving relationships. Although it may not be possible to totally eliminate sexual abuse
in society, agencies serving persons with developmental disabilities need to strive to provide that individuals who are supported within their agency are at not at greater risk because
they rely on care-giving services.

If abuse is to be reduced, it is critical that agencies commit to
the promotion of an *environment of healthy boundaries.* There
are several procedural levels that need to be addressed to create healthy boundaries. Finkelhor (1984) suggested that abuse
cannot occur if any one of four barriers are in place: motivation, justification or overcoming conscience, opportunity, and
overcoming victim resistance. Most agencies have addressed
this by only attempting to address the latter through consumer
education. However consumer education alone is insufficient.
The policies for reduction of abuse in agencies requires inter-

vention at many levels including consumer education and empowerment, staff awareness and training, alteration of personal care procedures, respect for privacy, and interviewing and screening upon hiring for staff attitudes and motivation.

Consent for Sexual Activity

Families, staff and agencies are often faced with the dilemma of advocating for the rights to sexual expression while ensuring that there is informed consent. Stavis (1996) suggests that agencies must make a reasonable professional determination of the individual's ability or lack of ability to consent to various types of sexual activity. Consent ability is assumed if the person understands that the body is private, knows the act is sexual, and that he or she can say "no" (ARC, 1998). Ames, Hepner, Kaeser, and Pendler (1988) similarly define consent as involving capacity (knowledge), that is informed and voluntary. However, other definitions have suggested that consent involves both expressed knowledge and ability to act on the knowledge through responsible interpersonal behaviour (Ames & Samowitz, 1995).

An adult with a developmental disability can legally consent to sexual activity, however a child (age defined in law) cannot. The Criminal Code says that children under 12 years of age are never capable of providing consent to sexual activity. Children between 12-14 years are not considered old enough to consent to sexual activity with the following exceptions: when two young people consenting to the sexual activity have no more than two years difference in their age and the older teenager is not yet 16 years.

Sexual activity without consent is a crime; it is also a crime if a person with authority over the person uses that authority to obtain the consent (ARCH, 1990). It is highly questionable whether true legal consent is possible when a consumer consents or submits to sexual activity with a person on whom they are dependent. In Canada, a person 14 years and over is protected from sexual exploitation by a person in power and authority over them or on whom the person is dependent (ARCH, 1990).

Consent is a much-debated issue in social services at this time. The issues appear to be very different in the United States and Canada. In the United States, there is a reliance on the right to personal autonomy; the Canadian approach appears to revolve around the exclusion of unwanted physical intrusion upon one's body. As a result, the approaches to assess competence for sexual activity have been very different on either side of the North American border.

Although American state laws vary, the ARC guidelines (using New Jersey law) have defined consent "as a person 18 years or older who demonstrates an understanding that his or her body is private, and that he or she has the right to say no, and that he or she knows that the conduct is distinctly sexual" (ARC, 1998, p. 4). In New York State, the regulations ensure the rights to sexual expression for persons with developmental disabilities but within the limits of consensual ability (Niederbuhl & Morris, 1993). As such, processes have been put in place in agencies to predetermine consent capacity for persons served in agencies in the state. Niederbuhl and Morris (1993) describe the process for their state operated facility. It involves formal testing using the Socio-Sexual Knowledge and Attitude Test (Wish, McCombs, & Edmonson, 1979), followed by a formal meeting involving the psychologist, social worker, the primary individual care plan representative, front line staff, nurse, and administrative staff. The outcome of the meeting is to determine if the person is capable of giving informed consent. The American policy in some states appears to require proof of informed consent capacity in order to be eligible to sexual rights.

In Canada, the precedent-setting case of "Eve" provided some important perspectives on the right of the person with a developmental disability to make decisions regarding her body (Rioux & Yarmol, 1987). Although Eve was not was considered competent to make a decision regarding non-therapeutic sterilization, the courts disallowed the consent of a *de facto* guardian to make such a decision on her behalf. There appears to be a presumption of capability, unless proven otherwise. This is evident in the sexual policy of Riverview Hospital in Vancouver, British Columbia. According to their policy, if a person chooses to engage in sexual behaviour, the person's capacity to consent is evaluated by completion of a questionnaire that is reviewed by the treatment team. Unless indicators of nonconsent are present, consent capability is assumed (Riverview Hospital, 1993). The Canadian presumption appears to be that persons with developmental disabilities have the same sexual rights as nondisabled persons; limitations to those rights can only be abridged if and when there is clear justification.

Creating Healthy Boundaries in Agencies

Contrary to popular myth, offenders against persons with developmental disabilities are not generally the stranger on the street. The offences often happen within the support network and by persons who have gained access to the person by virtue of the person's disability (Sobsey, 1994).

Persons with developmental disabilities *may* require 24 hour supervision, assistance with personal care and many different professionals and paraprofessionals in their lives for long periods of time. The personal and private nature of the interactions provides the opportunity for someone who is so inclined to offend. Staff are rarely taught how to respectfully perform personal care procedures. Staffing ratios are often so stretched that even if there were guidelines, staff are alone with consumers performing these personal care procedures. The lack of agency policies, procedures and staff training allow this boundary violation to go unguarded and unobserved.

Most theorists would further suggest that the high rate of sexual abuse of persons with developmental disabilities is intricately linked to power. Rutter (1989) examined the power dynamics involved in sexual abuse by people in positions of trust and found that the relationship usually is one that has great significance for the victim and that the sexual aspect of the relationship occurs because of the culture of compliance to authority that the victim has learned throughout their life. If a feature of the lives of people with developmental disabilities is a high rate of abuse particularly by people on whom they are reliant for care, it may be that this behaviour has come to be tolerated within the community of consumers.

There is a growing body of research that shows that persons with developmental disabilities may be more tolerant of abuse. The work of Flynn, Reeve, Whelan, and Speake (1985) supports this notion of cultural tolerance. These researchers found that consumers were equally tolerant of acceptable and unacceptable rules. Other authors have found that persons with developmental disabilities were less likely to have negative feelings towards abuse and more tolerant of personal touch especially from staff (McCabe, Cummins, and Reid,1994; Owen, Griffiths, Sales, Feldman, and Richards, 2000) . Given the intimate nature of the care provided in residential services, it is possible that interactions may become confused or distorted for some people. In this context, the sexual advances of staff and other caregivers toward a person with a disability may be tolerated or misinterpreted as appropriate social approach behaviour. In some cases, the person with a developmental disability may be unaware of the boundaries of acceptable staff behaviour beyond care-giving duties, and of their right of refusal. This lack of awareness of their rights and lack of self-efficacy were found in the work of McCarthy (1993) and Thompson (1994). Consumers also may feel intimidated and afraid to repel advances because of the control and power that they perceive that care-providers have over their lives.

There are many factors that may contribute to abuse tolerance including the social isolation of consumers, lack of access to sexual relationships, lack of sex education, and reliance on staff for personal care-giving. Consumers may also tolerate abuse because they need to rationalize the dissonance (Festinger, 1957; Dietrich & Berkowitz, 1997; Johnson, Kelly & LeBlanc, 1995) caused when people on whom they are reliant for personal care engage in behaviour that is unreasonable. It may be easier to rationalize that the behaviour is acceptable than that the much-needed caregiver is wrong.

Most staff would never think of taking sexual advantage of a person with a disability and if the thought occurred they would quickly correct the thought. So what is different with those who offend? What we know about persons who sexually offend is that they have developed a way of cognitively justifying their behaviour. They feel sexual arousal, yet they know that that is inappropriate given the circumstances. Therefore, the person experiencing dissonance must either control the arousal or change the thought that what they want to do is wrong. Unfortunately, society's negative attitudes toward persons with disabilities and the myths about the sexuality of persons with disabilities allows this justification to more easily occur. For example, if one believes people with disabilities don't feel pain the same way as others, or won't understand what has happened, then there will be less dissonance in justifying the offense. Other offenders may distort the offense by claiming that they are providing "hands on" sexuality training, despite the fact that breaches personal boundaries. In some cases, this faulty thinking occurs with a combination of alcohol or drugs, but not always.

Some agencies have developed hiring procedures to ensure that (i) individuals with a known history of abuse are screened out, (ii) the person's attitudes towards persons with disabilities is examined, and (iii) the nature of the staff person's response to stress and power situation can be explored. This procedure may not be fool-proof but it represents a positive move forward to creating healthy boundaries.

Investigation/Reporting

Staff members should be aware of the indicators of sexual abuse. The Advocacy Resource Centre for the Handicapped-ARCH (1990) suggests these include presence of an STD, underwear that is stained or torn, bruised genitalia or anus, sore throat, presence of semen on clothes or body, unusual odor, pain while walking or sitting, and significant change in sexual behaviour or attitude.

The staff should also be taught how to respond to an abuse disclosure. The procedure that staff employ following a disclosure is critical for both the emotional well being of the victim and to ensure that proper steps are taken toward responsible action. An improper response can create significant emotional distress for the victim and taint the case for court.

Staff members should be trained in the steps to follow. A list of steps should be available in procedure for easy reference. Here are some of the recommendations from ARCH (1990):

If a person with a developmental disability discloses abuse or there is evidence that abuse has occurred staff should:

✓ *speak to the person in private; be patient; avoid helping the person with your words*

✓ *allow the person to use their communication systems, or write or draw a picture*

✓ *accept the allegation without judgment*

✓ *let the person tell you what happened*

✓ *avoid leading questions which could destroy the case in court*

✓ *don't assume the person was frightened, did not enjoy the experience or that the victim likes or dislikes the abuser*

✓ *assure the person that he/she is not bad or responsible for what has happened*

✓ *make no promises to keep it secret, staff will need to report this to their supervisors*

✓ *if there is still danger, assist the victim to get out of danger*

✓ *try to get the name of the suspected abuser, but do not confront the person*

> ✓ *the victim should be taken to a hospital emergency department, sexual assault unit or family doctor for examination as soon as possible and before evidence is lost; if the person is unable to consent to treatment, a guardian should be contacted (unless the accused has some relationship to the guardian)*
>
> ✓ *follow the agency protocol for reporting the incident, however reporting to someone in the agency does not absolve a staff member from responsibility to ensure the police or child protection authorities are notified*
>
> ✓ *the person should be told what options are available (calling police, getting a lawyer, receiving counselling and post trial support), what will happen next, who will be told, and what action can be taken to avoid further abuse*
>
> ✓ *immediately after the interview, document everything*
>
> ✓ *keep the information confidential.*

Crimes, including sexual crimes, against persons with developmental disabilities are rarely reported (Wilson & Brewer, 1992). Sobsey (1994) has suggested that it is important to have procedures to ensure that abuse is reported to the police. However, it is critical to develop protocol for the police and agencies to work together to ensure that the rights of victims and accused with developmental disabilities are upheld throughout the process. A manual was developed by the Roeher Institute (1992) as a guide for the legal community in addressing the sexual abuse of people with developmental disabilities. However, many agencies have worked with the local police and the courts to develop their own unique protocols for reporting of sexual assault. For example, in the Niagara Region, Ontario, Canada, community agencies and the police have developed guidelines for reporting sexual assaults against persons with developmental disabilities (Richards, Watson, & Bleich, 2000). See Chapter 12 for a discussion of these guidelines.

Recommendation 5:

Agencies need a policy that clearly guards the healthy boundaries necessary to reduce abuse. It includes the following:

(1) consumer and staff abuse awareness and prevention training,
(2) staff-consumer relationships with regard to appropriate social approach behaviours, and respect,
(3) screening staff during hiring to eliminate those who may promote a culture of abuse, and
(4) attitude sensitization as part of ongoing training and practice.

Implications for policies go beyond sexuality issues alone but to the following issues of :

(1) privacy,
(2) respectful personal care procedures,
(3) consumer rights to self-determination and to refuse compliance to intolerable requests, and
(4) training for staff in abuse identification and reporting.

Relationship Development

Opportunity

In the United States, there was a litigation that required agencies to provide persons with developmental disabilities the opportunity to develop a range of relationships in their lives, including sociosexual relationships (Coleman & Murphy, 1980). Interestingly, although 95% of the agencies provided opportunity for people to meet and interact as a social group, only 15% of the agencies would ever let a heterosexual couple be alone together.

Opportunity for relationships is more than just making sure people are congregated and have the chance to meet. True opportunity for relationships requires the following: (i) development of social skills to enable individuals to form a range of meaningful relationships (i.e., relationship training), (ii) self-determination and freedom of choice regarding the expression of that relationship within socially-accepted parameters, and (iii) privacy to develop intimate relationships appropriately.

Privacy

One of the major controversies that often arise with regard to right to privacy is a parent or guardian claim of "right to know" about sexual matters. Ames, Hepner, Kaeser, and Pendler (1988) suggest that this claim has no greater substance in the area of sexual matters than in other privacy matters.

In the United States, right to privacy is constitutionally protected; this right has been interpreted by some to include sexual privacy. However in Canada, there is no such right enshrined in the Charter of Rights and Freedoms. However, the Charter does nonetheless provide for a reasonable degree of autonomy over important decisions affecting one's private life (Rowe & Save, 1988).

Range of Relationships

In North American society, sexual activity is more likely to be accepted if it occurs within the context of a relationship. Persons with developmental disabilities have the potential to engage in the same range of relationships as nondisabled persons. Some individuals may choose to date, others may marry and/or have children. Some persons may be heterosexual and others may be homosexual or bisexual. Some relationships may be monogamous and others polygamous or promiscuous. Just as with nondisabled persons, persons with disabilities have the right to self-determination and the freedom to choose their sexual lifestyle within the social standards imposed by the law or social framework (Ames & Samowitz, 1995). In some cases the choices that people make will not be in synchrony with those of the agency, however, the same range of relationships that exist in society in general will also exist among persons with developmental disabilities. Thus, persons with developmental disabilities should not be sanctioned in ways that contradict what is accepted in society. This does not imply that if a person with a developmental disability is engaging in a behaviour that is unsafe or unwise, that there would not be an obligation to provide the person counsel, education, and protection. In fact, there is an obligation to do so.

Recommendation 6:

Agencies serving persons with developmental disabilities have an obligation to provide opportunity and training for persons with developmental disabilities to develop a range of relationships in their lives, some of which may be sexual, and to provide an atmosphere of respect for self-determination in those relationships and opportunity for the relationships to develop.

Conference Deliberations

The conference participants in the session on Policy and Procedures agreed that Policies and Procedures on Sexuality are
essential for agencies that support persons with developmental
disabilities. When policies and procedures are carefully and
respectfully developed, they create an atmosphere of "healthy
and responsible sexuality". The following were the key components identified by our participants:

> ✓ *A consistent and person-centred value-base to en-
> sure an atmosphere of sexual responsibility while at
> the same time ensuring that individual rights are
> protected.*
> ✓ *Commitment to the education of consumers with re-
> gard to their sexuality, relationships, social skills,
> responsibility, protection from harm, and, where ap-
> propriate, parent training.*
> ✓ *Commitment to staff education in sexual policies and
> procedures that are consistent with the consumer
> education, and includes training in procedures for
> responding to both appropriate and inappropriate
> expressions of sexuality, abuse prevention and in-
> tervention, and attitude sensitivity.*
> ✓ *Ensuring access to relationship/couple counselling,
> victim counselling, and assessment/intervention for
> inappropriate or deviant behaviour.*
> ✓ *Access to medical services for sexual information,
> birth control, sexually transmitted disease, sexual
> dysfunction, and medication.*
> ✓ *Prevention of sexual abuse including procedures*

> *and training to ensure healthy boundaries, appropriate staff/consumer contact and power-relationships, respect of privacy, and provision of normalized support. Procedures to respond to reports of abuse and to support the individual through the courts and the aftermath as necessary.*
>
> ✓ *Provision of the opportunity for individuals to engage in meaningful relationships of their choosing.*

Summary

State of the Art

In 1978, Hall and Sawyer encouraged agencies to develop sexual policies that recognized the following elements:

1. Persons with developmental disabilities have the right to express their sexuality and develop appropriate sexual behaviours within their capabilities.
2. Sociosexual relationships are considered an essential part of normal development.
3. Sexual activity would be in private between consenting adults with no evidence of violence.
4. Healthy sociosexual expression requires sex education and family life planning programs; birth control measures would be recommended and made available to, but not imposed upon sexually active individuals.
5. Individuals with developmental disabilities are "entitled to the same rights, freedoms and restrictions of sexual expression as are granted in the population at large" (p. 42).

Although there are many aspects to their article that are now outdated, their essential message of respect is similar three decades later. However, there is far greater opportunity in this millennium to actualize this in both policy and practice. Today, persons with developmental disabilities are supported in their own homes or smaller group homes. The normalization movement that began in the 1970's has resulted in increased awareness of the potential of persons with disabilities to live full lives, including a sexual life. Consumer and staff training materials now are more readily available. Access to appropriate medical and clinical services continues to expand. Awareness of the rates of abuse, causes and potential system-wide strategies for change, now exist. Thus although the spirit remains similar to Hall and Swayze's (1972) recommendations, today's sexual policies go beyond discussion of the sexuality of the person with a disability, to a broader view of the person within the context of the culture and system of support.

Clinical Implications

There are several clinical implications that arise out of Policy and Procedures on Sexuality. If there is an obligation to provide appropriate staff and consumer education, then there must also be an obligation to develop appropriate resource personnel for an agency to perform training. Currently, many agencies do not have staff who are qualified to provide this type of training. Additionally, access to specialized clinical or medical treatment can also present a challenge. Persons with developmental disabilities may be rejected from mainstream services because they are deemed unable to benefit from treatment approaches for nondisabled persons, or because available resources have been devoted to programs designed for nondisabled people. There are insufficient and scattered clinical and medical expertise to ensure access to specialists who have training with persons with developmental disabilities. As a result, agencies with expertise with persons with developmental disabilities may need to team up with persons with medical and clinical expertise to ensure adequate resources are developed.

Agency Implications

The development of *Policies and Procedures in Sexuality* is a process. The acceptance of a Policy and the development of Procedures is only a beginning step. Implementation of the policies and procedures and monitoring for adherence is a vital commitment that must be made to this process. This will require staff time, development of equipment and expertise, accessing outside resources, and supervisory time to do this well and on an ongoing basis.

What Should Be Done Now

All agencies need to commit to begin the process of policy development or revision of outdated policies regarding sexuality. Administrators should involve all parties in the process: consumers, family members, advocates, clinical resource personnel, front-line staff and the Board of Directors. A small steering committee with representatives from these groups should be formed. One of the first steps of this group will be to gather information about existing policy and procedures both in their own agency and in similar agencies. Next, it is often helpful to gather real-life scenarios that have occurred in recent years in the organization, for which direction was necessary. It is important to gather these from all parties listed above. Often educational sessions provide a useful forum to ensure that all parties have basic information on rights, realities and the debunking of myths. There must be ample opportunity for dialogue and consideration of all perspectives. If all parties are invested in the *Sociosexual Policy and Procedures*, implementation will be less challenging.

The policy itself should be brief. It should include a purpose statement, a short policy statement, and then a list of the basic areas of policy. A good policy should fit on one sheet of paper. It should be general and identify the basic values of the organization including (i) the obligation to support the rights of persons with disabilities in the area of sexuality, (ii) a commitment to the provision of both consumer and staff training, (iii) promotion of opportunities to foster healthy relationships, (iv) recognition of the obligation to acquire effective treatment, counselling and medical services in the sociosexual realm as needed, and (v) creation of a healthy sociosexual atmosphere that minimizes the opportunity for sexual exploitation or abuse.

Once the Board of Directors has passed the policy, the next step is to develop procedures that can ensure that the policy is implemented consistently. Procedures give guidance to staff regarding various situations (examples might be "How to determine if a person is consenting." Or "Staff response to nonconsenting sexual behaviour" or "Steps to follow if abuse is suspected or reported"). The procedures are guidelines for staff to respond to the typical situations that might occur.

Implementation of the policy and procedures then requires that all interested parties be provided with the written guidelines, all staff are fully trained, and consumers are informed of the policies and procedures.

In many cases, agencies maintain an ongoing committee that is responsible for reviewing situations where there is ambiguity, disagreement or conflict. This resolution committee is known to all parties and accessible for not only staff and administrators, but consumers as well.

Final Consensus Statement

Wolfensburger (1972) suggested many years ago that persons with developmental disabilities should have the right to live life as normal as possible, including their sexual life. However, most community and institutional agencies serving this population have failed to address this issue in a proactive and constructive way. Persons with developmental disabilities are sexual beings. Agencies that support persons with developmental disabilities can no longer deny this by ignoring the issue of policy development. Sexuality policies must balance the need to respect the rights to sexual expression and physical integrity of each individual, while providing a healthy and safe environment where every one is protected from harm. It is only then that true normalization of the sexuality of persons with developmental disabilities can be achieved.

References

Advocacy Research Centre for the Handicapped–ARCH. (1990). *Responding to the abuse of people with disabilities*. Toronto, ON: Author.

American Psychiatric Association (1994). *Diagnostic and statistical manual of mental disorder (4th ed.)*. Washington, D.C.: Author.

ARC- Association for People with Developmental Disabilities (1998). *Policy on sexuality*. Arlington, Texas: Author.

Ames, H., Hepner, P. J., Kaeser, F. & Pendler, B. (1988). *Guidelines for sexuality education and programming for the next decade.* Prepared for the 1988 International conference on developmental disabilities: Employment, integration and community competence. New York.

Ames, H. & Samowitz, P. (1995, August) Inclusionary standard for determining sexual consent for individuals with developmental disabilities. *Mental Retardation,* 264-268.

Annon, J. S. (1976). *Behavioral treatment of sexual problems: Brief therapy.* New York: Harper & Row.

Coleman, E. M. & Murphy, W. D. (1980). A survey of sexual attitudes and sex education programs among facilities for the mentally retarded. *Applied Research in Mental Retardation, 1,* 269-279.

Deisher, R. (1973). Sexual behavior of retarded in institutions. In F.F. De La Cruz & G.D. La Veck (Eds.), *Human sexuality and the mentally retarded* (pp. 145-152). New York: Brunner/ Mazel.

Dietrich, D. & Berkowitz, L. (1997). Alleviation of dissonance by engaging in prosocial behavior or receiving ego-enhancing feedback. *Journal of Social Behavior and Personality, 12,* 557-566.

Edmonson, B., McCombs, K., & Wish, J. (1979). What retarded adults believe about sex. *American Journal of Mental Deficiency, 84,* 11-18.

Festinger, L. (1957). *A theory of cognitive dissonance.* Stanford, CA: Stanford University Press

Finkelhor, D. (1984). *Child sexual abuse: Theory and research.* New York: The Free Press.

Flynn, M. C., Reeve, D., Whelan, E., & Speake, B. (1985). The development of a measure: A tool to measure the mentally handicapped adult's tolerance of rules and recognition of rights. *Journal of Practical Approaches to Developmen-*

tal Handicap, 9, 18-24.

Foxx, R. M., McMorrow, M. J., Storey, K., & Rogers, B. M. (1984). Teaching social/sexual skills to mentally retarded adults. *American Journal of Mental Deficiency, 89,* 9-15.

Fresco, F., Philin, L., & Peters J, (1993). Sexual assault support groups for women with developmental disabilities. *The Habilitative Mental Healthcare Newsletter, 12(6),* 98-103.

Gilby, R., Wolf, L. & Golberg, B. (1989). Mentally retarded adolescent sex offenders: A survey and pilot study. *Canadian Journal of Psychiatry, 34,* 542-548.

Griffiths, D. (1999). Sexuality and developmental disabilities: Mythconceptions and facts. In I. Brown & M. Percy (Eds.). *Developmental Disabilities in Ontario* (pp. 443-451). Toronto: Front Porch Publishing

Griffiths, D. (in press) Sexual Aggression. In W. I. Gardner (Ed.), *Aggression.* New York: NADD Press.

Griffiths, D., Haslam, T., & Richards, D. (1994). Approaches to sexual situations: Caregiver and manager perspectives. Unpublished manuscript.

Griffiths, D., Quinsey, V. L., & Hingsburger, D. (1989). *Changing inappropriate sexual behavior.* Baltimore, MD.: Paul H. Brookes.

Haaven, J., Little, R., & Petre-Miller, D. (1990). *Treating intellectually disabled sex offenders.* Orwell, VT.: Safer Society.

Hall, J. E. & Sawyer, H. W. (1978). Sexual policies for the mentally retarded. *Sexuality and Disability, 1,* 34-43.

Hingsburger, D., Griffiths, D., & Qunisey, V. (1991). Detecting counterfeit deviance: Differentiating sexual deviance from sexual inappropriateness. *The Habilitative Mental Healthcare Newsletter, 10,* 51-54.

Howe, E. M. (1993). *Considerations for the development of*

agency policies concerning sexual contact and consent. State of New York: Office of Mental Retardation and Developmental Disabilities.

Johnson, R., Kelly, R. & LeBlanc, B. (1995). Motivational basis of dissonance: Aversive consequences or inconsistency. *Personality & Social Psychology Bulletin, 21,* 850-855.

Kempton, W. (1978). Sex education for the mentally handicapped. *Sexuality and Disability,* I, 137-145.

Kempton, W. (1988). *Life horizons I and II.* Santa Barbara, CA: Stanfield Publishing.

Kempton, W. (1993). *Sexuality and persons with disabilities that hinder learning: A comprehensive guide for teachers and professionals.* Santa Barbara, CA: James Stanfield Publishing.

Kramer Monat-Haller, R. (1992). *Understanding and expressing sexuality: Responsible choices for individuals with developmental disabilities.* Baltimore, MD: Paul H. Brookes

Lee, Y. K & Tang, C. S. (1998). Evaluation of a sexual abuse prevention program for female Chinese adolescents with mild mental retardation. *American Journal on Mental Retardation, 103,* 105-116.

Lindsay, W. R., Bellshaw, E., Culross, G., Staines, C., & Michie, A. (1992). Increases in knowledge following a course of sex education for people with intellectual disabilities. *Journal of Intellectual Disability Research, 36,* 531-539.

Lumley, V. A., Miltenberger, R. G., Long, E. S., Rapp, J. T. & Roberts, J. A. (1998). Evaluation of a sexual abuse prevention program for adults with mental retardation. *Journal of Applied Behavior Analysis, 31,* 91-101.

Lunsky, Y. & Konstantareas, M. M. (1998) The attitudes of individuals with autism and mental retardation toward sexuality. *Education and Training in Mental Retardation and Developmental Disabilities, 33,* 24-33.

Mansell, S., Sobsey, D. & Calder, P. (1992). Sexual abuse treatment for persons with developmental disabilities. *Professional Psychology: Research and Practice, 23,* 404-409

McCabe, M. P., & Cummins, R. A. (1996). The sexual knowledge, experience and feelings and needs of people with mild intellectual disability. *Education and Training in Mental Retardation and Developmental Disabilities, March,* 13-21.

McCabe, M. P., Cummins, R. A. & Reid, S. B. (1994). An empirical study of the sexual abuse of people with intellectual disability. *Sexuality and Disability, 12,* 297-306.

McCabe, M. P. & Schreck, A. (1992). Before sex education: An evaluation of the sexual knowledge, experience, feelings and needs of people with mild intellectual disabilities. *Australia and New Zealand Journal of Developmental Disabilities, 18,* 75-83

McCarthy, M. (1993). Sexual experiences of women with learning difficulties in long-stay hospitals. *Sexuality and Disability, 11,* 277-285.

Miltenberger, R. G.., Roberts, J. A., Ellingson, S., Galenski, T., Rapp, J. T., Long, E. S. & Lumley, V. A. (1999). Training and generalization of sexual abuse prevention skills for women with mental retardation. *Journal of Applied Behavior Analysis, 32,* 385-388.

Niederbuhl, J. M. & Morris, C. D. (1993). Sexual knowledge and the capability of persons with dual diagnosis to consent to sexual contact. *Sexuality and Disability, 11,* 295-307.

Owen, F., Griffiths, D., Sales, C., Feldman, M. & Richards, D. (2000). Perceptions of acceptable boundaries of persons with developmental disabilities and their caregivers. *Journal of Developmental Disabilities, 7(1),* 34-49.

Page, A. C. (1991). Teaching developmentally disabled people

self-regulation in sexual behavior. *Australia and New Zealand Journal of Developmental Disabilites, 17*, 81-88.

Polk Center (1998). *Policy and Procedures Manual.* Common-
wealth of Pennsylvania, Department of Public Welfare:
Author.

Pringle, H. (1997). Alberta Barren. *Saturday Night.* 30-74.

Razza, N. A., & Tomasulo, D. J. (1996). The sexual abuse
continuum: Therapeutic interventions with individuals with
mental retardation. *The Habilitative Mental Healthcare
Newsletter, 15*, 84-86.

Richards, D., Watson, S., & Bleich, R.. (2000). Guidelines and
practices for reporting sexual assault. *Journal of Developmental Disabilities, 7(1)*, 130-140.

Rioux M., & Yarmol, K. (1987). The right to control one's
own body: A look at the "Eve" decision. *Entourage, 2, 26-
30.*

Riverview Hospital (1993). Policy on patient sexuality. Vancouver, B.C.: Author.

Roeher Institute (1994). *Violence and people with disabilities:
A review of the literature.* Ottawa, Ontario: National Clear-
inghouse on Family Violence.

Roeher Institute (1992). *No more victims: A manual to guide
the legal community in addressing the sexual abuse of people with a mental handicap.* Toronto: Author.

Roeher Institute (1988). *Vulnerable: Sexual abuse and people
with an intellectual handicap.* Toronto, ON: G. Allan Roeher Institute.

Rowe, W. S. & Savage, S. (1988). *Sexuality and the developmentally handicapped: A guidebook for health care professionals.* Lewiston, NY: Edwin-Mellan Press.

Rutter, P. (1989). *Sex in the forbidden zone: When men in
power– therapists, doctors, clergy, teachers and others–
betray women's trust.* Los Angeles: Jeremy Tarcher.

Ryan, R. (1994). Post-traumatic Stress Disorder in persons with developmental disabilities. *Community Mental Health Journal, 30*, 45-54.

Sandowski, C. (1993). Responding to the sexual concerns of persons with disabilities. *Journal of Social Work and Human Sexuality, 8,* 29-43.

Scheerenberger, R. C. (1983). *A history of mental retardation.* Baltimore, MD: Paul H. Brookes.

Scotti, J. R., Speaks, L. V., Masia, C. L., Boggess, J. T., & Drabman, R. S. (1996, June). The educational effects of providing AIDS-Risk information to persons with developmental disabilities: An exploratory study. *Education and Training in Mental Retardation and Developmental Disabilities,* 115-122.

Shore, D.A. (1978) Special populations: The next sexual frontier. *Journal of Sex Education and Therapy, 4,* 25-36.

Sobsey, D. (1994). *Violence and Abuse In The Lives Of People With Disabilities.* Baltimore: Paul H. Brookes.

Sobsey, D. & Doe, T. (1990). Patterns of sexual abuse and assault. *Journal of Sexuality and Disability, 9,* 243-259.

Sobsey, D. & Varnhagen, C. (1991). Sexual abuse, assault and exploitation of individuals with disabilities. In C. Bagley & R. J. Thomlinson (Eds*.), Child sexual abuse; Critical perspectives on prevention, intervention and treatment* (pp. 203-216). Toronto, ON: Wall and Emerson.

Stanfield, J. & Cowardin, N. (1992). *LifeFacts: Sexuality.* Santa Barbara, CA: James Stanfield.

Stiggall-Muccigrosso, L. (1991). *Policies: Why bother, who does it help?* AAMR Annual Conference, Washington, DC.

Stavis, P. F. (1991). *Harmonizing the right to sexual expression and the right to protection from harm for persons with mental disability.* New York State Commission on

Quality of Care.

Strong, C. (1989). *A conceptual look at empowerment.* Calgary: The Vocational and Rehabilitation Research Institute

Szymanski, L. S. & Tanguay, P. E. (Eds.) (1980*). Emotional disorders of mentally retarded persons: Assessment, treatment and consultation.* Baltimore, MD: University Park Press.

Thompson, D. (1994). Sexual experiences of men with learning disabilities having sex with men: Issues for HIV prevention. *Sexuality and Disability, 12,* 221-241.

Valenti-Hein, D. C., Yarnold, P. R., & Mueser, K .T. (1994). Evaluation of the dating skills program for improving heterosocial interactions in people with mental regartaion. *Behavior Modification, 18,* 32-46.

Walker-Hirsch, L. & Champagne, M.P. (1991). Circles revisted: Ten years later. *Sexuality and Disability, 9,* 143-148.

Ward, K. M., Heffern, S. J., Wilcox, D., McElwee, D., Dowrick, P., Brown, T.D., Jones, M. .J., & Johnson, C. L. (1992). *Managing inappropriate sexual behavior: Supporting individuals with developmental disabilities in the community.* Anchorage, Alaska: Alaska Specialized Education and Training Services.

Whitehouse, M. A. & McCabe, M. P. (1997, Sept.). Sex education programs for people with intellectual disability: How effective are they? *Education and training in mental retardation and developmental disabilities,* 229-240.

Wilson, C. & Brewer, N. (1992). The incidence of criminal victimization of individuals with an intellectual disability. *Australian Psychologist, 2,* 114-117.

Wish, J. R., McCombs, K. F., & Edmonson, B. (1979). The socio-sexual knowledge and attitude test. Wood Dale, IL.: Stoelting.

Wolfensburger, W. (1972). *The principle of normalization in human services*. Toronto, ON: National Institute on Mental Retardation.

Chapter 4

Consent for Sexual Relations

Stacey Sheehan

Introduction

Providers of care for persons with developmental disabilities are placed in the unenviable position of balancing seemingly irreconcilable interests when faced with the issue of consent to sexual relations. They have a duty to protect those whom they serve from sexual abuse and its potentially extreme psychological and physical consequences. How are they to accomplish this in the context of the fundamental principles upon which our society is based? We have fought hard for and honour the rights and freedoms now guaranteed to us, including the right of personal privacy in sexually related matters and of the equality of individuals. Our society values the principles of personal choice, self-determination and independence for persons with developmental disabilities. Isn't it contrary to these principles to 'evaluate' a person's competence to make choices and decisions regarding their sexual behaviour? What should be the standard of 'informed consent' in the context of sexual relations, who should decide, and how are the criteria to be constituted? Can we afford to err on the side of rights and freedoms when depression, pregnancy, and death from a sexually transmitted disease are swinging in the balance? Yet won't too stringent a standard fail to provide sufficient sexual freedom to persons with developmental disabilities and inhibit the fulfillment of their personal pleasure, personal growth, and sense of identity? There seems to be little or no policy guidance to individuals entrusted with the care of persons with developmental disabilities to provide a framework with which to approach this not so delicate balance. Presently, policies appear to be black or white: either there is a 'no sex' policy being applied throughout a residence or, alternatively, there is the informal 'do your utmost to educate and hope for the best' policy. Neither is appropriate. Providers of care must be equipped with a sound appreciation of the dynamics of consent as it relates to sexual activity before any framework can be applied to maximize the potential for the personal fulfillment of those they serve while minimizing their exposure to undue risks. Concepts of consent are reviewed below from the criminal law as a starting point for a principled approach to developing a framework regarding the capacity of persons with developmental disabilities to consent to engage in sexual relations.

Elanore was a 62 year old woman living in a supported independent living facility. Although she was not capable of handling her own financial affairs, she was able to take the bus to her part time job at the florist and enjoyed socializing with people. For the past 18 months, Elanore had enjoyed a meaningful relationship with a retired "higher functioning" 67 year old male. Elanore was deeply in love with her boyfriend. She was happy with how well he treated her: he would call her, pick her up in his van, and they would go out on dates.

Sometimes, arrangements were made for Elanore to spend the weekend at her boyfriend's home. A subsequent criminal investigation revealed that on a number of occasions, Elanore's boyfriend's two grandsons, ages 7 and 9 years old, also spent the weekend with them. They would watch pornographic videotapes together. Elanore's boyfriend would perform sexual acts with her in front of the boys. He also orchestrated sexual acts to take place between Elanore and his young grandsons, including mutual oral sex and attempted intercourse. He engaged in sexual activity with his own grandsons as well. Some of the sexual acts were recorded on videotape. Elanore was devastated when her boyfriend was charged with sexually assaulting his grandsons. She failed to appreciate how the police did not understand that what took place with the boys was "fun, natural, loving, and perhaps educational". "I love Robert and Henry and would never do anything to harm them," she emphasized. The matter came to the attention of the authorities after the grade 4 student called the AIDS hotline as advertised in a television commercial to see if he and his little brother were going to die as a result of their sexual activity.

Case Study
Literature Review

Introduction

The criminal law enunciates the minimum standard of conduct that will be tolerated by society in human relations. It consists of the delicts in the Criminal Code of Canada, the Common Law that has developed in the interpretation and application thereof, and must be consistent with The Canadian Charter of Rights and Freedoms. It is fluid and continues to change to reflect societal attitudes and social mores in prioritizing social values. The concept of 'consent' is like a piece of driftwood being polished in the refining swirls of case law, each decision and/or amendment influencing the shape of future ones to come, in situations which may not as yet have been contemplated. The evolution of the law of consent as it pertains to sexual relations in the criminal context shows that the minimum standard of conduct tolerated by our society may be a prohibitively high standard for some persons with developmental disabilities.

Age of Consent

a) Sexual Interference

It is illegal to engage in sexual activity with a person under 14 years of age and it is no defense to a charge that the minor 'consented' to the activity (Criminal Code of Canada, s. 150.1, 1985). This presumption of incapacity to consent may not be rebutted, no matter how much the minor may wish to engage in the activity. Thus, it is illegal for a 19-year old to engage in sexual activity with a person just shy of his or her 14th birthday, even if the child appears to understand the nature and consequences of the activity. The Supreme Court of Canada had occasion to consider the "pressing and substantial concern" of protecting, in that case, female children from premature sexual intercourse in R. v. Nguyen; R. v. Hess, (1990). Parliament had considered it so important to protect girls under 14 years of age from intercourse that they made it illegal to engage in it whether or not the person believed that the female was over 14 years of age. The constitutionality of this section, which was the predecessor of the present section, was challenged because men who held an honest and reasonable belief that the female was over 14 years of age could be convicted of a criminal offence and sent to jail even though they did not have criminal intent. The court considered the purpose of the legislation as protecting children from the grave physical harm and permanent psychological harm that could result from sexual intercourse at such an early age. It presupposed that children are ill-equipped to deal with the physical, emotional and economic consequences of pregnancy. Counsel had argued that society must bear the increased medical and social costs, as well as the decreased productivity that result from juvenile pregnancies and prostitution. Only two members of the court agreed that a further purpose of the legislation was to protect girls under 14 years of age from the exploitation by those who would enlist them to a life of prostitution and related nefarious undertakings. The majority of the court held that a defense of due diligence should be permitted, with two members dissenting that the problems addressed by the section were so serious that it should be an absolute liability offence. They saw little hardship in refraining from engaging in sexual relations with a young female until knowing her well enough to be absolutely certain of her age. The discussion had some insightful comments about the nature of consent, though subtle and not specifically defined. Wilson (cited in R. v. Nguyen; R. v. Hess, 1990) in her concurring decision in the result indicated:

> Moreover, it seems to me that if the legislature is of the view that children under a given age are not in a position to make an *informed decision* about whether to expose themselves to the hazards of premature sexual intercourse, then it

is logical for it to eliminate the defence of consent. (p. 173)

As one set of authors explains: "… a minor, it is reasoned, no
matter how willing or eager, has not given consent because she
is below the age at which she has the legal right or the *social
maturity* to offer it" (MacNamara & Sagarin, 1977, p. 80).

Madam Justice McLachlin (cited in R. v. Nguyen; R. v. Hess,
1990) in her dissenting reasons indicated, "A child of 13 or
younger cannot be presumed to *meaningfully* consent to intercourse" (p. 200).

Case law has never gone into great detail to explain what characteristics specifically make people under 14 years of age inherently incapable of giving their consent to engage in sexual
activity with an adult. In 1872, an accused was convicted of
indecently assaulting 8 year old boys despite their lack of resistance in the case of Reg. V. Lock (1872) where it was held
that the children did not resist as they were ignorant of the nature of the act. The Supreme Court of Saskatchewan applied
these criteria in The King v. Walebek (1913) where a man was
charged with having sex with a 21 year old woman known to
him to be an "imbecile". The complainant was described as
being able to count to ten, feed the horses, and run messages.
She was not able to dress herself or comb her hair, had not
gone to school, and did not have sufficient awareness to be
sworn. The accused argued that he obtained her consent by
offering to pay her 25 cents, an obligation which he fulfilled.
The court referred to the principle in Lock (supra) that there
must be an appreciation of the *moral nature* of the act and indicated at page 135 that "the very nature of the bargain goes to
show that from mere imbecility on her part she was incapable
of exercising any judgment on the matter."

Besides the fact that children may not experience sexual activity as wrong or harmful, we are left to common sense to identify other relevant ways in which they differ from adults. Although the 13 ½-year old and the 20-year old both may consume the same pop-culture sexually explicit diet of *Seinfeld, Friends, 90210,* and *The Spice Girls,* there is an enormous difference in their social interactions. The 13 ½-year old must obey and follow the rules set down by his parent who provides the necessities of life for him. His responsibilities are likely to include keeping his room straight, helping with the dishes, and attending school. He is likely to succumb to peer pressure and/or simply acquiesce in activities due to the limited personal experience available with which to exercise his judgment. On the other hand, the twenty year old's responsibilities are likely to include working, paying rent, and food preparation. She will have established the ability to argue, debate, and criticize based on her own experience. Perhaps young teens are more likely to act on infatuation or sheer impulse in perceiving love as the fulfillment of immediate desires or wishes. For instance, they may perceive that their rule-imposing custodial parent 'hates' them because they insist the children eat their vegetables, bathe and brush before bed, and go to sleep at a decent hour. Alternatively, they may perceive the steady diet of chocolate and Happy Meals fed to them while visiting the non-custodial parent on weekends, and watching TV till all hours of the night as 'love'. While children under 14 years of age may be able to describe that sexual intercourse involves the male putting his penis in the female's vagina; that women can become pregnant if they don't use birth control, and that people can get herpes or AIDS from engaging in sexual intercourse, it is unlikely that they are able to apply those abstract concepts to their own personal experience and needs. Lack of perspective and undeveloped choice-making abilities, in conjunction with the significant possible consequences of sexual relations are critical factors in explaining why children under 14 years of age are not entitled to rebut the presumption that they are incapable of consenting to sexual activity with adults.

However, the presumption of the lack of capacity of persons under 14 years of age to consent to sexual relations is not absolute. Presently, youths between 12 and 16 years of age who are less than two years older than the complainant are entitled to rely on the defence of consent. The British Columbia Court of Appeal considered whether it was a violation of the charter right to equality to provide adolescents with a defence to which adults were not entitled in R. v. Le Gallant (1986). The court reviewed the relevant principles surrounding the right to equal treatment and acknowledged that "[t]here are many cases where the needs of society and the welfare of its members dictate inequality for the achievement of socially desirable purposes." The court affirmed the principle that the interests of true equality may require differentiation in treatment between groups. In this case, it is part of normal development for adolescents to explore their sexuality together. However, adolescents are in a different position than adults. The court explains:

> In relation to an adolescent, an adult is generally in a position of much greater *sexual experience, authority, and persuasive and coercive potential* than another adolescent. Adults and adolescents are not similarly situated in this respect. It is therefore neither unreasonable nor unfair to treat them differently (p. 300).

With this section in mind, it may be that one of the more important elements of consent as it relates to minors engaging in sexual activity is the position of the parties in relation to one another and the ability to act freely of manipulation. This trend is expanded in the next section of the criminal code considered below.

b) Sexual Exploitation

Although, generally speaking, the age of consent to engage in sexual relations is 14 years, there are special provisions in the Criminal Code which make it illegal to have sex with a young person between the ages of 14 to 18 years if the person is in a position of trust or authority towards a young person or with whom a young person is in a relationship of dependency regardless of the young person's consent, wishes or desires (Criminal Code of Canada, s. 153, 1985). The Supreme Court of Canada had the opportunity to analyze the meaning and scope of the section for the first time since it came into force January 1st, 1988 in R. v. Audet (1996). LaForest (1996), writing for the majority at paragraph 14 indicated, "It is evident that Parliament passed s.153 of the criminal code to protect young persons who are in a vulnerable position toward certain persons because of an imbalance inherent in the nature of the relationship between them." The phrases 'position of trust', 'position of authority', and 'relationship of dependency' are not defined in the Criminal Code of Canada. The court abstracted the following elements of the definition of these phrases throughout paragraphs 33 and 34 of the decision: 1) It involves more than a legal right over the young person and may include an actual power to command the youth which the adult has acquired under the situation; 2) It invokes the notions of power and the ability to hold in one's hands the future or destiny of the young person; 3) It creates an opportunity for all of the persuasive and influencing factors which adults hold over children to come into play; and 4) It includes the power to influence the conduct and actions of others by enforcing obedience or containing a superiority of merit that compels unconstrained obedience, respect, and trust. The purpose of the section is to vitiate apparent consent in circumstances where, by definition, the young person has lost his or her independence and freedom of action in choosing.

The existence of this section shows the emphasis Parliament has placed on the free exercise of will from undue influence in determining sexual relations. A young person's vulnerability and weakness to persons with whom they are in a position of trust, power or relationship of dependency supercedes all other considerations pertaining to informed consent. Presumably, an individual just shy of his or her 18th birthday is well aware of the physical, medical, social and moral consequences of engaging in sexual activity, and indeed may be sexually experienced. The section underscores the significance of *voluntariness* to engage in sexual activity. In R. v. Audet (1996), the 22 year old physical education teacher was convicted under this section after he engaged in oral sex with a fourteen year old student, despite the fact that it was summer holidays; he had no idea she was going to be at the club he went to that evening; he did not buy her alcohol; it was someone else's suggestion that the entire group go back to the cottage; the fourteen year old was in the care of her two cousins in their early twenties; he went to bed without making any sexual advances to the teen; she entered the bed in which he was sleeping despite the fact there was another available to her; and he immediately stopped when she advised him she was becoming uncomfortable. The court held at paragraph 20:

> The relative positions of the parties have always been relevant to the validity of consent under Canadian criminal law. The common law has long recognized that exploitation by one person of another person's vulnerability towards him or her can have an impact on the validity of consent (p. 493).

The court held that teachers will, apart from exceptional circumstances, be in a position of trust and authority towards their students having regard to the considerable influence they exert over their students and the role society has entrusted them regarding the development of its children. In addition to teachers; parents, coaches, counsellors, psychiatrists and spiritual leaders may all be precluded from engaging in sexual activities with persons in their care under 18 years of age.

Often, people with developmental disabilities are described as having a mental age substantially less than their chronological age. Many times, the mental age is estimated to be less than 14 years. The issue arises as to whether or not it could be argued that these sections apply to mental age, thus removing from accuseds charged with sexually assaulting persons with developmental disabilities with a mental age of less than 14 years the defence of consent and mistaken belief in consent. While this would simplify prosecutions and thereby perhaps increase protection to persons that fit in that category, it would be undesirable and unduly restrictive to persons with developmental disabilities. While there are no reported cases where this argument was made in the context of a sexual assault, a similar argument was considered in OGG-MOSS v. THE QUEEN (1984). In that case, the accused was a residential counsellor at a hospital for persons with developmental disabilities, having direct daily care of the residents. He was charged with assaulting a 21-year old person with severe developmental disabilities after he struck the resident in response to the resident purposefully spilling his milk on the table. The counsellor relied on the defence of corrective measure by force, which is available to teachers, parents and persons standing in the place of a parent in the application of force to a child under their care for purposes of correction. Diskson (1984) indicated:

> ... there is a qualitative difference between immaturity, childishness or childlike behaviour and the behaviour of a mentally-retarded adult, especially of a severely retarded adult as in this case. A mentally retarded adult is not a child in fact, nor for the purposes of the law in general nor for the purposes of s.43 of the criminal code (p. 127).

The court decided that the defence was unavailable to the accused, indicating:

> A farther important consideration is that chronological childhood is a transitory phase, and for a child in the chronological sense the suspension of the criminal law's protection against certain kinds of assault is a temporary phenomenon. For the mentally retarded person the definition of "childhood" proposed by the appellant is a life sentence and the consequent attenuation of his right to dignity and physical security is permanent (p. 127).

Thus, while it is likely that the age of consent provisions in the criminal code relate simply to chronological age, the principles enunciated therein are relevant when applied to the elements of consent in other areas of the law, particularly the latest definition of consent to sexual relations which includes a reference to an 'incapability' of consenting. These principles include the notions of informed and voluntary decision making by a person of social maturity who appreciates the moral context of the activity and is free of undue or coercive influence.

Sexual Assault

a) Evolution of Legislation

Bryant (1989) provides a brief historical perspective of the legislation in the Criminal Code of Canada designed to specifically protect persons with developmental disabilities from sexual abuse. Much of the language used in our judicial statutes and decisions is offensive as terminology continues to evolve over time. From 1892 until its repeal by the new sexual offence legislation in 1980/81/82, the criminal code made it an offence to have sexual intercourse with a female who was known or there was good reason to believe, was 'feebleminded, insane, an idiot or an imbecile'. 'Deaf and dumb' females were added to the list in later amendments. Essentially, there was a presumption that persons with developmental disabilities could not consent to sexual relations. No doubt, such protection was deemed necessary as a result of conflicting decisions from England regarding the nature of consent as it applied to persons with developmental disabilities (See R. v. Fletcher, 1859; R. v. Charles Fletcher, 1866). The Crown was required to prove that the intercourse took place against the female's will, which seemed to require evidence of resistance. This was difficult since the female may not have offered resistance not knowing the sexual or moral nature of the act or being incapable of exercising her will due to the developmental disability. In addition, the Crown was required to prove the sexual relations were committed without her consent, although 'strong animal instincts might exist notwithstanding her imbecile condition' which would prevent the act from constituting rape. The court held in R. v. Charles Fletcher (1866) that if "Parliament intended to protect 'idiots' as being incapable of consent, then it could specifically do so as it did in the prohibition to having sexual relations with children of tender years" (p. 249).

It took a lengthy period of time for the courts to acknowledge that the section designed to protect persons with developmental disabilities from sexual abuse was unduly restrictive on their individual rights. It was not until 1943 that the Saskatchewan Court of Appeal held that the inquiry must go beyond merely determining if the complainant had a developmental disability, and that the inquiry must extend to whether in fact consent was given. In Rex v. Probe (1943), the court described the purpose of the legislation as follows:

> The gravamen of s.219 appears to consist in the act by a man of having carnal knowledge of a woman or girl who, by reason of one of the infirmities mentioned therein, must be deemed ***mentally and morally incapable*** of resisting his solicitation to do so. To put it colloquially, the object of the enactment is to prevent such females from being taken advantage of and made

'easy marks' by morally unscrupulous men (p. 293).

In applying the section to the facts of the case, the court held:

> It would seem to me unreasonable to hold however that just because a woman is proved to be deaf and dumb she is ipso facto incapable of lawfully consenting to carnal knowledge. Common experience tells us that not infrequently women and girls so afflicted are unquestionably moral and highly intelligent, with the ability to take and utilize an advanced education (p. 294).

The court relied upon a legal presumption in favour of sanity as was applied in other areas of the law. While this presumption may exist in law, it is important that caregivers to persons with developmental disabilities do not absolve themselves of their responsibilities to protect those in their care by deferring to this legal fiction. Most often, it is readily apparent when a resident is at risk, and providers of care should not hesitate to act in accordance with any guidelines in place to assist them. They should seek direction from the administration and even the court if there are no guidelines in place. Instead of approaching the issue from a 'presumption' perspective, it is more beneficial to simply examine all of the surrounding circumstances known to the parties at the time to establish whether, in fact, the parties were capable of consenting to sexual activity. This has been the approach taken in the Criminal Code since the early 1980's.

b) Legislative Definition

Prior to August 15th, 1992, the issue of consent as it related to physical and sexual assaults was dealt with solely in s.265(3) of the Criminal Code of Canada which enumerates a series of conditions which negate the apparent consent and/or participation of the complainant. The conditions flow from the legal principle that to be legally effective, consent must be freely given. The vitiating factors include submission or lack of resistance by reason of force, threats, fear of force or threats, fraud, or the exercise of authority. Judicial interpretation of this section remained somewhat limited in the application of the enumerated conditions particularly as they applied to sexual assault cases. With the enactment of Bill C-49 came a

s.273.1

Subject to subsection (2) and subsection 265(3), "consent" means, for the purposes of (the sexual assault sections), the *voluntary agreement* of the complainant to engage in the sexual activity in question. (Emphasis added)

1. No consent is obtained, for the purposes of (the sexual assault sections), where
2. the agreement is expressed by the words or conduct of a person other than the complainant;
3. the complainant is incapable of consenting to the activity;
4. the accused induces the complainant to engage in the activity by abusing a position of trust, power or authority;
5. the complainant expresses, by words or conduct, a lack of agreement to engage in the activity; or
6. the complainant, having consented to engage in sexual activity, expresses, by words or conduct, a lack of agreement to continue to engage in the activity.

Nothing in subsection (2) shall be construed as limiting the circumstances in which no consent is obtained; (Criminal Code of Canada, 1992, c. 38, s.1.).

more specific definition of consent to reflect the power imbalances that often exist between the sexual aggressor and the complainant in sexual assault cases.

The first important point to be made is that consent is communicative conduct. There is a two pronged approach to determining consent to sexual relations: 1) Was agreement to engage in sexual activity communicated? If so, 2) Were the words or conduct of agreement communicated voluntarily? This section protects or precludes persons with developmental disabilities who are unable to communicate their consent to another from engaging in sexual activity. Case law has developed to confirm that silence, non-resistance, failure to escape, acquiescence and compliance only indicate a failure to object or resist, they do not constitute consent. (See R. v. M. (M.L.), 1994); R. v. Wills, 1992; R v. Ewanchuk, 1999). This is important to keep in mind for those caregivers who resort to "the smile test" as coined by Stavis (1999). This refers to situations where the caregiver retroactively interprets a pleasurable response to sexual activity as consent to it. Pleasure is not a criteria from which to infer consent. No doubt, Elanore in the case example believed the activity was pleasurable while quite clearly she was incapable of giving meaningful consent. Consent must be communicated prior to the touching, and as the Supreme Court of Canada held in R. v. Ewanchuk (1999), one sexual assault is not a reasonable step to ascertain whether or not the complainant is consenting to further sexual contact. A person must be able to point to factors of the complainant's communication that led him to believe she was consenting to a sexual touching. It is not sufficient to believe in his own mind that she needs it or might enjoy it. McLaughlin (1999) resorted to the dictionary definition to clarify the elements of consent in her dissenting reasons in R. v. Esau, (1997) at paragraphs 64 and 65:

> Webster's Third New International Dictionary
> (1986), defines consent as "capable, deliberate,
> and voluntary agreement to or concurrence in
> some act or purpose implying physical and
> mental power and free action." (p. 309)

Furthermore, s.273.2 places a positive duty on the sexual aggressor to "take reasonable steps, in the circumstances known
to the accused at the time, to ascertain that the complainant
was consenting" (Criminal Code of Canada, 1992) if he wishes
to rely on the defence of mistaken belief in consent. Since the
reasonableness of the steps depends upon the particular circumstances of the complainant known to the accused at the
time, it would be reasonable to make greater efforts to ensure
that a person known to the accused to have developmental disabilities is truly consenting to the activity, as opposed to simply just going along with it or not resisting it. The Supreme
Court of Canada has made it clear that the action of giving or
withholding consent is determined solely by reference to the
complainant's subjective internal state of mind toward the
touching at the time it occurred. In R. v. Ewanchuk (1999),
the court indicated at paragraph 26 that lack of consent is established purely from the complainant's perspective that in her
mind she did not want the sexual touching to take place, no
matter how strongly her conduct may contradict that claim.
This is very important to protect persons with developmental
disabilities whose conduct may be misinterpreted by members
of society who are unfamiliar with them and who may rely on
stereotypes to interpret their behaviour. For instance, some
persons with developmental disabilities are extremely vulnerable to sexual assault as they are far more open and demonstra-
tive in the expression of affection than the general public at

large. A sexual aggressor who was aware of this fact would have to take reasonable steps to ensure that the kissing, hugging, and sitting on his lap were actually sexual 'come-ons' by the complainant before jumping to that conclusion. Also, the complainant's assertion that in his mind he was only being affectionate and was not consenting to sexual relations would be respected. Furthermore, conduct arising from the consequences of being institutionalized, such as that arising from a diminished sense of privacy, or a tendency to be compliant and submitting to routines, would not be relevant to the issue of whether the complainant, in his own mind, withheld consent. Major (cited in R. v. Ewanchuk, 1999) explained why the approach to consent is purely subjective:

> The rationale underlying the criminalization of assault explains this. Society is committed to protecting the personal integrity, both physical and psychological, of every individual. Having control over who touches one's body, and how, lies at the core of human dignity and autonomy. The inclusion of assault and sexual assault in the Code expresses society's determination to protect the security of the person from any nonconsensual contact or threats of force. The common law has recognized for centuries that the individual's right to physical integrity is a fundamental principle, "every man's person being sacred, and no other having a right to meddle with it in any the slightest manner": See Blackstone's Commentaries on the Laws of England (4th ed. 1770), Book III, at p. 120. It follows that any intentional but unwanted touching is criminal.

c) Informed Consent

Clearly, from the research thus far, any consent given must be informed to be valid. What is the appropriate scope of the informational component to engage in sexual relations? In the United States, each State is responsible for its own laws and the standard of knowledge required varies from State to State. Stavis (1999), advises that the New Jersey rule set forth in State v. Olivio (1991) is that a person is competent to consent to sex if in the context of all of the surrounding circumstances, the person is able to understand the distinctly sexual nature of the conduct and the right to refuse to engage in that conduct with another. Understanding the risks and consequences of the activity is not required. Stavis advises that New York State is at the other end of the spectrum requiring some understanding by the complainant of the implications of sexual relations, including societal mores on the appropriateness of engaging in the conduct, for example, if one was married or not. The standard is enunciated in People v. Cratsley (1995). Hawaii has an extremely stringent standard as enunciated by the Court of Appeals of the State of Hawaii in The Interest of John Doe, (1996):

> In determining whether a complainant is mentally defective, the court evaluates whether the complaining witness understands the physiological elements of the sex act, as well as the moral, societal, and medical consequences of the sex act. Do they appreciate the taboos to which a person will be exposed, including the

capacity to appraise the nature of the stigma, ostracism, or other non-criminal sanctions associated with sexual intercourse outside of marriage, or with a married person. The court will evaluate the complainant's ability to appraise the risk of sexually transmitted diseases which are components of the normal person's decision to participate in sexual intercourse (Court Syllabus).

The standard to be applied in Canadian law seems to have moved from the New Jersey standard closer to the Hawaii standard. This is evident in the Supreme Court of Canada decision R. v. Cuerrier (1998), which explored the scope of fraud that would vitiate consent. Prior to the 1983 amendments, the Criminal Code stipulated that consent was vitiated in indecent assaults where it was obtained "by false and fraudulent representations as to the nature and quality of the act". 'Nature and quality of the act' received constrained and narrow judicial interpretations such that it was limited to the sexual character of the act. Thus, the type of fraud that would vitiate consent usually involved sexual relations under the guise that they were necessary to a medical procedure and engaged in solely for medical purposes (See R. v. Harms, 1944; R. v. Maurantonio, 1968). It was held in R. v. Clarence (1888) that a husband's failure to disclose that he had gonorrhea was not a fraud as to the nature and quality of the act and therefore did not vitiate his wife's consent to sexual relations. In Bolduc v. The Queen (1967), the Supreme Court of Canada held that the fraud perpetrated by a properly qualified medical intern on the female patients he was examining by passing off a third person watching the procedure as bona fide medical personnel when, in fact, he was really just a voyeur, did not go to the nature and quality of the act. The court decided the women had consented to a proper medical examination and they got one, despite the fact that the women testified that they would never have given their consent if they were aware of the true identity of the third person.

Courts continued to narrowly define fraud as relating to the 'nature and quality of the act' even after those qualifying words were removed in the 1983 amendments to the criminal code which stipulated that "no consent is obtained where the complainant submits or does not resist by reason of 'fraud'". (Criminal Code of Canada, s.265(3)(c), 1985). In 1987, the British Columbia Court of Appeal held that the fraud perpetrated by a man who falsely obtained sexual services by agreeing to pay the complainant $100 when he never intended to pay her, was insufficient to vitiate consent because it did not relate to the nature and quality of the sexual act (See R. v. Petrozzi, 1987).

The trend of these cases would suggest that persons with developmental disabilities need only appreciate the physical and/ or sexual nature of the act in order to be able to consent to it. However, R. v. Cuerrier (1998) put an end to the trend concluding that "it is no longer necessary when examining whether consent in assault or sexual assault cases was vitiated by fraud to consider whether the fraud related to the nature and quality of the act." (paragraph 108). In considering whether there would be a valid consent in the absence of disclosure of an HIV-positive status, the court acknowledged the complexity of sexual relationships:

> It cannot be forgotten that the act of intercourse
> is usually far more than the mere manifestation

of the drive to reproduce. It can be the culmi-
nating demonstration of love, admiration and
respect. It is the most intimate of physical relations and what actions and reactions led to mutual consent to undertake it will in retrospect be
complex. (p. 50)

The court did not follow the common law principles applied
and developed since R v.Clarence (1888) and held at paragraph 127:

Without disclosure of HIV status there cannot
be a true consent. The consent cannot simply
be to have sexual intercourse. Rather it must be
consent to have intercourse with a partner who
is HIV positive. True consent cannot be given
if there has not been a disclosure by the accused
of his HIV positive status. *A consent that is
not based upon knowledge of the significant
relevant factors is not a valid consent.* (p. 50)

However, it is important to note that the four member majority
of the Supreme Court of Canada held that the existence of
fraud should not vitiate consent unless there is a significant
risk of serious harm. They held at paragraph 135 and 137 that
while the standard is sufficient to encompass other sexually
transmitted diseases that constitute a significant risk of serious
harm in addition to the risk of HIV infection, that detriment in
the form of mental distress suffered on account of lies told
about the party's age; wealth; extent of his affection, fidelity or
sexual prowess would not be sufficient to meet the standard to
vitiate consent.

In a separate judgement, Madam Justice L'Heureux-Dube would have maximized the individual's right to determine by whom, and under what conditions, he or she will consent to physical contact by another by not limiting the types of fraud to those that only place the complainant at significant risk of serious harm. She indicates that the provisions are aimed more generally at protecting people's physical integrity, promoting people's physical autonomy and by recognizing each individual's power to consent, or to deny consent, to any touching – however serious. She contends in paragraph 12 of her judgment that consent is only legally valid if the voluntary agency of the person being touched is not negated. She argues at paragraph 15 that the purpose of s.265(3) is to ensure that when consent is obtained, it is a true reflection of the person's autonomous will.

> The focus of the inquiry into whether fraud vitiated consent so as to make certain physical contact non-consensual should be on whether the nature and execution of the deceit deprived the complainant of the ability to exercise his or her will in relation to his or her physical integrity with respect to the activity in question (p. 16).

She questions why the court would define fraud more broadly in the commercial context of protecting people's property interests where the degree of the risk or harm is not a factor, than for sexual assault which she deems as "one of the worst violations of human dignity" by limiting it to significant risk of serious harm.

> ...it is not for the Court to narrow this protection because it is afraid that it may reach too far

> into the private lives of individuals. One of
> those private lives presumably belongs to a
> complainant, whose feeling of having been
> physically violated, and fraudulently deprived
> of the right to withhold consent, warrants the
> protection and condemnation provided by the
> Criminal Code (p. 19).

While L'Heureaux-Dube went further than the majority, two
members of the court would not have gone as far as the majority. They held that the fraud in this instance did go to the nature and quality of the act and therefore it was not necessary to
expand the definition of fraud from its common law interpretation. They questioned how psychological harm might fit into
the new test of 'significant risk of serious harm' when a sexual
relationship induced by fraudulent representations may lead to
depression, self-destructive behaviour or suicide? McLachlin
canvassed other situations that may arise at paragraph 47:

> For example, pregnancy may be regarded as a
> deprivation in some circumstances, as may be
> the obligation to support a child. It follows that
> lying about sterility or the effectiveness of birth
> control may constitute fraud vitiating consent.
> To take another example, lies about the pros-
> pect of marriage or false declarations of affec-
> tion inducing consent, carry the risk of psycho-
> logical suffering, depression and other conse-
> quences readily characterized as deprivation.
> The proposed rule thus has the potential to
> criminalize a vast array of sexual conduct. De-
> ceptions, small and sometimes large, have from
> time immemorial been the by-product of ro-

> mance and sexual encounters. They often carry
> the risk of harm to the deceived party. Thus far
> in the history of civilization, these deceptions,
> however sad, have been left to the domain of
> song, verse and social censure. Now, if the
> Crown's theory is accepted, they become
> crimes (p. 26).

Clearly, issues surrounding the standard of 'informed consent'
raise exceedingly difficult moral, ethical, social, and political
considerations in which well-intentioned and well-educated
people may never reach a consensus. Risk of harm is obvi-
ously an important factor in determining which of competing
equal values is to take precedence over the other. While it
may be easier to quantify the risk of harm to persons with developmental disabilities of contracting HIV infection or becoming pregnant, how do we quantify the risk of harm to the
human spirit if one is condemned by operation of the criminal
law to an asexual existence? This question becomes even
more interesting when examined in the constitutional context.

4) The Constitutional Context

In assessing whether or not the principles reviewed in this
chapter set an appropriate standard to ensure that people are
consenting to sexual activity, it is important to bear in mind
that bodily integrity, sexual autonomy, and control over psychological integrity attract Charter protection pursuant to s.7 of
the Charter which guarantees the right not to be deprived of
life, liberty, and security of the person except in accordance
with fundamental justice (See <u>Rodriguez v. British Columbia</u>
(Attorney General), 1993; <u>R. v. Morgentaler, Smoling & Scott</u>,
1988).

It is significant because the courts have applied an exceptionally high standard of consent when it involves the waiver of a Charter right. For instance, in R. v. Wills (1992), the Ontario Court of Appeal held that an individual must make a voluntary and informed decision to waive a constitutionally protected right, such as consenting to investigatory search and seizures. At page 546 the court explained the broad extent of the 'informed' decision in those circumstances. One must be aware of what he is doing, the significance of his act and the use the police can make of the consent. The police must advise individuals of their right to refuse to consent to the search and that anything seized may be used in the event of a prosecution. The person asked for his or her consent must appreciate in a general way what his or her position is with respect to the investigation (ie. whether she is an accused, a suspect, or simply a potential witness) and must understand the nature of the

- An understanding of anatomy and physiology such that sex involves more than penile penetration of the female including that women can have orgasms and receive pleasure from the stimulation of various erogenous zones (McCarthy, 1993).
- That sex is usually an act between two people engaged in private.
- That it is not proper to have sex with animals, children, or immediate blood relations, or to have sex for money.
- That sex can lead to pregnancy, and that pregnancy requires a substantial emotional and economic commitment.
- That methods of birth control, when used properly, may reduce the risk of pregnancy.

- That there is an ability to obtain birth control from a drug store, clinic, or dispensary at the residence.
- That sex can lead to sexually transmitted disease which could include pain, discomfort, or death, together with an understanding of methods to reduce the risk of sexually transmitted diseases and identifying high-risk partners.
- That some people believe that sex is only gratifying in a loving, respectful, monogamous relationship.
- That you can refuse to engage in sexual activity with someone even if you have agreed to engage in it before with that same person, and that it is enough to just say 'no' without having to provide a good justification for the refusal.

potential charges he or she is facing. Applying the same broad extent of an 'informed decision' to consent to sexual relations, the following factors may play a role:
While it is not necessary for persons to conform and adhere to all of the above components of 'informed consent', it is necessary that there be an appreciation of each and every factor to establish having the capacity to consent to sexual relations.

It may be that applying a constitutional standard to the informational component of consent is so onerous when it comes to persons with developmental disabilities, that it could be argued that the ensuing preclusion of sexual activity is also in violation of the right to life, liberty, and security of the person. For instance, the Supreme Court of Canada, in its landmark decision regarding non-therapeutic sterilization of incompetent persons in E. (Mrs.) v. Eve (1986) relied on some interesting factors when examined under the rubric of consent as it has evolved since that time. For instance, the court indicated at p. 54 that "...the implications of sterilization are always serious. As we have been reminded, it removes from a person the great privilege of giving birth, and is for practical purposes irreversible." The court went on to consider the significant negative psychological impact that non-consensual sterilization has on the 'mentally handicapped', quoting from the Law Reform Commission of Canada (1979):

> It has been found that, like anyone else, the mentally handicapped have individually varying reactions to sterilization. *Sex* and parenthood hold the same significance for them as for other people and their misconceptions and misunderstandings are also similar. Rosen maintains that the removal of an individual's procreative powers is a matter of major importance and that no amount of reforming zeal can remove the significance of sterilization and its effect on the individual psyche. (p. 55)

This is significant because Eve clearly is not capable of consenting to sexual relations applying the standard of consent as it has evolved to date. Anyone having sex with Eve would be committing a criminal offence provided he had sufficient development to form the mens rea to commit the act. In the judgment, Eve was described as having no concept of the idea of marriage, or the consequential relationship between intercourse, pregnancy, and birth. She was also described as suffering from expressive aphasia wherein she was unable to communicate outwardly thoughts or concepts which she might have perceived. The paradox is that the court upheld the "importance of maintaining the physical integrity of a human being ... particularly as it relates to the privilege of giving life" (page 63), in a situation where that very human being would be precluded from engaging in sexual activity to protect her physical integrity from unconsented sexual touchings. While a flexible approach to the balancing of interests on a case by case basis is necessary when it comes to sexual relations of persons with developmental disabilities, it is likely that any residence would be liable if it failed to protect its residents from criminal sexual touching or if it knowingly enabled a resident to be exposed to undue risks associated with sexual activity, regardless of a noble intention to respect the resident's personal autonomy.

Conference Deliberations

Conference participants appeared to be frustrated with the lack of policy and/or lack of guidance in applying any policies that did exist surrounding this issue, which arises constantly in their day to day dealings with persons with developmental disabilities. A significant degree of stress was evident in their attempt to protect residents from undue harm while respecting their privacy and autonomy in the absence of clear criteria to delineate when and how intervention is appropriate. While participants were willing to accept the responsibility of attempting to balance these interests, a common theme was expressed in asking the question, "Who am I to make such an important decision?" Participants recognized the need for further education and training to enable them to carry out this duty.

Consensus was reached that a committee should be set up immediately to develop clear policies to guide staff and oversee the continuing educational and training component required by staff. The participants were unable to agree on whether this committee would be a more centralized committee establishing professional standards on a regional or provincial basis, or simply an internal committee per residence. Participants did agree that government regulation was not the best approach to establish and enforce the appropriate guidelines, as it was thought to be cumbersome, impersonal, general, and inflexible. Guidelines and criteria developed by the proposed committee would ensure an appreciation of the practical considerations in applying such criteria. As well, the committee was thought to be in a position to exercise familiarity and flexibility in the application of the guidelines to particular parties and issues as they arise. There was a consensus that the specific policies should be made known to residents and their families upon admission.

It was felt that such a committee could not only establish clear policy and guidelines with specific criteria to provide staff with a framework to approach this issue, but it could also accept referrals from staff to assist in applying the policy in difficult or unclear situations. This would ensure a consistent and principled approach to the application of the policy, free of any biases or misconceptions on behalf of the caregiver. While high-risk activity engaged in by a person with severe developmental disabilities would be more clear cut, it would be beneficial to have more than simply the caregiver's assessment of situations involving less risky or less complex sexual touchings between persons who may not fully appreciate all of the relevant factors. Participants envisioned a flexible standard where a resident could be found incapable of consenting to certain activity with certain individuals under certain conditions while being found capable of consenting with the same or other individuals as the variables of activity and circum-

stance shifted. The other benefit of such a committee was that
it would be an identifiable and accountable body to which residents could formally address their needs and concerns regarding the content and application of the policy.

There was no consensus as to how the committee should be
constituted. While there were some benefits to having representation from the residents, their families, and the administrators in addition to the counsellors and caregivers, some participants expressed fear that those members might not be able to
deal with the issues objectively. Administrators have an interest in minimizing their exposure to liability, thus the current
'no sex' policies. Residents were seen to have an interest in
erring on the side of personal freedoms.   Family members
were seen as superimposing their will upon the situation instead of allowing residents to exercise voluntary and informed
poor judgment. While it is important to ensure that the committee has the benefit of broad experience from diverse perspectives, it is unclear how to accomplish that goal without
undue politicization of the committee.

Participants recognized the need for individual clinical evaluations of competency to be conducted to determine residents'
capacities to give and receive consent.   Given the dynamics
of consent, it would be just as important to identify aggressive
individuals who may not be capable of appreciating the language and behaviour of non-consent. Such evaluations would
assist in designing an appropriate program for each resident
and in flagging high-risk relations that would require more supervision.   Evaluations would include examples from daily
observations of the resident's choice making abilities (for example, can the resident choose appropriate clothing or indicate
recreational preferences?); the resident's ability to exercise his
will in declaring or asserting his needs (for example, has the

resident demonstrated a capacity to say "no" to someone or refuse to participate in something?); any previous sexual experience known to the caregiver, including prior victimization or current high-risk behaviour such as failure to use condoms; the clinical assessment of the resident's current functioning level; and the level of sexual education achieved by the resident, including knowledge about the use of contraceptives, factors surrounding sexually transmitted diseases, and the moral context of certain activity.

Some participants acknowledged the need to talk to those in their care and ask them questions regarding what they do when they are alone with another and how they feel about it. While no doubt, this is prying into their private lives, it may be the only way to detect the abuse described in the case example. Open dialogues between residents and caregivers or open forums encouraging communication between residents will provide residents with a designated means of obtaining help, clarification, and guidance with respect to any activity they have engaged in or are in contemplation of engaging. They will have the benefit of learning through others' experience and perspective.

Some participants seemed uncomfortable in applying such a stringent standard of consent and felt it was unrealistically high to apply the Hawaii standard for example. It was felt that residents with attention deficits and memory limitations were not particularly receptive candidates for the extensive sexual education required. The discomfort of applying such a high standard seemed to turn to sadness and regret in examples where the resident clearly was not capable of consenting but seemed nonetheless to take pleasure in the touching. Another complicating factor for participants was how they should deal with reckless behaviour by a resident. On the one hand, consenting adults may do whatever they please. They may throw caution to the wind and engage in indiscriminant, unprotected sex with multiple partners in high-risk categories regardless of their marital status, or how well they know them, or how well they are treated by them. On the other hand, it is tempting to cite the above examples of behaviour as indicators that the resident may not comprehend the nature and quality of her behaviour. Consensus was reached that the exercise of poor judgment was not the equivalent to a lack of capacity to consent.

Summary

The State of the Art

Capacity to consent to sexual relations includes the ability to appreciate the nature of the sexual activity together with its risks and methods of reducing those risks. It includes the ability to understand there is a choice to refuse to engage in any activity and in fact, the ability to exercise that choice at any time. It also includes the ability to make decisions involving the social context of the activity in accordance with personal values. The risks of engaging in sexual activity not only encompass the possibility of pregnancy or infection, but may also include the emotional risks of rejection, guilt, or embarrassment arising from the partner's motives, the circumstances, or society's perception of the event. Caregivers need to know what verbal and non-verbal behaviour constitutes communication in sexual encounters between persons with developmental disabilities and must be able to assess the voluntariness of the communication.

The fundamental principle of human dignity in individual autonomy over sexual relations has shaped this definition of consent. The standard of consent is designed to protect persons from the violation of unwanted touchings. However, as the standard is applied to persons with developmental disabilities, the issue arises as to whether protection from violation has evolved to the point of violation in and of itself? Applying the same standard of capacity to consent to sexual relations as is used for the general population may exclude persons with developmental disabilities from the ability to engage in sexual relations altogether, while failing to apply the same standard would deprive them of the same degree of protection from potentially horrendous consequences enjoyed by the general population.

The standard is necessarily high. Not only is it to avoid for example, the rampant spread of HIV amongst residents, but as the case example underscores, there is no dignity in engaging in sexual activity in the absence of meeting the high standard of capacity. Presumptions of incapacity are also not appropriate, and agencies that enforce a 'no sex' policy are likely to be liable for the undue restrictions placed on a resident's right to sexual autonomy. Presumptions of capacity are not appropriate, and agencies will be liable for failing to protect residents from undue harm. The size of the space between this rock and this hard place must be determined on a case by case basis.

The biggest weakness in this area is the lack of clear guidelines to assist caregivers in determining when and how intervention is necessary and the absence of specific criteria to be applied by them in making such a determination. It is unfair and dangerous, both to caregiver and resident, that the reality of sexual relations among residents continues to go unacknowledged in a formal way. Surely, once reduced to writing on a page, the policy will come under attack. How is any policy to balance the equal yet competing moral, social, medical, political, ethical and religious values subsumed by this issue? Accountability has a high price, but the bid has to open somewhere. Clear policies need to be put in place immediately, and resources need to be committed to the education and training of caregivers in this area.

Clinical Implications

One option to deal with this issue is for caregivers to continue to make ongoing inquiries of those in their care to ensure that there is a capacity to consent to sexual relations while acknowledging the changing nature of significant variables. Caregivers may be loathe to pry into the personal lives of the persons in their care when it comes to romantic or sexual encounters. After all, we all appreciate privacy in such matters and prying offends normalization efforts. Furthermore, such proactive inquisitions may provide caregivers with the opportunity of misusing their influence by supplanting their own judgments in situations rather than permitting a resident to exercise their own judgment, even though the resident meets the standard of capacity. Caregivers may feel it is unrealistic to expect a caring, well-intentioned individual to stand by and watch disaster strike when a calculated "abuse of authority" is likely to save the day. While the world might be a safer place if everyone had someone to watch over them, it would not necessarily be a better place. The fact remains that consenting adults can and will often do whatever they please. Of course, sexual activity engaged in with a person who is not capable of consenting is not a private matter at all, and is nothing short of criminal. As is evident from the case example, caregivers must be vigilant in following up and ensuring residents appreciate their actions. It is not enough to simply ask, "How was your weekend?" It may be necessary to ask, "What did you do? How did that make you feel? Did you use any protection? Why not? Was anyone else there? Was it recorded? Is that what you wanted? Where is the recording now? ..." Caregivers must be willing to accept the stress and responsibility involved in ascertaining these important sex facts in a nonjudgmental fashion. They must be committed to not interfering in situations where the resident is deemed to have the capacity to consent to the sexual relations, however ill-advised. Persons who have the capacity to consent to sexual relations are entitled to make mistakes, whether they have developmental disabilities or not. The temptation to interfere would be removed from caregivers in the second option of dealing with this issue, which is for the caregivers to intervene only when they are presented with a situation they cannot ignore. This still offers residents some protection from apparent abuse while maximizing residents' personal privacy. However, having regard to the potentially devastating consequences of nonconsensual sexual relations, it would be unfortunate to afford persons with developmental disabilities less protection out of a fear that caregivers will abuse their authority. With proper education and appropriate policies in place to assist caregivers, it is possible to achieve a greater balance between these competing interests.

Agency Implications

Agencies have responded to this ethical issue by either having no sex policy in place to assist their staff in dealing with the issue in a principled manner, or by instating a 'no sex' policy hoping to eliminate the issue altogether. While at least 'no sex' policies make the agency's obligation, and therefore the appropriate course of conduct, clear to caregivers, it places them in the position of either turning a blind eye to consensual relations between consenting adults or unnecessarily restricting those relations. This restriction is compounded because generally, residents are already experiencing limited access to appropriate sexual relationships. Any blind eye approach is dangerous because it is arbitrary and minimizes the importance of the policy and the reasons why it is necessary. If they are strictly applied, 'No sex' policies rob residents of the self-determination the agency is there to support, and no doubt, residences will be sued for arbitrarily restricting the rights of the persons with developmental disabilities under their care. If the policy is not applied strictly and a pattern develops of turning a blind eye for what the caregiver determines to be the right reason, agencies are inviting disaster. Agencies will not avoid liability by failing to instate any policy by leaving it up to the caregivers to act in the resident's 'best interests' on an ad hoc basis. While it is harder to shoot a target you can't see, once it is too late and a resident is pregnant or infection sweeps the residence, no one will be able to hide from their share of the responsibility. This issue is a mine field for agencies, who are recommended to approach it from a top priority/ bottom line perspective. Agencies must ensure that caregivers receive proper training to appreciate the principles underlying the formation of policies as well as potential consequences of both following policy and not following policy. Agencies are responsible to create an atmosphere of compliance with policy and must not condone caregivers looking the other way. It is necessary that policies be continually reviewed and updated to reflect the fluid nature of consent as it relates to sexual relations and persons with developmental disabilities.

What Should Be Done Now

The agency needs to acknowledge the issue in a mission statement articulating its responsibility to ensure the rights of the individuals in its care and to protect those who cannot protect themselves. A hierarchy of values should be prioritized to act as a framework to approach the development and application of any policies. Clinicians should take stock to recognize and write down the manner in which the issue arises for them and how they chose to deal with it and why. If a policy is presently in place, they should record instances where the policy was followed and the outcome, or state reasons why the policy was not followed and the outcome. Upon review, these reports may be of assistance in identifying the role that stereotypes played, or areas lacking in education, or it may identify the impracticality of the present policy. Open dialogues should be engaged with other agencies and caregivers to take advantage of a broader base of successful and tragic experiences in dealing with this issue. Perhaps a web page could be dedicated to this issue inviting all agencies to submit their policies for comparative purposes and encourage clinicians to share their experiences.

Committees should be established to develop a comprehensive policy consistent with the agency's mission statement. The policy should acknowledge resident rights, and establish criteria upon which residents would be evaluated to establish a capacity to give consent or receive consent, and indicate how those incapable of giving or receiving consent are to be treated by staff. The policy should indicate that under no circumstances is a member of staff to engage in sexual relations with a resident. The policy also needs to detail the procedure for staff to investigate and report sexual abuse to the appropriate agency and legal authorities.

The committee must also prepare educational materials with which to train staff in implementing the sexual policy. Staff should be updated on the potential liability residences face in various scenarios. Residents must receive ongoing education with respect to sexuality and the related issues of values, pregnancy and health-related issues. The sexual instruction should have easily identifiable components so that the resident's level of sexual education can readily be ascertained by reference to the resident's file.

Residents should be placed inside the residence to maximize their security by keeping those who are more likely to be sexual aggressors furthest away from those who are less likely to be capable of consenting. Increased supervision must be afforded to residents in greater need of protection. Space should be available to provide residents with the opportunity to explore sexual relations in a safe and neutral environment in privacy but with caregiver awareness.

Final Consensus Statement

The complexity of the issue of consent to sexual relations must not stop agencies from developing and implementing clear policies to provide caregivers with a consistent and principled framework with which to approach the dilemmas they face. The effort is necessary to reduce the stress and uncertainties experienced by caregivers in fulfilling their dual obligation of protecting those who are not able to protect themselves while honouring the freedoms of those who can in a consistent manner having regard to relevant fundamental principles.

References

Bolduc v. The Queen, 3 C.C.C..294 (S.C.C.) (1967).

Bryant, A. (1989). The issue of consent in the crime of sexual assault. (1989) 68 Can. Bar Rev. 94.

Criminal Code of Canada. S. 150.1 (1985).

Criminal Code of Canada. S. 153. (1985).

Criminal Code of Canada. S. 265(3) (1985).

Criminal Code of Canada. S 273.1. (1992).

Criminal Code of Canada. S. 273.2. (1992).

E. (Mrs.) v. Eve 2 S.C.R. at 428 (1986)

Law Reform Commission of Canada (1979*). Sterilization: implications for mentally retarded and mentally ill persons*. Working Paper 24.

MacNamara, & Sagarin, (1977). *Sex, crime, and the law*.

McCarthy, M. (1993). Sexual experiences of women with learning difficulties in long-stay hospitals. *Sexuality and Disability, 2(4)*, 277.

OGG-MOSS v. The Queen, 14 C.C.C. (3d) 116 (S.C.C.) (1984).

People v. Cratsley, 86 N.Y. 2d 81, 629 N.Y.S. 2d992 (N.Y. Ct. App. 1995).

R. v. Audet, 1106 C.C.C. (3d) 481 (S.C.C) (1996).

R. v. Charles Fletcher, 10 Cox 248 (1866).

R. v. Clarence, 22 Q.B.D. 23 (1888).

R. v. Cuerrier, 127 C.C.C. (3d) 1 (S.C.C.) (1998).

R. v. Esau (1997) 116 C.C.C. (3d) 289 (S.C.C.).

R. v. Harms, 81 C.C.C. 4 (1944).

R. v. Le Gallant, 29 C.C.C. (3d) 291 (B.C.C.A.) (1986).

R. v. Maurantonio, 1 O.R. 145 (1968).

R. v. Nguyen; R. v. Hess, 59 C.C.C. (ed) 161 (S.C.C.) 1990.

R. v. Petrozzi, 35 C.C.C. (3d) 528 (1987).

R. v. Wills, 7 O.R. (3d) 337 (Ont. C.A.) (1992).

Reg. V. Lock, 12 Cox CC 244 (1872).

Rex v. Probe, 79 C.C.C. 289 (Sask. C.A.) (1943).

State v. Olivio, 123 N.J. 550, 589 A. 2d 597 (N.J., May 1, 1991).

Stavis, P. (1999). Recent developments in law and recent data on sexual incidents: Policy considerations for providers. [On-line]. Available: www.cqu.state.ny/cc66a.htm#3.

Stavis, P. (1999). Cases and trends. [On-line] Available: www.cqc.state.ny.us/cc55htm.

The Interest of John Doe, FC-J No. 91-56090 (HI Ct. App. 1996)

The King v. Walebek, 21 C.C.C. 130 (1913).

Chapter 5

Sex Education

Shelley L. Watson, Dorothy M. Griffiths, Debbie Richards, and Len Dykstra

Introduction

Individuals who have a developmental disability need skills to enable their successful transition from childhood into adulthood and require knowledge to be able to enjoy the rights and responsibilities as a member of adult society. An important but traditionally neglected transitional learning area is sexuality education. However, in recent years, sexuality education has both gained considerable attention and sparked great controversy.

Although sexuality education is a primary issue for the integration into the community of individuals who have a developmental disability, there are great disadvantages in this area of learning (McCabe & Cummins, 1996). McCabe (1999) states that "it is clear that sexuality is not an integral part of the lives of people with either intellectual or physical disability" (p. 168). Throughout the 1980's, the disparity between curriculum and life-transitional goals for persons with developmental disabilities has become increasingly apparent (Lawrence & Swain, 1993). Although most professionals agree that sexuality education is important for persons with developmental disabilities, often the agreement ends there. Opinions differ on content, explicitness of materials, teaching approaches, morality, and values.

In this chapter, some of the ethical dilemmas regarding sexuality education will be explored. Let's examine the following case examples that depict some common dilemmas faced by those who work in this field.

Case Study #1

Bill is a 29-year-old man with a mild developmental disability who lives semi-independently in a supported independent living situation. Each weekend he is a patron of two of the local bars in town. He will often meet up with a female he may or may not know, and they may have sex during the course of the evening. Most recently, he has been diagnosed with Genital Herpes. When support staff talked to him about the importance of using condoms and possibly informing his partner about the Herpes virus, he said that he did not want to do that, since it had never been an issue in the past.

Support staff have talked to him repeatedly about this issue and have ensured that he has condoms in his wallet. They do know that he uses condoms on some occasions, but believe this is not being done 100% of the time.

- What is the obligation of Bill's support staff?
- Should formal sex education be provided for Bill?
- Is the agency responsible for allowing Bill to infect individuals in the community?
- Is Bill solely responsible for his actions?

Case Study #2

Tom and Sally are a couple that have a moderate degree of developmental disability along with minor physical limitations. They have been seeing each other exclusively for the past four years, and their relationship appears to be positive. Most recently, the couple asked if they could become more intimate (i.e., sexual intercourse). They explained that up to this point they have been kissing and hugging, with occasional petting. After counselling, it was determined that Tom was unable to get an erection; yet, sexual intercourse was very important to Sally for her in the relationship. Medication for sexual dysfunction was suggested as an option by the counsellor. Both agreed this would be a possibility. Support staff are opposed to the couple engaging in sexual intercourse, stating that Sally does not understand the consequences of sex. The counsellor determined that Sally is very aware of what her decision involves, and feels that staff do not need to know the details of the couple's sexual relationship.

- Should we teach Sally and Tom about the possibility of treatment?
- Should Sally and Tom be taught alternative methods to be intimate?
- Should we discourage sexual intimacy?
- Is intimacy part of sexuality training?
- Should the staff be involved in sex education training?
- Do staff need to know intimate details of couples' sexual relationships?

Case Study #3

An 8-year-old girl named Sarah has cerebral palsy and uses a wheelchair for mobility. She is reliant on caregivers for bathing, toileting, weekly swimming lessons, and physical education at school. Due to Sarah's trusting nature and dependency on caregivers, the teacher's assistant at the school believes that Sarah should have sociosexual education. In particular, issues of boundary violations and sexual abuse need addressing. Her parents are opposed to this teaching, saying their daughter will become fearful of people that help her daily. They say she has trusting, caring people around her who would not abuse her.

- Is it necessary to teach Sarah about good touch/bad touch?
- What should be taught? How far should the teaching go?
- Is Sarah vulnerable to sexual abuse?
- Is she too young to be involved in sex education? At what age should training begin?

Case Study #4

Justin is a sixteen-year-old male who attends high school Monday to Friday. Fifty percent of his classes are segregated special education classes, while the other fifty percent are integrated regular classes (one being gym class). Most recently, there have been three complaints by students from the gym class, saying Justin was in the bath-

- Could Sarah's parents be involved in the training?
- Do her parents have the final say?
room masturbating after physical education class.

Justin has a girl friend, Lisa, who is 15 years old, and who also attends the same school. Lisa and Justin have been dating for approximately six months. In the beginning of their relationship, they would hold hands at the school. Justin and Lisa only see each other at school; their families do not approve of their children dating because of their ages and disabilities. Teachers have recently observed the couple becoming more intimate (i.e., holding each other for long periods of time in the hallways, as well as hugging and kissing one another several times throughout the day.)

When approached about this, they have responded with:
1. He/she is my boy/girlfriend
2. I really love him/her
3. I like to do that
4. All of the other students at school are doing it

- Should sociosexual training be done with this couple?
- Should it be done in the integrated or segregated class setting?
- Should they be taught separately or together?
- What should be taught?
- Should instruction about sexual intimacy be part of the curriculum?
- Would information about sexual intimacy encourage them to explore their sexuality further than present behaviours?
- Do the families need some type of training?

- Should staff receive additional training in order to deal with this issue more effectively?

Case Study #5

Tom is a 35-year-old male who lives in a group home with four other males. Tom recently told staff he likes Susan, who lives in another group home across town. He wishes he could take her out on a date. Over the past several years, Tom has been intimately involved with Joe (one of his roommates). Support staff do not think that Tom is gay; however, he does not have any intimate relationships with females. His lack of opportunity with females is believed to be the reason for his homosexual relationships. Every time he has had a girlfriend, their times together have been supervised by support staff and they have never been given opportunity to be alone, except on one occasion, two years ago. At that time, Tom was found on top of his girlfriend in the living room of her home. Staff felt Tom was too aggressive and the female was non-consenting. Therefore, the relationship was terminated. Staff is now hesitant to condone Tom's wishes to have Susan as a girlfriend due to this previous behaviour.

- Does Tom need sociosexual training?
- What does he need to be taught?
- If he is not gay, then why is he intimate with Joe?
- Does he need education about safe sex in a gay relationship? Is staff promoting his homosexual actions if they teach this?
- Could he and his new girlfriend be involved together in the social/sexual training from the beginning of the

relationship? Or is that too presumptuous?
- Should Susan be taught about safe sex?

Literature Review

The following literature review will address many of the critical questions regarding sexuality training. These are: Should sexuality education be taught? What should be taught? How should it be taught? Who should receive sexuality education? This review will also cover evaluation and accountability regarding sexuality education.

Should sexuality education be taught?

Individuals who have developmental disabilities are sexual beings with gaps in knowledge and experience and unmet needs in the sexual and relational aspects of their lives (Adams, Tallon, & Alcorn, 1982; Whitehouse & McCabe, 1997). McCabe and Schreck (1992) found the sexuality knowledge of individuals who have mild intellectual disabilities was limited, inaccurate, inconsistent, and even improbable. In two recent studies, researchers concluded that individuals who have an intellectual disability have lower levels of sexuality knowledge and experience in all areas except menstruation and body part identification when compared to a typical student population (McCabe & Cummins, 1996; Szollos & McCabe, 1995). See Table 1 for a review of research on the sexual needs and knowledge of individuals who have a developmental disability.

Formal sexuality education is, however, not generally provided to individuals who have a developmental disability. Persons without disabilities receive sex education from parents, friends and other sources (i.e., school, community agencies). People

Table 1 - Summary of Sexual Needs and Knowledge Research

Article	Participants	Assessment	Findings	Limitations	Comments
Fischer & Krajicek (1974)	16 children (8 boys and 8 girls) with developmental disabilities (DD) and their parents	Interview involving questions and pictures concerning sexual identification, body parts, body functions, emotional functions, pregnancy, and birth	For the most part, children demonstrated a considerable range of awareness around sexuality, however, there was little comprehension of sexual situations such as intercourse, pregnancy, and childbirth	Small sample size No discussion of questions used in interview No demographic data presented	Parents were surprized at the level of knowledge of sexuality of their children
Edmonson & Wish (1975)	18 men with DD	Semi-structured interview in conjunction with realistic drawings or photos	Average correct response was 28% with highest being 65% and lowest being 10%.	No discussion of reliability or validity of interview	Discussion of characteristics of participants (i.e., embarrassment, prone to guess)
Hall & Morris (1976)	61 non-institutionalized participants with DD 61 institutionalized participants with DD	Instrument created by researchers to assess knowledge and attitudes regarding self and sexuality (revised from Hall, Morris, & Barker, 1973)	Institutionalized participants demonstrated considerable less knowledge on socio-sexual topics	Only institutionalized participants received new scale No reliability or validity data on old or new scale	Concluded that amount of knowledge tends to decrease with increasing months in institution
Edmonson, Wish, & McCombs (1979)	25 institutionalized men & women with mod MR; 25 institutionalized men & women with mild MR 50 males and 50 females with mild-moderate levels of MR living in the community	SSKAT (Socio-Sexual Knowledge and Attitudes Test)	IQ was positively related to knowledge scores on 7 of 14 sub-tests Institutionalized females had the highest level of knowledge Institutionalized men had the lowest level of knowledge	To preserve time, not all participants received the same sub-tests; All received testing on anatomy/terminology, but 3 additional sub-tests were randomly assigned to each participant	

Study	Sample	Measure	Findings	Limitations	Comments
Watson & Stainton-Rogers (1980)	194 children with a DD from 4 schools; 61 children without DD	SAFER (Sex Attitudes and Facts for the Educationally Retarded) measure created by researchers	On all 10 scales of SAFER, students with disabilities had significantly lower knowledge and more conservative attitudes than control group		40 middle-class children had significantly lower sexual knowledge than the 154 working-class children.
Gillies & McEwen (1981)	554 participants between 14 & 16 yrs old; 79 who have a DD and 475 without	Questionnaire created by the researchers	Students without disabilities had a significantly higher level of sexual knowledge than students with disabilities	Very uneven sample sizes	Advise that generalization from results should be made with caution due to large sample size
Timmers, DuCharme & Jacob (1981)	25 adults with DD living in normalized apartment setting	Questionnaire created by researchers- semi-structured interview	Participants had quite good knowledge of body parts, sexuality, and dating	No reliability or validity data for interview	Attitudes reflected cultural norms
Schultz & Adams, (1987)	97 participants from 10 randomly selected schools (62 female and 35 male) 37 respondents from the pilot test school	Family Life Information Inventory modified to accommodate the reading comprehension level of participants	Concern for decisions regarding pregnancy- high need Concern about marriage, child care, and parenthood Decision making and goal setting	Does not explain how inventory was modified Limited demographic data	Used descriptive statistics Need Index and Not Met Index calculated for each need statement
Niederbuhl & Morris (1993)	32 individuals (16 men and 16 women) living in an institution for individuals who have a dual diagnosis	SSKAT Staff perceptions of ability to give consent	Capability status correlated significantly with all other variables of interest (SSKAT, level of MR, adaptive behaviour age, completion of sex education course, psychiatric diagnosis, ability to give consent in other areas)	Each author tested 8 males; social worker tested all of the females but 2, who were tested by first author No discussion of criteria for "critical knowledge"-determining competence to consent	Even if participants had strong SSKAT scores, many were still deemed unable to give consent because they lacked what the team considered to be "critical knowledge" Some agencies had policies against sexual relations between unmarried persons
McCarthy (1993)	60 women with learning difficulties (LD) ages 20-63	Semi-structured in-depth interviews	Men and women with LD experience sex very differently- sex was for men's pleasure and men took their pleasure at the expense of the women's	Does not describe methodology- what questions were asked? No criterion for inclusion/exclusion	Based on 4 years' practical experience of work with women with DD on the AIDS Awareness/Sex Education project

(table continues)

Article	Participants	Assessment	Findings	Limitations	Comments
Thompson (1994)	19 men with LD who have sexual activities in public areas ages 16-67	Qualitative interviews- do not state questions asked	Identified 3 ways would meet men for sex	Discuss limitations Difficulty in accuracy-relating time and frequencies, particularly of event with may have occurred many months previously	Discussion of ethics and ethical issues when researching individuals who have a DD Rich data and personal experience, but do not outline questions asked
Szollos & McCabe (1995)	25 participants with mild intellectual disability (ID) 10 volunteer staff 39 students in first-year students (GP)	Sex-Ken (ID and GP) Sex-Ken-C (for caregivers)	Women generally had a higher level of knowledge than men, except in masturbation; Men expressed a greater need to know and need to experience than women	Uneven sample sizes Uneven distribution between males and females	University students showed greater knowledge than participants with ID, except in body part identification and dating & intimacy
McCabe & Cummins (1996)	30 people with mild ID 50 first-year psychology students	Sex-Ken (ID & GP)	Individual with ID had lower levels of knowledge in all areas except menstruation and body part identification	Uneven sample sizes Uneven distribution between males and females	Individuals with ID were less experienced in areas of intimacy & sexual intercourse, but higher experience of pregnancy, masturbation, & STD
Konstantareas & Lunsky (1997)	31 individuals with autistic disorder (AD) 16 with DD	Composite test comprising of SSKEAI (Socio-sexual knowledge, experience, attitudes, and interests) test; SSKAT; & Vocabulary knowledge	Ability to define a sexual activity was lower in people with AD Ability to select through pointing out sexually relevant body parts was not different by level of functioning, group, or gender	40% decline in participation rate- limits generalization	Females with AD reported having more sexual experiences than their DD peers Negative correlation between knowledge and endorsement of sexual activities
McCabe (1999)	60 people with mild ID 60 people with physical disability (PD) 100 people from GP	Sex-Ken (ID; PD; and GP)	People with ID had lower levels of sexual knowledge and experience, more negative attitudes to sex, stronger sexual needs than people with PD		People with PD showed these same trends when compared to "general population"

with disabilities are likely to receive their sex information from "other" sources. According to McCabe (1999), this demonstrates that there is less discussion of sexual issues among people with disabilities with family (parents or siblings) or friends. McCabe (1999) suggests that individuals who have developmental disabilities have very little opportunity to learn about sexuality from sources other than the media and formal sex education classes. Like parents everywhere, those with an adolescent who has a disability may well express a non-specific, positive view regarding sex education. However, they are unlikely to actually provide this education in the home or to seek assistance from government or volunteer agencies (McCabe & Cummins, 1996). Fischer and Krajicek (1974) suggest that professionals who work with individuals who have a developmental disability must find appropriate bridging points where training techniques can be made available to parents or significant others so that they can provide appropriate sociosexual information.

Persons with developmental disabilities experience limited discussion about sexuality, develop negative feelings in relation to their sexuality, and consequently, demonstrate low levels of sexual expression. Although there is limited available information on the sexual attitudes of individuals who have a developmental disability, it has been reported that they are poorly informed and hold largely negative attitudes toward the expression of their sexuality (Szollos & McCabe, 1995). Persons with developmental disabilities also hold many misconceptions about sexuality, including the belief that sexual intercourse is intended to hurt the female, that women can give birth without being pregnant, and that masturbation causes harm. Other misconceptions included the belief that men have periods, and that in heterosexual intercourse, the penis generally goes into the woman's anus (Szollos & McCabe, 1995).

The development of sex education programs specifically designed for this population is essential in order to enhance quality of life (McCabe & Schreck, 1992). By filling gaps in sexual knowledge, an educational program may ultimately improve the social and personal adequacy of the young adult who has a developmental disability. According to Gillies and McEwen (1981), this is accomplished by decreasing his or her level of social disorganization and generally contributing to an improvement in the quality of life experienced.

In recent years, there has been an increased acceptance of the value of sexuality education for persons with developmental disabilities. There appear to be four factors that have influenced this change in acceptance. These factors are deinstitutionalization, the increased awareness of sexual abuse of people with intellectual disability, the advent of AIDS, and the interest that people with intellectual disability have expressed in learning more about sexuality (Whitehouse & McCabe, 1997). Each of these will be briefly explored in the following sections.

Community Living and Deinstitutionalization

With the movement to the community of individuals who have a developmental disability, it became essential that adequate information be provided so that individuals were equipped to make informed choices about sexual behaviour (Szollos & McCabe, 1995). There was also concern that many persons in institutions had not learned socially appropriate sociosexual interaction, and hence, needed to learn new social roles.

The increased awareness of sexual abuse

Without proper sex education, individuals run the risk of being sexually exploited or rejected by others (Edmonson, 1980). Sobsey and Mansell (1993) contend that denying individuals who have disabilities access to sex education may increase the vulnerability of people with disabilities to potential abuse by those who will exploit their lack of knowledge about sexuality. Carmody (1991) asserts that an understanding of sexual behaviour is a crucial requirement in ensuring that people with an intellectual disability are protected from sexual assault. If individuals who have a developmental disability are not made aware of their own sexual feelings and their rights to choose or not to choose sexual partners, confusion and the possibility of sexual exploitation is increased. A lack of sex education and opportunities to develop a sexual identity result in confusion and uncertainty about what is acceptable behaviour from other people. Carmody (1991) further contends that it is not possible to protect people from sexual assault unless they have an understanding of their own bodies and human anatomy.

HIV/AIDS

Society has experienced a critical shift regarding the value of sexuality education because of the discovery of the HIV virus (Griffiths & Lunsky, 2000). Sexual ignorance became rapidly recognized and became a life threatening risk.

However, according to Bartel and Meddock (1989), the Centre for Disease Control cannot release its data to indicate what percentages of young people with AIDS have disabilities.

Young people are at an increasingly high risk for contracting AIDS; adolescents who have disabilities are a group potentially at high risk for contracting HIV and AIDS (Bartel & Meddock, 1989).

Because students with disabilities are rarely included in large-scale studies of adolescent risk behaviours, little is known about their risk behaviours and their access to comprehensive health education, including HIV/AIDS education components (Blanchett, 2000). Recent studies in this area have primarily focused on the HIV/AIDS knowledge and risk behaviours of incarcerated youth (e.g., Kanterbury, Clavet, McGarvey, & Koopman, 1999). Consequently, little is known about the HIV/AIDS knowledge and risk behaviours of adolescents with disabilities (Blanchett, 2000).

This increased risk was substantiated in a study by Scotti, Speaks, Masia, Boggess, and Drabman (1996), who discussed factors that may contribute to the risk of HIV infection in individuals who have developmental disabilities. These included their rate of sexual activity and the failure of service providers to acknowledge their sexuality or to provide appropriate sex education. For most students, but especially for students who have developmental disabilities, questions exist about whether mediating variables such as impulsivity, awareness of disease causality and control, and perception of self-efficacy affect the risk behaviours known to be associated with transmitting AIDS (Bartel & Meddock, 1989). Blanchett (2000) also discussed characteristics of some students with disabilities that placed them at risk for HIV/AIDS, including a lack of information about issues of sexuality, lack of opportunity to have myths and misinformation corrected, poor social skills, and poor decision-making and problem-solving skills. Furthermore, research suggests that students with disabilities may be more vulnerable to sexual abuse and drug abuse, which could impact the probability of contracting HIV (Prater & Serna, 1999). Scotti et al. (1997) found in their study of AIDS education for persons with developmental disabilities that on average, participants engaged in 1.2 different forms of HIV-risk behaviour. Furthermore, 77% of the participants reported believing that they were at risk for HIV infection at the time of the pretest, with this figure remaining consistent across the study.

Students with special needs cannot be ignored when designing and implementing of HIV education programs. As demonstrated by the above research, students with disabilities may be more vulnerable to contracting HIV than their peers (Prater & Serna, 1999). However, despite this increased vulnerability, research has shown that people with developmental disabilities know very little about HIV/AIDS and how to minimize their risk (McGillvray, 1999).

Much attention in AIDS prevention has been rightfully directed toward groups that are considered to be at high risk; however, individuals who have disabilities have been virtually ignored in the current AIDS crisis (Bartel & Meddock, 1989). As evidence of this, few credible special curricula exist for teaching adolescent students who have disabilities about AIDS. Scotti et al. (1997) state that a discussion of sexually transmitted diseases is notably lacking in many of the sex education programs and few educational packages exist to help this population cope with the threat of AIDS infection. Furthermore, Scotti et al. (1997) contend that despite the clear need for behavioural skills training programs for persons with developmental disabilities, an investigation of the published literature and two recent bibliographies failed to uncover a single outcome study on the effects of providing AIDS education to this population.

Interest from Persons with Developmental Disabilities for Education

Heshuis (1982) conducted a literature review and participant observation study involving persons who have a developmental disability. He found several common themes including enjoyment, desire, or anticipation of sensual/sexual contact, fear or anxiety about sexual contact, desire for more intimate degrees of physical contact, the belief that sex belongs with marriage, and ignorance of basic facts on sexual relations. His data indicate that individuals who have a developmental disability have a desire for more knowledge and skills regarding sexuality. McCabe (1999) found similar results. In a recent study, she concluded that the respondents with disabilities indicated higher levels of sexual needs than respondents who did not have a disability. She suggested that participants who had disabilities had a strong need to experience dating, intimacy, and sexual interaction, but because of their lack of knowledge, their negative feelings about sexuality, and conceivably because of their lack of opportunity for sexual expression, they are currently unable to participate in these experiences.

Thus, the trend toward deinstitutionalization and the awareness of potential risk of abuse or life threatening disease, coupled with the increasing interest in sociosexual education among persons with developmental disabilities, have created a shift in the value that the field has placed on sociosexual education.

What should be taught?

Early sex education programs focused on behavioural control of inappropriate sexual activities, particularly inappropriate masturbation (Mitchell, Doctor, & Butler, 1978) and neglected issues such as "dating, relationships, gender security, and exploitation" (Rowe & Savage, 1987, p.11). In 1979, Wish, McCombs and Edmonson, reported that the most important topics for sex education were birth control information, intercourse, venereal disease (how to contract, symptoms and who to tell), and pregnancy (how to get and prevent). Avoiding street pick-ups and inappropriate physical contact were also ranked as very important. The number ten spot on the list of topics of importance was identification of body parts and dating, which received equal ratings.

Kempton (1975) and Gordon (1971) were among the first to develop sex education curricula that provided information, not just about sexual biology, but about relationships, marriage, dating and parenting. Significant shifts in attitudes toward the sexuality of persons with developmental disabilities began in the seventies and eighties. Parents became less conservative toward sexuality, recognizing the importance of sex education as protection for their children (Johnson & Davies, 1989; Pueschel & Scola, 1988). Staff attitudes as well became more generally accepting. There was stronger approval of sexual behaviour between consenting adults in a private setting (Adams et al., 1982), but uncertainty toward issues of abortion, sterilization, and homosexuality (Johnson & Davies, 1989). Sex education became more focused on the sociosexual learning needs of persons with developmental disabilities. In addition to education about anatomy, birth control, sexual intercourse, hygiene and venereal disease, educators incorporated into their curricula an increased emphasis on relationships, social behaviour, self esteem, decision-making, sexual lifestyles, and abuse (See Kempton, 1993).

Recently, Griffiths and Lunsky (2001) conducted a replication of the 1979 Wish, McCombs and Edmonson study, and found subtle but significant changes in attitudes toward the sexuality of persons with developmental disabilities in the past 20 years. In their comparative study on the changes in importance on various topics for sexuality education as rated by professionals and parents between 1979 and 1999, Griffiths and Lunsky (2001) reported that the shifts in topics included:

✓   increased emphasis on body parts
✓   increased recognition in the importance of relationships (going steady, extramarital contact/limits, dating, engage-ment), but decreased recognition of the importance of marriage or premarital sexual contact
✓   increased awareness of vulnerability issues (rape, incest and other inappropriate sexual contact) and understanding that the risk is not necessarily a vulnerability in the indi-vidual (suggestibility to dares), nor primarily found in stranger situations (street-pickups)
✓   increased recognition of sexual diversity (masturbation, homosexuality, and adult movies and literature).

Griffiths and Lunsky (2001) suggested that recent changes in the sexuality curricula reflect the increased awareness and knowledge in the field of sexuality and disability. The four most critical changes in sociosexual awareness for persons with developmental disabilities were as follows:

❑   the rates and nature of abuse and exploitation of persons with developmental disabilities
❑   the nature of sexually inappropriate behaviour of persons

with developmental disabilities
- ❑ the discovery of HIV/AIDS and its presence in this population
- ❑ recognition of the importance of preventive health education and care for this population.

These issues address the importance of comprehensive programs of sex education that incorporate training, not only on matters related directly to sex, but also on social relationships and enhancement of self-esteem (McCabe, 1999). According to McCabe and Schreck (1992), sex education was generally provided to address problems, not to develop sexuality as an integrated part of the person's life. Therefore, many areas of sexuality are never considered in such programs. Foley (1995) asserts that the absence of a well-designed curriculum may result in delivery of a human sexuality program that lacks comprehensiveness and cohesiveness.

In order to plan effective curricula for individuals who have a developmental disability, it is important to first determine what information individuals need (Goldman, 1994). Whitehouse and McCabe (1997) assert that the real challenge is to assist individuals who have a developmental disability to gain a sense of sexual identity. This would be vital for heterosexual or homosexual relationships, or for having sex without a partner. In order to accomplish this, educators must develop an understanding of the actual sexual needs of the participants. Only then can they tailor programs to address these needs, rather than imposing the values of the non-disabled culture on people with disabilities (Whitehouse & McCabe, 1997).

Lumley and Miltenberger (1997) contend that for adults who have developmental disabilities, education regarding sexuality should be more extensive than usually is provided. They suggest that too often, sexuality education is rudimentary. Monat-Haller (1992) contends that sexuality education should include the teaching of anatomy and physiology as well as maturation and body changes.

Kempton (1993) also supports teaching of body parts and physiology in her curriculum, *Life Horizons 1 and 11.* She believes sexuality education should include discussion of male and female anatomy, including reproduction, the sexual life cycle, and human sexual response. Kempton (1993) also contends that curricula should include a discussion of sexual health, including the care of sex organs. This would entail a discussion of good habits of cleanliness, as well as the importance of medical examinations for men and women.

Although the basics of sex education are crucial to any curriculum, when teaching sex education, it is advisable to avoid a narrowly defined concept of sexuality, such as coitus and reproductive physiology (Cole & Cole, 1993). Reproduction and sexual behaviour are not synonymous. Men and women must learn not only about sexuality, but they must also learn about sexual relationships. Add to this the need to learn about love, and it becomes apparent that this develops into a complex task. Beyond sexual love is the more generic love for humankind, a love not implying sex, involving personal interaction and charm (Cole & Cole, 1993). In sex education programs, although it is necessary to convey explicit information about sexual behaviour, choices, and risks, it is also important to reach beyond the biological and address the social and emotional aspects of sexuality (Sobsey & Mansell, 1993). Sobsey (1994) echoes this statement, and declares that the important social and emotional contexts of sexuality are often carefully

withheld from sex education. He goes on to say that unfortunately, these are not only among the most enjoyable aspects of
sexuality, they are also among the most essential ones (Sobsey,
1994).

Moreover, because adults have the right to engage in consensual sexual relationships, education about what constitutes appropriate and inappropriate sexual relationships is also necessary (Lumley & Miltenberger, 1997). Griffiths (1999) agrees
and asserts that an essential part of sociosexual education is
teaching about the responsibilities that come with sexual expression. This includes education about contraception, consent,
and sexually transmitted diseases.

Monat-Haller (1992) further asserts that complex legal issues
need to be confronted and resolved, working toward *responsible* choices that are in the best interest of the individual. Programs should help students to explore values and attitudes as a
basis for developing responsibility for their own behaviours
and health, as well as those of others. Education programs
must provide opportunities for students to develop positive
behaviours and to practice interpersonal and social skills (i.e.,
decision making, communication, negotiation and refusal
skills, stress management, and goal setting) that help them to
identify, avoid, escape, and/or manage high-risk situations
(Prater & Serna, 1995).

Brantlinger (1992) discusses "family life education" and its
importance for the individual who has a developmental disability. Family life education is broader in scope than sexuality education. In addition to sexuality education, it includes
such components as decision-making skills related to sexual
and intimate social behaviours and communication within the

context of intimate social relationships. Also included in family life education is assertiveness in expressing personal feelings and desires, assuming responsibility for behaviours related to sexuality, developing sensitivity to the feelings and attitudes of others, and living harmoniously with others in domestic situations (Brantlinger, 1992). If students who have developmental disabilities are to be better prepared for the intimate social, sexual, and parental roles they aspire to and generally assume, then teachers must provide a comprehensive and meaningful family life education (Brantlinger, 1992).

Page (1991) discusses the importance of managing potential consequences of sexual activity, including sexually transmitted diseases and pregnancy. Individuals who have a developmental disability should be taught clearly the consequences of sexual behaviour (Whitman, 1990). Further, Timmers, DuCharme, and Jacob (1981) found that 50% of males in their normalized sample wanted children, although they had only vague plans about achieving this aim. Therefore, the message that children are a consequence of sexual intercourse needs to be conveyed, alongside the concept of what child-rearing involves.

Individuals who have a developmental disability must also be provided with accurate and explicit information regarding the prevention of STD's, including HIV and AIDS (Cole & Cole, 1993). Avoiding unwanted pregnancy and sexually transmitted diseases is crucial.

With regards to education regarding sexually transmitted diseases, Jacobs, Samowitz, Levy, and Levy (1989) propose an extensive HIV education program and declare that participants must learn several things. Their recommendations are as follows:

✓ People must perceive HIV infection as a personal threat
✓ Emphasize that HIV infection is preventable
✓ Individuals must be convinced that they can manage the behavioural changes that may be necessary
✓ Reassure individuals that they can still be sexually satisfied (pp. 235-236)

These researchers go on to state that it is clear that before a significant reduction in HIV-risk behaviour can be expected, HIV/AIDS programs for persons who have developmental disabilities will need to target the modification of specific risk behaviours. This can be accomplished by providing direct skills training and adequate support for the utilization of those new skills.

Hylton (1993) discusses SAFE: *Stopping AIDS Through Functional Education*, designed for use with people with mild to moderate developmental disability, but which has also been used with people who have serious learning problems, head injury, or mental illness. Hylton (1993) states that part of SAFE's success lies in its adaptability.

Scotti et al. (1996) conducted a study of AIDS-Risk information and the educational effects for individuals who have a developmental disability. Following their involvement in an HIV/AIDS education program, participants who had mild developmental disabilities demonstrated statistically significant increases in HIV/AIDS knowledge. Participants in the moderate range did not demonstrate any significant changes. However, the researchers stated that despite the encouraging increase in HIV/AIDS knowledge, it is highly unlikely that the program had a significant impact on the actual sexual behaviour of the participants, such as condom use and decreased frequency of high-risk behaviours. Scotti et al. (1996) concluded that before a significant reduction in HIV-risk behaviour can be expected, HIV/AIDS programs for persons with developmental disabilities will need to target the modification of specific risk behaviours by providing direct skills training and adequate support for the use of those new skills.

Cole and Cole (1993) contend that accurate and explicit information regarding the prevention of STD's, including AIDS, must be available to all children and adults in our society. They also posit that there needs to be a greater understanding and consideration of the problems imposed by physical disabilities on sexual functioning. In discussing reproductive options and birth control, one must assess whether the disability influences fertility and fertility options. Moreover, an individual with a physical disability may have alterations of body functions that interfere with the timely and accurate recognition of symptoms of sexually transmitted diseases (Cole & Cole, 1993).

Furthermore, some birth control methods may be contraindicated for women who have specific disabilities. There may also be unrecognized and ongoing medical conditions that may affect fertility, such as irregular menses and chronic infection that must be discussed in sexuality education classes for individuals who have a developmental disability (Cole & Cole, 1993). Reproductive choices that are suitable for women who have a disability must be taught.

Independence, personal esteem, positive body image, and positive sex messages should also be emphasized (Cole & Cole, 1993). These individuals need to learn about their rights and need to be granted the opportunity to refuse or question approaches that they believe inappropriate. Sobsey and Varnhagen (1991) assert that sex education providers need to review the philosophy of curricula to increase focus on assertiveness, choice, discrimination of appropriate and inappropriate requests, and improved sex education. This includes learning decision making skills, the freedom to choose, and the responsibility for those choices. Such practices will promote self-esteem and problem solving mastery (Goldman, 1994).

Furthermore, existing curricula need to consider placing more emphasis on marriage, the decision to parent, and parenting. These are areas that are generally not being addressed in education programs for individuals who have a developmental disability (Schultz & Adams, 1987).

Whitehouse and McCabe (1997) contend that few programs have been concerned with the enhancement of positive attitudes towards sexuality. However, these researchers declare that programs that focus solely on increasing the positive attitudes of people with intellectual disability with regards to sexuality ensure that people have information but not the permission to use the information. Although the message of sexuality education should be generally positive, Fifield (1986) suggests that there is an ethical responsibility to teach about negative aspects of sexuality such as abuse, harassment, and assault. Muccigrosso (1991) concurs with this and states that at the very least, instructional content should include relationships and rules, as well as private information and details about body parts. However, it must also include "OK" and "not OK" touching, assertiveness skills, an understanding of common ploys used by exploitative people, and reporting skills. It is insufficient to merely teach about these topics. Educators must also provide the participants with the knowledge of how to respond in preventing or reporting such situations. Sexual abuse is often not reported because the individual has no knowledge that his behaviour is inappropriate or that there is action that can be taken to prevent or respond to abuse.

Individuals with and without disabilities have the same rights to information, services, and to health service providers with adequate knowledge, sensitivity, and experience in areas of sexual development (Cole & Cole, 1993). Self-empowerment, life skills, parenting, and medical concerns are common to everyone, but these are issues that may need special attention in individuals who have developmental disabilities.

As individuals mature, new problems may be added to under-lying disability issues. Some examples of this might include further confusion of gender role, stigma, need for more adap-tive equipment, societal expectations of the aging adult, and the anticipated transition from health to illness (Cole & Cole, 1993).

Diaeger and Wong (1994) also note that most sex education programs have tended to assume a heterosexual perspective, teaching heterosexuality as the only sexual option available to people with an intellectual disability, rather than actually ad-dressing the needs and circumstances of the individual. Sex educators must also understand that women who have disabili-ties possess the sexual desires and actions of women in gen-eral, as well as their specific concerns related to their disabili-ties (Corbett, Shurberg Klein, & Bregante, 1989).

How should information be taught?

Adams et al. (1982) state that there is a need for a validated sex education curriculum that is incorporated into the everyday living environment. A sex education program cannot simply be "tacked on". It requires considerable curriculum development and staff co-ordination (Coleman & Murphy, 1980). Griffiths (1999) echoes this and states that learning about one's sexuality does not take place in six one-hour sessions, nor is it restricted to one period in one's life. She asserts that learning about sexuality is a lifelong process. This means that people with developmental disabilities, just like individuals who do not have disabilities, will learn about sexuality throughout their life development, when it has meaning to their lives. She goes on to state that these individuals need access to accurate information when it is age appropriate and contextually relevant for them to know this information (Griffiths, 1999).

Because persons with developmental disability have such limited sexual knowledge, this may suggest that formal sex education classes are largely ineffective. McCabe (1999), however, asserts that it is not sufficient for people who have disabilities to receive information on sexual issues. It is important that the information changes their knowledge about sexuality, both short term and long term, and improves their experience of sexual interactions. As stated by Edmonson (1980), such a program requires good facilitators, support provider participation, resources, and time. This type of education is most effectively offered in a long-range and comprehensive manner (Muccigrosso, 1991).

Sexuality education entails discussing many topics that most people would rather avoid. Therefore, the first principle for developing a sex education program is to make the trainers and the participants comfortable. Individuals who have a developmental disability must always be consulted and involved in the development and delivery of any education and services they receive (Sobsey & Doe, 1991).

Educators must be made aware that if the training information is to be meaningful, then messages about sexuality should be tailored for the specific audience (Jacobs et al., 1989). Sex educators must take into account the sexual desires and actions of the participants in general, as well as their specific concerns related to their disabilities (Corbett et al., 1989). Corbett et al. (1989) further caution that existing sex education curriculum rarely includes either images or concerns of persons who have a disability. This exclusion merely contributes to the problems outlined previously. Persons who have disabilities need to be represented, in their diversity, in all printed materials, all visual aids, and all video materials (Corbett et al., 1989).

The location of the training is important (e.g., in a classroom, the educator's office, and the recreation room of a group home). The setting should be culturally appropriate and not provide confusing messages (i.e., use of a bedroom). If a group is formed, individuals who have similar levels of functioning should be grouped together. It must also be determined if a group or individual session would be most appropriate for the specific person (Jacobs et al., 1989).

Educators must also ensure confidentiality and build trust. When teaching people with a developmental disability, it is especially important to prepare them for each session (Jacobs et al., 1989). Distributing an agenda, telling them what the topic is, and what is going to happen will help ease the tension. Facilitators must also ensure that participants understand what is going to be discussed.

Jacobs et al. (1989) suggest using the person's vocabulary to encourage questions and discussion. Facilitators must be as non-judgemental as possible, avoiding value-laden words. Jacobs et al. (1989) argue that someone may consider promiscuity to be sex with two persons in 20 years; others may feel very differently. Also, what is "dirty" to one person may be quite acceptable to another. The program must be simple, using plain language, and should involve much repetition over a lengthy period of time to be as effective as possible (Muccigrosso, 1991). It is also important not to go too fast (Jacobs et al., 1989). All the relevant information will probably have to be covered over a series of sessions.

Muccigrosso (1991) also contends that the particular learning styles of most persons with developmental disabilities dictate that the instruction be participatory as opposed to lecture format. Role plays and dramatization are excellent techniques for educating as well as for checking learning. Sobsey (1994) suggests drawing on a variety of resources and techniques. He suggests an eclectic approach to education, although community-based training and learning methods are absolutely necessary for some of the learning goals essential to risk reduction. Nonetheless, the infrequency of certain natural learning opportunities, along with some of the associated risks, makes it impossible to teach all of these skills in their natural contexts. Therefore, simulation, vicarious learning through stories or audio-visual materials, and a variety of other formats for instructional delivery must be included in the educational program. For many teaching objectives and for many students, generic personal safety materials designed without consideration of disability are valuable educational resources, but for most students with disabilities, additional instruction and support will be necessary and some of the materials will require modification. For other participants, programs specifically designed for individuals who have disabilities will be the best resources.

Visual aids are also essential to help the participant to understand and remember. When using visuals, however, Jacobs et al. (1989) suggest to keep in mind the importance of being as concrete as possible. "If you put a condom on a banana, so might the person with a developmental disability" (p. 235). Monat-Haller (1992) states that sex education for individuals who have developmental disabilities must be explicit. Verbal content needs to be in simple language suited to students' vocabularies and learning styles. Visual aids such as pictures, videotapes, books, and dolls are also essential.

Hylton's (1993) SAFE program demonstrates many of these points, since it is not meant to be followed in a rigid, lock-step fashion. Rather, it offers an array of lessons, videos, take-home brochures, slides, and illustrations from which instructors may assemble approaches for meeting the needs of different learners. The videos, take-home brochures, slides, and illustrations in SAFE help make the lesson more concrete. The videos employ a variety of formats: interview, demonstrations, and soap opera-like dramatization to prompt learners to discuss their concerns, and to role play coping skills related to HIV prevention. SAFE uses a pre-test, post-test, strategy to compare the level of information and skills learners demonstrate before training with what they demonstrate after instruction. It employs a variety of learning strategies, including modelling, role playing, guided practice, and teaching regular skills in regular environments. Hylton (1993) asserts that it is unique because it pays special attention to developing a context that can support both learning and the practice of HIV/ AIDS prevention behaviour and it offers strategies for doing this.

Who should be taught?

The field has very little empirical evidence regarding the type of participant who benefits most from a general sexuality education course (Lindsay, Bellshaw, Culross, Staines, & Michie, 1992). As well, it is not known whether different methods of instruction are more effective with different participants.

Sexuality training is best if provided proactively or preventatively (Griffiths, 1999). Too often, individuals with developmental disabilities are provided sexuality education only if there is a problem. They are provided reactive education when they have been abused, have become pregnant, have contracted a disease, or have acted in a risky or inappropriate manner. The objective of sexuality education is to teach responsibility for one's sexual feelings and desires, not to eliminate sexual interest and responses (Griffiths, 1999). Therefore, the simple answer to *who should be provided sexuality education?* is that all individuals who have a developmental disability should be provided the opportunity for sexuality education suited to their interests and needs.

Ames (1991) contends that the developmental years prior to puberty are a time when sexual rehearsal play is both a natural and healthy preparation for later adult sexual adjustment. It is also a time of vulnerability to distortion and trauma executed through ignorance, situation, or with intention. This can result in adult paraphilias of which little is understood, or seldom properly treated. For these reasons, good sexuality education ought to begin at birth, outlined in a framework of positive, healthy attitudes and responses from nurturing caregivers.

Although education is crucial for individuals who have a developmental disability, it is also imperative that sex education programs be developed for the staff as well as persons with developmental disabilities (Jacobs et al., 1989). Sex education programs have a greater likelihood of success if care providers (family, staff) are also involved. It is important for generalization that the individuals in the natural environment support the learning objectives of the program, and support the implementation of program learning (McCabe & Cummins, 1996).

How can effectiveness be determined?

Educators have long suggested that an inventory or a test is crucial to determine where to begin with sociosexual instruction, and what has been learned consequent to instruction (Edmonson et al., 1979). In teaching sex education, it is important to assess the participant's skills before, during, and after the intervention as a means of evaluating progress (Lumley & Miltenberger, 1997). In a multicomponent program, this may entail assessing progress at the completion of a number of different phases. For example, for a program containing sex education and social skills training components, it is important to assess the participant's skills in these areas after the specific training has taken place through use of a comparison to baseline. This is required in order to ascertain whether training has been successful. Lumley and Miltenberger (1997) assert that evaluating progress in this way allows training to be modified or reinstated as necessary.

Minimally, Griffiths (2001) advocates the use of a pre and a post evaluation of sexual knowledge and attitudes. The Socio-

Sexual Knowledge and Attitudes Test (Wish, Edmonson, & McCombs, 1980) and the Sex Ken-ID (McCabe, 1994) are among the few evaluation tools available that measure change in both knowledge and attitude. Whitehouse and McCabe (1997) stress the need for evaluation of sexual attitudes. They state that future programs need to consider the use of both checklists and transcript analysis to cover both the more accurate but more limited assessment of sexual facts, as well as the more complex analysis of feelings and attitudes. These measures provide an individually administered evaluation, using a picture book to which participants answer questions that require minimal verbal demands. The Sex Ken-ID is a much more updated version for assessment; however, it differs significantly from the SSKAT in that it also requests information about experiences. This latter difference may move the Sex Ken-ID past a point of evaluating educational knowledge and attitude, and into a clinical range that may not be appropriate for general educational purposes.

Edmonson and Wish (1975) found that a test of body terminology is not the equivalent of inferential comprehension of sexual activity. It is also more important to measure the skills the individual actually utilizes in a target situation (Lumley & Miltenberger, 1997). Remember that in evaluating behavioural skills training procedures, the outcome measure should be an increase in actual behaviours and skills, rather than merely increasing knowledge (Lumley & Miltenberger, 1997).

Evaluation of training effectiveness is common practice in the field of developmental disabilities. Coleman and Murphy (1980) reported that only one-third of the institutions they surveyed lacked formal evaluation of their sex education program. The remaining two-thirds were evaluated by a variety of

measures, including surveys of staff reactions, pre-post questionnaires, or behavioural measures of the residents. However,
79% of the evaluation results were not available. This latter
statistic reflects what typically happens in the field. Valid and
reliable outcome evaluation of the impact of training is often
lacking. In addition, evaluation of generalization of learning is
typically non-existent.

The field is now inundated with sexuality education programs;
however, there is little research to support that persons with
developmental disabilities benefit from most of these courses
(Lindsay et al., 1992). Although countless sexuality education
programs have now been developed, they have generally not
been evaluated (McCabe, 1999). Even among the sexuality
programs that are commercially available, few provide empirical evidence to demonstrate that they are effective in teaching
persons with developmental disabilities knowledge or skills
that will maintain and generalize to their lives. Lindsay et al.
(1992) report that there is very little evidence that clients will
acquire and retain this knowledge. In addition to the cost of
materials, extensive and expensive staff time is being spent on
sexuality education that cannot often be demonstrated to be
effective. Additionally, people with developmental disabilities
are being taught, and it is assumed therefore that they have acquired knowledge and skills. However, without pre and post
training evaluation, this assumption may be both erroneous
and dangerous. Unverified assumptions that people have
knowledge and skill after training which is sufficient to protect
them can leave both the individuals and agencies vulnerable.

Whitehouse and McCabe (1997) further assert that research
that has examined the effectiveness of sex education programs
has had a number of methodological flaws. Some of these

flaws have included a lack of adequate measures, a lack of control groups, and no follow up data. However, the most obvious flaw of a large number of studies is the lack of quantitative data (Whitehouse & McCabe, 1997). Of the research that has reported evaluation data, none has reported the effectiveness of sex education in relation to increasing sexual knowledge and enhancing positive attitudes toward sexuality (Whitehouse & McCabe 1997). In order for effective sex education programs to be developed, there needs to be greater emphasis on the evaluation of sex education programs and not just their development.

The lack of evaluation of sexuality education and its implications for the lives of persons with intellectual disabilities is finally being realized. Agencies are beginning to recognize the critical importance of evaluating and documenting the effectiveness of their sociosexual educational programs (e.g., Jacobs et al., 1992; Scotti et al., 1997) and the need for accountability regarding the quality of sexuality education (see Kastner, DeLotto, Scagnelli, & Testa, 1990). It is now insufficient to provide people with developmental disabilities sexuality education unless it can be demonstrated that the education leads to increased knowledge and the ability to apply that knowledge where appropriate (See Chapter 3).

The validity of sexual abuse prevention training is another area of particular concern. Whitehouse and McCabe (1997) note that the field is demanding sexuality education as a means of decreasing the vulnerability of persons with disabilities to sexual assault. However, there is very little evidence that sex education does in fact decrease the vulnerability to people with intellectual disabilities to sexual assault (Whitehouse & McCabe, 1997). Hard (cited in Senn, 1989) presented a correlational study that showed that men and women with disabilities who had received sex education had experienced less rates of abuse than those who had no sex education. However, no long term study that could demonstrate causality has been initiated.

Of particular importance to the topic of sexual abuse prevention training is the issue of in situ assessment, which is the use of a naturalistic setting in which the participant is unaware that he or she is being evaluated. This method of assessment has been used by a number of researchers to evaluate the outcomes of training programs on the lives of the persons trained when they are in the *"real"* world (Collins, Schuster, & Nelson, 1992; Haseltine & Miltenberger, 1990; Lumley, Miltenberger, Long, Rapp, & Roberts, 1998). Haseltine and Miltenberger (1990) demonstrated this form of assessment for teaching self-protection skills to individuals who have a developmental disability. In this study, assessment probes occurred in situ in settings that the participants were likely to inhabit on a frequent basis, such as on the sidewalk in front of the participant's group home, the parking lot by the group home, or in the vicinity of a nearby convenience store. The researchers developed a pool of 12 role-plays depicting potentially abusive situations. Due to ethical concerns, the role plays did not depict sexually abusive situations, but instead depicted potential abduction scenarios using authority or incentive lures. Each role play consisted of two inducements for the participant to leave with the confederate abductor. The confederate may have approached the individual on foot or by car, but in each case, he greeted the participant in a friendly manner, and offered the participant some inducement to leave with him.

Participants were assessed on a 0 to 3-point scale. A score of

0 was given if the participant went with the abductor regardless of vocalization, and a score of 1 was given if the participant did not go with the abductor, but did not move away or provide any verbal refusal. A score of 2 was given if the participant verbally refused the solicitation or moved at least 6.5 metres away from the abductor and initiated the movement within three seconds. A score of 2 was also assigned if the participant failed to say no or move away, but did inform a staff person of the solicitation within two minutes after the abductor left the scene. A score of 3 was given if the participant told a staff person about the incident within two minutes after refusing the solicitation or getting away.

Collins et al. (1992) also employed a similar assessment format for their analysis of teaching a generalized response to the lures of strangers to individuals who have a developmental disability. In their study, settings included sites along the street of the community satellite centre where the participants received vocational training and sites where the participants received community-based instruction, such as shopping malls or the library. Domestic training sites were also included, such as an apartment complex. Three basic types of lures were used in the investigation. These included authority, general, and incentive. An example of an "authority lure" would be "{name of supervisor} said for you to go with me". A general lure would be "Would you like to go for a ride in my car?" and an example of an incentive lure would be "Would you like to go get a soda?"

Lumley et al. (1998) also employed the use of in situ probes. In their study, prior to meeting with the participants in the first training session, a male confederate unknown to the participant was introduced as a new staff member. Within 15 minutes after becoming acquainted with the participant, the confederate presented one of the lures. There was never any physical contact between the confederate and the participant during the assessment. If the participant agreed to the requested behaviour, a staff person from the group home who was listening at the door interrupted immediately or the confederate made an excuse to leave. If the participant said "no", or asked the confederate to leave, he did so immediately. If the participant made no response to the request, the confederate made an excuse to leave after 15 seconds.

The ethical issues surrounding the use of in situ evaluation present a significant challenge for researchers. As Lumley and Miltenberger (1997) discuss, the use of in situ probes is likely to be effective in evaluating sexuality education programs, whereas attempts to assess the acquisition of skills using interview or paper and pencil measures cannot evaluate how an individual will actually respond in an abusive situation. However, most researchers chose not to use this method due to concerns about exposing an individual to seemingly real, albeit simulated, sexual abuse lures.

Thus evaluation, although critical to determination of effectiveness, is often missing and based on training response or pre-post data only. Moreover, more valid evaluation of effectiveness is fraught with ethical challenges.

Conference Deliberations

Conference participants raised many valid questions throughout the meeting. Emphasis was placed on four primary areas including:

1. The obligation and responsibility of the agency and staff,
2. The rights of individuals who have a developmental disability to be informed,
3. The legal issues stemming from one's choices of their sexual lifestyles,
4. The liability of the agency and staff to provide education.

The group went on to say that the rights of an individual who has a developmental disability may be violated if the agency is not obligated to develop and teach sex education. A question was then posed: "Should sex education be voluntary or mandatory?" If it is not voluntary, and becomes mandatory due to the obligation of the agency, the individual's rights again are being compromised.

With that in mind, participants decided that a clear and practical policy would be the key factor in addressing these concerns. That policy should include: a) the role of the agency to promote healthy sexuality, and b) the opportunity for all individuals to be provided accurate information to allow for healthy and safe choices.

Session attendees agreed that much of the responsibility for sexuality issues tends to be placed on frontline staff. The general feeling of session attendees was that the overwhelming expectation of their agency's administration, families, and the community was that the frontline person was ultimately responsible.

It was unanimously agreed that agencies need to commit to the ongoing training of support staff to ensure that they are able to conduct themselves from a philosophically agency-guided policy in promoting and teaching sexuality to the individuals be-

ing supported. The group discussed other significant questions, such as "Are those of us in the field of developmental
disabilities presenting two very confusing views? Are we perhaps perpetuating dependence in the area of sexuality and yet
encouraging independence in all other areas of life?" The dilemma frontline staff often face is whether to provide opportunities for people to take personal risks that are possibly a risk
to others (i.e., vulnerable people, community, peers, agency).

Conference participants cautioned that regardless of ongoing
staff training, staff might still have difficulty not imposing its
own values and morals onto the individual. With that in mind,
agencies need to be aware of this challenge and ensure safeguards are put into place and the rights of the individuals who
have a developmental disability are not being compromised or
devalued in any way.

The group discussed the responsibility, liability, and legal aspects of sexuality training with individuals who are currently
at risk of developing a sexually transmitted disease. After
much debate, the group was able to come to consensus. The
group believed there should be a policy statement that ensures
accurate information is being provided to support individuals
to make healthy and safe choices. The conference attendees
did not feel that service providers can assume liability because
they are unable to force individuals to use protection who either have, or are at risk of a sexually transmitted disease.
However, to reduce the risk of STD's, the agency should support and encourage the use of condoms, provide medical expertise and encourage the individual to inform the partner.
From a legal perspective, the group believed reporting was essentially the decision of the person who has a sexually transmitted disease, not a service provider. Furthermore, session

attendees recognized that if staff, parents, or others take responsibility from persons who have a developmental disability, they would not and/or could not learn to take responsibility for themselves. Agencies need to move from protection models to support modes. At this time, there are differing views among parents, educators, frontline staff, and others regarding protection and risk.

Although the group was able to identify several relevant issues, it also recognized that other important topics were not discussed (i.e., birth control, pregnancy). However, this did not in any way denote their importance. The group did, however, believe that any sexually related issue should be built into a sexuality training curriculum.

The final outcome of the deliberations concluded that there are several critical factors in developing an effective training package. Consensus concluded that recognition of accurate and appropriate information needs to be provided for all people who have a developmental disability. Agencies need to develop policies and sex education programs to meet the needs of individuals on all fronts related to sexuality. Staff training should be prioritized by agencies to increase the likelihood that consistent and appropriate information is given to individuals. Lastly, individuals who have a developmental disability should not only be provided with good sex education, but should also be supported and given opportunities for intimate sexual relationships that are respected by all. However, with rights come responsibility, and taking away freedom is a natural consequence for everyone in the community.

Summary

Sexuality education is a greatly needed and greatly neglected area of training for persons with developmental disabilities. There is widespread and growing recognition of the importance of sociosexual education; however, few agencies provide ongoing access to proactive and preventative training. Moreover, the quality of such programs has been questioned and is without empirical support. Thus, sexuality education in the field of developmental disabilities is in a state of paradox. It is considered to be a primary feature to the promotion of sexual health and prevention of sexual diseases; however, it is generally limited, reactive, and without evidence of effectiveness.

State of the Art

Agencies have an obligation to provide opportunity for sexuality education to ensure that individuals with developmental disabilities have knowledge and skills that will enable them to be involved, to the largest extent possible in all aspects of life, including their sexual life. Additionally, sexuality education is required to prevent challenging behaviours and unwanted pregnancy, reduce the risk of abuse, reduce the threat of HIV and AIDS, and to encourage sexual health.

A state of the art sexuality program should have several components such as:

- empirically or at least consensually validated sexuality education materials that cover a comprehensive breadth of topics,
- be based on person-centred evaluation and adapted to the individual sensitivities and special needs, beliefs and values, and educational or learning needs,
- provide training that both teaches and models appropriate

socially accepted standards of conduct,

- provide training using a variety of mediums such as pictures, group discussion, role modelling, repetition, and use of concrete materials,
- be evaluated, following training for knowledge, attitude and skill acquisition, and provide follow-up as needed.

Clinical and Agency Implications

As discussed in Chapter 3, agencies must commit in policy and practice to provide proactive, quality sexuality education within their agency. As such, it requires ongoing commitment from management and staff who are interested in learning how to teach sexuality education. It requires opportunities and materials for staff education and ongoing resources to ensure implementation and continuity of training.

There are several steps for agencies to ensure that sexuality programs are teaching what is needed (to whom and when), teaching it well, and ensuring that what was taught is learned and able to be applied.

First, the sexuality training materials that are selected must be valid tools for teaching the necessary knowledge and attitudes regarding sexuality. Agencies should determine if there has been evidence that the materials they are purchasing have been researched or field tested. The topics should cover a range of topics (i.e., from anatomy to parenting), and options (i.e., from sexual intercourse to abstinence), and include current issues (i.e., safer sex practices). Sexuality training requires appropriate audio-visual materials to ensure that the topics can be properly taught.

Second, controversy regarding sexuality education can take place because of content and the explicitness of the medium used to teach about sexuality. However, it is important to use a variety of mediums such as pictures and concrete materials. The materials must be appropriate to the age, special needs, sensitivities, and values of the person. Sexuality education should be a gradual educational process; age appropriate topics should be introduced at age appropriate times in the person's life. The participants may require special adaptations for learning (i.e., for persons of different functioning levels or types of disability, such as vision or hearing). The materials and teaching approaches may also need to be adapted to the sensitivities, interests, and values of the individuals (for example with persons who have been abused, or for individuals who have strong moral or religious beliefs regarding specific areas of sexuality).

Third, sexuality training should be conducted by persons who have the knowledge and skill to do so. Although there are qualified sex educators, the reality is that most persons with developmental disabilities are taught by interested persons within agencies who have seen an unmet need for education in their agency and have pursued independent study or courses to learn how to provide the training. It is, however, important that the program that is developed within any agency be reviewed by others within the agency for both content and teaching approach to ensure that the educator both teaches and models appropriate socially accepted standards of conduct.

Fourth, sex education is most effective if it is taught using a variety of instructional methods such as direct instruction, movies or slides, group discussion, group exercises (i.e., create a collage of appropriate hygiene products), role playing of social skills, repetition of topics in different ways and the use of concrete materials (i.e., birth control devices).

Fifth, the effectiveness of the training program needs to be evaluated for each participant to determine if the desired increase in knowledge and skill acquisition was achieved. If not, further training would be required. Sexuality education should adhere to the same standards that are placed on other training programs. There should be educational goals, training steps and outcome evaluation.

Final Consensus Statement

There is a growing interest in providing sexuality education for persons with developmental disabilities. However, for the most part, agencies have not implemented sexuality education as a proactive part of their training for persons with developmental disabilities. It was the consensus of the conference participants that there should be an obligation for agencies to provide training or access to this type of training for the persons in their agencies. Moreover, there was a consensus that to ensure quality, sexuality programs should be carefully developed, conducted in an appropriate and value-based manner, evaluated for effectiveness, and monitored by the agency.

References

Adams, G. L., Tallon, R .J., & Alcorn, D. A. (1982). Attitudes toward the sexuality of mentally retarded and nonretarded persons. *Education and Training of the Mentally Retarded, 17(4)*, 307-312.

Ames, T. R. (1991). Guidelines for providing sexuality-related services to severely and profoundly retarded individuals: The challenges for the 1990s. *Sexuality and Disability, 9(2)*, 113-122.

Bartel, N. R. & Meddock, T. D. (1989). AIDS and adolescents with learning disabilities: Issues for parents and educators. *Reading, Writing, and Learning Disabilities, 5*, 299-311.

Carmody, M. (1991). Invisible victims: Sexual assault of people with an intellectual disability. *Australia and New Zealand Journal of Developmental Disabilities, 17(2)*, 229-236.

Cole, S. & Cole, T. M. (1993). Sexuality, disability, and reproductive issues through the lifespan. *Sexuality and Disability, 11(3)*, 189-204.

Coleman, E. M. & Murphy, W. D. (1980). A survey of sexual attitudes and sex education programs among facilities for the mentally retarded. *Applied Research in Mental Retardation, 1*, 269-276.

Collins, B. V., Schuster, J. W., & Nelson, C. M. (1992). Teaching a generalized response to the lures of strangers to adults with severe handicaps. *Exceptionality, 3*, 67-80.

Corbett, K., Shurberg Klein, S., & Bregante, J. L. (1989). The role of sexuality and sex equity in the education of disabled women. *Peabody Journal of Education, 64(4)*, 198-212.

Edmonson, B. (1980). Sociosexual education for the handicapped. *Exceptional Education Quarterly, 1(2)*, 67-76.

Edmonson, B., McCombs, K., & Wish, J. (1979). What retarded adults believe about sex. *American Journal of Mental Deficiency, 84(1)*, 11-18.

Edmonson, B. & Wish, J. (1975). Sexual knowledge and attitudes of moderately retarded males. *American Journal of Mental Deficiency, 80(2)*, 172-179.

Fifield, B.B. (1986). Ethical issues related to sexual abuse of disabled person. *Sexuality and Disability, 7(3/4)*, 102-109.

Fischer, H.L. & Krajicek, M. (1974). Sexual development of the moderately retarded child: level of information and parental attitudes. *Mental Retardation, 12(3)*, 28-30.

Foley, R. M. (1995). Special educators' competencies and preparation for the delivery of sex education. *Special Services in the Schools, 10(1)*, 95-112.

Gillies, P. & McEwen, J. (1981). The sexual knowledge of the "normal" and mildly subnormal adolescent. *The Health Education Journal, 40*, 120-124.

Goldman, R. L. (1994). Children and youth with intellectual disabilities: Targets for sexual abuse. *International Journal of Disability, Development, and Education, 41(2)*, 89-102.

Gordon, S. (1971). Missing in special education: Sex. *Journal of Special Education, 5*, 351-354.

Griffiths, D. (1999). Sexuality and people with developmental disabilities: Mythconceptions and facts. In I. Brown & M. Percy (Eds.), *Developmental disabilities in Ontario* (pp. 443-451). Toronto, ON: Front Porch Publishing.

Griffiths, D. & Lunsky, Y. (2000). Changing attitudes towards the nature of socio-sexual assessment and education for persons with developmental disabilities: A twenty-year comparison. *Journal on Developmental Disabilities, 7*, 16-33.

Haseltine, B. & Miltenberger, R. G. (1990). Teaching self-protection skills to persons with mental retardation. *American Journal on Mental Retardation, 95(2)*, 188-197.

Heshusius, L. (1982). Sexuality, intimacy, and persons we label mentally retarded: What they think- what we think. *Mental Retardation, 20(4)*, 164-168.

Jacobs, R., Samowitz, P., Levy, J. M., & Levy, P. H. (1989). Developing an AIDS prevention program for persons with developmental disabilities. *Mental Retardation, 27(4)*, 233-237.

Johnson, P. R., & Davies, R. (1980). Sexual attitudes of members of staff. *The British Journal of Mental Subnormality, 35*, 17-21.

Kastner, R., DeLotto, P., Scagnelli, B., & Testa, W.R. (1990). Proposed guidelines for agencies serving persons with developmental disabilities and HIV infection. *Mental Retardation, 28*, 139-145.

Kempton, W. (1975). *Sex education for persons with disabilities that hinder learning.* North Scituate, MA: Duxberry Press.

Lawrence, P. & Swain, J. (1993). Sex education programmes for students with severe learning difficulties in further education and the problem of evaluation. *Disability, Handicap, and Society, 8(4)*, 405-421.

Lindsay, W. R., Bellshaw, E., Culross, G., Staines, C., & Michie, A. (1992). Increases in knowledge following a course of sex education for people with intellectual disabilities. *Journal of Intellectual Disability Research, 36 (6)*, 531-539.

Lumley, V. A. & Miltenberger, R. G. (1997). Sexual abuse prevention for persons with mental retardation. *American Journal on Mental Retardation, 101(5)*, 459-472.

Lumley, V. A., Miltenberger, R. G., Long, E. S., Rapp, J. T., & Roberts, J. A. (1998). Evaluation of a sexual abuse prevention program for adults with mental retardation. *Journal of Applied Behavior Analysis, 31(1)*, 91-101.

McCabe, M. (1999). Sexual knowledge, experience, and feelings among people with disabilities. *Sexuality and Disability, 17(2)*, 157-170.

McCabe, M. & Cummins, R. (1996). The sexual knowledge, experience, feelings, and needs of people with mild intellectual disability. *Education and Training in Mental Retardation and Developmental Disabilities, 31(1)*, 13-21.

McCabe, M. & Schreck, A. (1992). Before sex education: An evaluation of the sexual knowledge, experience, feelings, and needs of people with mild intellectual disabilities. *Australia and New Zealand Journal of Developmental Disabilities, 18(2)*, 75-82.

McGillivray, J. A. (1999). Level of knowledge and risk of contracting HIV/AIDS amongst young adults with mild/ moderate intellectual disability. *Journal of Applied Research in Intellectual Disabilities, 12*, 1113-126.

Mitchell, L., Doctor, R. M. & Butler, D. C. (1978). Attitudes of caretakers toward the sexual behavior of mentally retarded persons. *American Journal of Mental Deficiency, 83,* 289-296.

Monat-Haller, R. K. (1992). *Understanding and expressing sexuality: Responsible choices for individuals with developmental disabilities.* Baltimore, MD: Paul H. Brookes Publishing Company.

Muccigrosso, L. (1991). Sexual abuse prevention strategies and programs for persons with developmental disabilities. *Sexuality and Disability, 9(3)*, 261-271.

Page, A. C. (1991). Teaching developmentally disabled people self-regulation in sexual behaviour. *Australia and New Zealand Journal of Developmental Disabilities, 17(1)*, 81-88.

Pueschel, S. M. & Scola, P. S. (1988). Parents' perceptions of social and sexual functions in adolescents with Down's Syndrome. *Journal of Mental Deficiency Research, 32*, 215-220.

Rowe, W. S. & Savage, S. (1987). *Sexuality and the developmentally handicapped.* Queenston, ON, Canada: Edwin Mellen Press.

Schultz, J. B. & Adams, D. U. (1987). Family life education needs of mentally disabled adolescents. *Adolescence, 22 (8)*, 221-230.

Scotti, J. R., Nangle, D. W., Masia, C. L., Ellis, J. T. Ujcich, K. J., Giacoletti, A. M. Vittimberga, G. L., & Carr, R. (1997). Providing an AIDS education and skills training program to persons with mild developmental disabilities. *Education and Training in Mental Retardation and Developmental Disabilities, 32*, 113-128.

Scotti, J. R., Speaks, L. V., Masia, C. L., Boggess, J. T., & Drabman, R. S. (1996). The educational effects of providing AIDS risk information to persons with developmental disabilities: An exploratory study. *Education and Training in Mental Retardation and Developmental Disability, 3 (12)*, 115-122.

Senn, C. (1989). *Vulnerable: Sexual abuse and people with an intellectual handicap.* Downsview, ON: G. Allan Roeher Institute.

Sobsey, D. (1994). *Violence and abuse in the lives of people with disabilities: The end of silent acceptance?* Baltimore, MD: Paul H. Brookes Publishing.

Sobsey, D. & Varnhagen, C. (1991). Sexual abuse, assault, and exploitation of Canadians with disabilities. In C. Bagley & J. Thomlinson (Eds.), *Child sexual abuse: Critical perspectives on prevention, intervention, and treatment* (pp. 203-216). Toronto, ON: Wall & Emerson.

Szollos, A. A. & McCabe, M. P. (1995). The sexuality of people with mild intellectual disability: Perceptions of clients and caregivers. *Australia and New Zealand Journal of Developmental Disabilities, 20(3)*, 205-222.

Timmers, R. L., DuCharme, P., & Jacob, G. (1981). Sexual knowledge, attitudes, and behaviors of developmentally disabled adults living in a normalized apartment setting.

Sexuality and Disability, 4, 27-39.

Whitehouse, M. A. & McCabe, M. P. (1997). Sex education programs for people with intellectual disabilities: How effective are they? *Education and Training in Mental Retardation and Developmental Disabilities, 32(3)*, 229-240.

Whitman, T. L. (1990). Self-regulation and mental retardation. *American Journal on Mental Retardation, 94*, 347-362.

Thanks to Michael Barrett and Susan Ludwig for their input into this very important topic.

Chapter 6

Sterilization and Birth Control

Robert King and Debbie Richards

Introduction

"The deadly mixture of moral chauvinism, pseudoscience and class politics developed into the eugenic fervor" (Sobsey, 1995, p. ix). Sexually segregated institutions and (involuntary) sterilization became the chosen methods of eliminating people with disabilities from society (Sobsey, 1995). The right of the state to protect itself from future generations of delinquents and the 'feeble-minded' was evoked at the expense of the rights of individuals with developmental disabilities.

In the century following the onset of the eugenics movement, issues of control, power, self-determination, individual and collective rights, social structure, the attitudes of the general population to sexuality and professional expertise have all entered the ethical debate regarding involuntary sterilization of individuals with developmental disabilities (Rioux, 1990). More recently, advocacy efforts to allow individuals with developmental disabilities to fully express their sexuality have promoted the development of sexual education programs, providing individuals with information to develop competencies to provide informed consent in sexual relationships. Legislation designed to prevent involuntary sterilization has also been established. A perceived need by caregivers and parents of children and adults with developmental disabilities to protect vulnerable individuals against exploitation and abuse has countered these advocacy efforts. In addition, caregivers and agencies providing support to individuals with developmental disabilities have been challenged to ethically balance their dual obligations of protecting individuals from abuse and exploitation while supporting individuals in developing all aspects of their lives, including their sexuality.

The following are examples of ethical dilemmas arising when addressing the issue of sterilization and birth control in individuals with developmental disabilities.

Case Study #1

Jessie is a 25 year old female with a mild to moderate developmental disability. She lives in her own apartment with supports from a local agency. She has had several heterosexual relationships beginning at age 19. Jessie has participated in sex education classes that had special emphasis on birth control.

Her support staff took her to the local public health unit for birth control pills. At age 20, she had a child after discontinuing this form of contraception. After the birth of her first child, her doctor suggested Depo Provera as a method of contraception. She received birth control pills as an added precaution for the first three months to ensure efficacy.

Jessie was provided with transportation to appointments during the first six months that Depo Provera was prescribed. She subsequently made a decision to go alone. Within two years, Jessie was again pregnant. She said she had missed past injections. Her child was removed from her care at birth by the Children's Aid Society, as recommended by her doctor.

It is now one year since the birth of her second child. Community Living staff continue to provide supports. Jessie often chooses to go to appointments with her gynecologist alone. People involved in Jessie's' life fear that she will become pregnant again. Many strategies have been attempted to have Jessie consider the implications of her sexual behaviour. She has been provided ongoing counselling regarding choosing a tubal ligation as a contraception option. She has refused due to her fear of surgery. Consequently, a third child was born and was also removed from Jessie's care at birth. Nursing staff and Jessie's parents have pressured Jessie's support agency to have Jessie undergo a sterilization procedure with or without Jessie's consent.

Support staff have provided intense education regarding birth control and healthy relationships and sexually transmitted diseases. Jessie's gynecologist has explained the sterilization procedure to her. She still refused the surgery, stating that she understood all of the implications. She stated again she would stay on birth control pills and promised to go for regular Depo Provera injections. It has now been two years since the birth of Jessie's third child.

- What are Jessie's rights?
- What are the ethical obligations of the agency?
- Is there any recourse for the physician?

- Should the agency further intervene?
Case Study # 2

Betty is a 29-year-old female who has a mild developmental disability and lives in her own apartment with a roommate. They receive approximately 10 hours of staffing support per week. Betty's mother sees her daughter frequently and they appear to have a healthy relationship. Her mother has expressed concern over her daughter's vulnerability to being sexually abused. Betty has begun dating a man and has told staff in confidence she and her partner are having a sexual relationship. Betty has been taking birth control pills since she was 18 years old, however, has forgotten to take her pills on occasion. Previous she was not sexually active; this was not a significant concern. However, things have changed.

Betty's mother has requested that her daughter have a tubal ligation to ensure Betty does not have a child. Her mother stated she is getting on in age and would not be able to assist her daughter should Betty have a child. When staff discussed this option with Betty, she stated she did not think she wanted to have children but said she would like to defer a decision to have a sterilization procedure done.

- Should this subject be pursued further with Betty?
- Does Betty's mother have legitimate concerns?
- Are there any interventions the agency could have put into place?
- Should Betty be given a deadline regarding the finalization of this decision?
- Should staff be insisting on administering her

medication to ensure there is no pregnancy?

Case Study # 3

Lily is a 35 year old female who has a profound developmental disability, with limited verbal and nonverbal communication skills. She also has cerebral palsy and consequently uses a wheelchair for mobility. In addition, she is a Hepatitis B carrier. Her menstrual cycle is very irregular. When she is menstruating Lily experiences heavy bleeding and is irritable due to cramping. Due to her physical limitations, she is unable to care for her menstrual hygiene. Due to the heavy bleeding, Lily's doctor has performed two Dilatation and Curettages (D & C) within the past two years. Lily has continued to have difficulty with her menstrual cycles, although these have lessened in intensity. She continues to display erratic mood swings which are believed to be symptoms of a Premenstrual Syndrome (PMS).

Support staff have set an appointment up with a gynecologist as they believe a hysterectomy should be performed to eliminate concerns regarding transmission of Hepatitis B, heavy bleeding, cramping and mood swings.

- Is this an ethical dilemma or a straight forward procedure?
- To what ethical standards should the physician be held, in considering the prescription of this permanent procedure?
- Is the agency putting their personal concerns regarding Hepatitis B ahead of Lily's medical vulnerabilities?

Case Study # 4

Joe and Sarah have been seeing each other for two years and are planning on getting married within the next two years. They live in semi-independent settings apart from one another with staffing supports from a local agency for individuals with developmental disabilities. Joe and Sarah have a moderate developmental disability.

Prior to marriage, Sarah's parents have stipulated that either Joe or Sarah have to be sterilized to prevent them from having to raise a child. Joe's parents are in agreement with this idea.

Joe and Sarah are involved in couple counselling and have been informed of the opinion of their families in regards to sterilization. When the topic of children was discussed, both Joe and Sarah said they had not made a decision as of yet, and would like to think about it further. Sarah's family would not accept their decision and told the counsellor to (1) explain the medical procedures of both vasectomy and tubal ligation and; (2) inform them they are to choose one of these procedures. The counsellor was very reluctant, however, with the insistence of both families, he did follow their direction. After two months of pressure from his family, Joe decided he would have a vasectomy.

Support staff were uncomfortable setting up the medical appointment with the physician, believing Joe was coerced (he feared he would no longer be allowed to see his family if he didn't get a vasectomy). When staff did not set the appointment up, the family went ahead and did this. Joe responded appropriately to questions posed in the medical appointment and a vasectomy was performed.

- Should the agency have intervened? When and how?
- Were the rights of this couple violated?
- What additional education could have been provided to this couple?
- Would an impartial guardian have been able to better assist this couple?

Literature Review

In 1986, in the case of Eve, the Supreme Court of Canada ruled that the non-therapeutic sterilization of individuals with developmental disabilities could not be authorized by any third party. In doing so, the Canadian Supreme Court, for the first time in Canadian history, proclaimed that the natural rights of all women, disabled or non-disabled, took precedent over society's right to enable sterilization to be performed without consent of the woman involved. Through asserting that the best interests of women should be framed in terms of the preservation of their right to bear children, as opposed to exercising the right of society to interfere with procreation through the construct of parental power, a history of bias and gross misunderstanding of the sexuality of individuals with developmental disabilities was challenged. In contrast however, a subsequent decision by the British House of Lords rejected the Eve decision, ruling that from a best interest perspective, the right to bear children was limited depending on the ability to exercise this right, including the ability to provide adequate parenting, despite not holding any other class of people to this standard (Rioux, 1990).

These decisions arose in the context of a tradition in both countries (and throughout the world) of systematic social neglect and gross misunderstanding of the sexual needs of individuals with developmental disabilities. Involuntary sterilization, punishment of expressions of sexuality through social isolation, and gender segregation (via institutionalization) has occurred in blatant opposition to principles more recently articulated by Held (1992). These principles include:

- Each human is unique and not interchangeable. It is normal to be different.
- Each individual has, according to his or her own uniqueness, different mental abilities and talents.
- In the realm of mental disability, no one is exclusively disabled.
- Sexuality is a fundamental need and integral part of being human.

The roots of the prejudice and sexual stigmatization to which individuals with developmental disabilities have been exposed can be traced to the Eugenics movement (1880-1940). In 1883, British scientist Sir Francis Galton initially proposed that only the most intellectually brightest women and men in society should procreate. Individuals with developmental disabilities were assumed to be genetically defective and at risk of conceiving children who would inevitably victimize the rest of society through criminal acts and sexual promiscuity. Segregation and involuntary sterilization arose as society's response to this theory. Indeed, in 1912, the Eugenics Section of the American (cattle) Breeders Society reported that "sexually segregated institutionalization and sterilization were the only acceptable means of eliminating people with mental retardation from society" (Sobsey, 1995). In advance of this, a law authorizing involuntary sterilization was passed in 1907 in Indiana, to be joined by similar laws in thirty-one additional states by 1948.

In Canada, the principles of the Eugenics movement were initially embraced with enthusiasm. Helen MacMurchy, first chief of the Federal Division of Maternal and Child Welfare, emphasized the special dangers of "feeble-minded borderline cases" who would 'pass as normal' in society despite carrying 'chains of hateful vice'" (Pringle, 1997, p. 34).

In 1927, in the case of Buck V. Bell, 274 U.S. 200 (1927), the United States Supreme Court upheld the constitutionality of involuntary sterilization, accepting the premise that mental retardation is genetically transmittable despite existing scientific evidence at the time to the contrary (in fact, only 15% of all individuals diagnosed with developmental disabilities have etiologies of their disability which are attributable to genetic causes) (Abramson, Parker & Weisberg, 1988). The majority opinion of this court was delivered by Oliver Wendel Holmes, who wrote, "We have seen more than once that the public welfare may call upon the best citizens for their lives. It would be strange if it could not call upon those who already sap the strength of the state for these lesser sacrifices, often felt to be much by those concerned, in order to prevent our being swamped with incompetence. It is better for all the world if instead of waiting to execute degenerate offspring for crime or to let them starve for their imbecility, society can prevent those who are manifestly unfit from continuing their kind … Three generations of imbeciles are enough" (Buck v Bell, 274 U.S. 2000, 1927).

By 1928, the United Farmers of Alberta Government drafted its Sexual Sterilization Act, which granted an appointed board the authority to order sterilization of any person suffering from a mental defect, initially with their consent. A similar act was subsequently passed in British Columbia. By 1937, the Alberta Provincial Government dispensed with the need for the Board to obtain consent. Despite world opinion, as expressed in the post-World War II Nuremburg trials that forced sterilization was a crime against humanity, in the 50's and 60's the Alberta Program proceeded at an accelerated rate. Ultimately 4,728 sterilizations were performed until the Sexual Sterilization Act was repealed in 1971 (Pringle, 1997).

In 1995, a former client of the Alberta Provincial Training School for Mental Defectives, Leilani Muir, sued the Alberta Government for wrongfully admitting her to this institution, classing her as a moron and presenting her in 1959 to the Eugenic Board for sterilization. She was falsely told after her sterilization that she had had an appendectomy. A ruling in her favour by the Provincial Court of the Queen's Bench in January of 1996 passed judgment on the years of rights suppression and segregation perpetrated on the clients of this institution (Pringle, 1997).

In the 1960's, principles of Normalization as espoused by B. Nirje and Wolfsenberger (cited in Kempton & Kahn, 1991) advocated the recognition of individual choice and desires of people with developmental disabilities and their right to live with, work with and love people of both sexes. In this context, the concept of dignity of risk was introduced and the process of de-institutionalization commenced. A recognition of the need for sexual education for individuals with developmental disabilities began. Improved access to specialized sexual education resources and the need for agency policy development regarding sexuality issues in the 1970's were primarily motivated by a systemic desire to prevent pregnancy amid concern for the welfare of potential children. Sexual rights and the fulfillment of needs of adults with developmental disabilities were rarely cited as an issue in this era.

The battle against compulsory sterilization laws, which continued to exist in twenty-three states in 1973, was accelerated by the United States Supreme Court guarantee of the right of women to abortion (Rowe vs. Wade, 1973). The ethical debate regarding the balance of rights of individuals with developmental disabilities vs. the rights of their prospective children to adequate care continued.

The unmasking of the vulnerability of individuals with developmental disabilities to sexual abuse and exploitation and the AIDS epidemic promoted further expansion of sexual education programs for individuals with developmental disabilities in the 1980's. This included the development of the widely used Circles Program, for example, by Champagne and Walker-Hirsch (cited in Kempton & Kahn, 1991).

A number of issues have arisen over the past thirty years regarding access to information concerning contraception and the prescription of contraceptive methods to individuals with developmental disabilities. The concept of informed consent has evolved over several decades from the assumption that individuals with developmental disabilities are universally incapable of making informed treatment decisions, to an acceptance legally that capacity to make informed treatment decisions is treatment-specific and requires individual assessments if concern regarding incapacity is raised. Problems regarding informed consent commonly arose due to a lack of access to comprehensive sexual education; while ironically, opponents to sexual education argued that access to sexual education programs would prompt individuals with developmental disabilities to act in socially inappropriate irresponsible manners. In addressing this dilemma, advocates have argued that as a legal concept, consent was designed to protect against sexual coercion rather than to deny individuals their right to sexual expression (Abramson et al., 1988).

The concept of consent and its relationship to the right to choose contraception in the context of the expression of sexuality became a key component in the debate regarding the dual obligation of service providers to promote and facilitate the development of individuals with developmental disabilities, while at the same time protecting them from harm in the context of their expressed sexual behaviour. Sundrum and Stavis (1994) have suggested:

1. It is the absence of consent that turns otherwise normal sexual behaviour between adults into criminal activity and a potential source of criminal liability.
2. It is the inability to provide consent due to a mental impairment that triggers a provider's obligation to protect from harm the individual who is incapable of self-protection.

Provider agency liability in this context can include:

a) criminal liability - facilitating or encouraging an

      incapable person to engage in sexual activity,

b) constitutional liability - substantially deviating from professionally recognized standards in failing to protect individuals in their charge from harm, and

c) tort liability - this requires three criteria: (i) the existence of a duty of one person to another, (ii) the occurrence of an injury, and (iii) proof that the breach of duty was the approximate cause of the injury.

In Canada, legal approaches to consent, as discussed elsewhere in this volume, are mandated by:

1. The Substitute Decisions Act (1992)
2. The Health Care Consent Act (1996)

These laws established general rules applicable to a broad set of circumstances. Concern has been expressed that the strict application of this legal framework by health practitioners ignores particular challenges that individuals with developmental disabilities face that relate to consent. These challenges include communication deficits, concurrent mental health concerns, limited life experiences, learned helplessness producing excessive compliance, and finally, the impact of negative past experiences on willingness to consent to future treatment recommendations (Sullivan & Heng, 1999).

An ethical approach to consent attempts to establish a basis for judgment about what to do in particular conditions, while also considering what it means for competent people to choose responsibly. This approach has been cited as requiring four essential elements (Sullivan & Heng, 1999):

1. Sufficient information on which to base the decision.

2. An understanding of this information.
3. Competency to give or withhold consent, including an ability to weigh the risks and benefits of the proposed treatment, alternatives and the choice of no treatment.
4. Voluntariness.

The importance of mediation and negotiation skills offered by caregivers and health practitioners to assist individuals with developmental disabilities in making decisions they are capable of making has been stressed. This emphasis rejects the idea that decisions based on personal values are arbitrary or matters of personal whim. The need to exercise skills to allow individuals to deliberate carefully about health issues and be connected to appropriate resources in this process has been highlighted.

Choice of contraceptive method optimally should be based on an understanding of the effectiveness, convenience, ability to offer protection from sexually transmitted diseases (STD's), reversibility and cost of the method under consideration. Multiple methods are currently available with varying degrees of suitability correlating with the degree of cognitive impairment of the individual involved, the presence of physical disabilities, access to supervision to ensure compliance and education in advance of use.

Table 1 – Female Birth Control Options

Method	Description	Success Rate/ Comments	Side Effects
Natural Methods	Please see Male chart		
Barriers and intrauterine devices Diaphragm	Shallow, dome-shaped cup that blocks the cervix	18% failure rate Must be used in conjunction with spermicidal cream or jelly	Risk of urethritis, cystitis, and yeast infections Possible allergy to latex or spermicide
Cervical cap	Smaller than the diaphragm, fitting more tightly over cervix	18% failure rate Must be used in conjunction with spermicidal cream or jelly	Risk of toxic shock syndrome (TSS) Possible allergy to latex or spermicide
Vaginal pouch (female condom)	Loose-fitting pouch with a closed end, inserted like the diaphragm or cervical cap	Inconvenient, but offers increased protection from STDs	Possible allergy to latex
Contraceptive sponge		18-20% failure rate	Possibility of allergic reactions to spermicide
Jellies and creams	Inserted into the vagina	21% failure rate Spermicide containing non-oxynol 9 is effective at killing HIV	Possibility of allergic reactions
Intrauterine device (IUD)	Prevent implantation of a fertilized egg in the uterine wall	3% failure rate, but a 2-20% expulsion rate in the first year of use; Offers no protection against STDs Life expectancy 1-5 years depending on type	Risk of pelvic inflammatory disease, perforated uterus, ectopic pregnancies, and uterine bleeding

(table continues)

Method	Description	Success Rate/ Comments	Side Effects
Chemical contraception Oral contraceptives	Known as "the pill", medication taken daily, containing estrogen and progestin to prevent ovluation	3% failure rate No STD protection	Diabetes, hepatitis, and breast cancer. Possible risk of multiple potential adverse effects, including weight gain, depression, nausea, and headaches. It decreases the risk of pelvic inflammatory disease and may ameliorate premenstrual symptoms
Norplant	6 small plastic rods containing a hormone are implanted in the upper arm to inhibit ovulation and increase cervical mucus	3.9% failure rate Norplant must be removed after 5 years or before, if desired	Long-term effects are unknown. There is a possible interaction between this method and anticonvulsants. Some women experience disruptions to their menstrual cycle
Depo Provera	Injected every 12 weeks to suppress ovulation, alter uterine lining, and increase cervical mucus	Offers long-acting protection (3 months) from pregnancy Approved in Canada in 1997 99% effective	Similar to oral contraceptives Irregular and unpredictable bleeding Not to be used if planning on becoming pregnant within 1-2 years
Surgeries Tubal ligation	Known as "tubes tied", procedure in which the Fallopian tubes are cut and tied	Sexual functioning remains the same Failure rate is 0.04% Permanent method	Complications may include bleeding, infection, negative reaction to anesthetic
Hysterectomy	Surgical removal of the uterus	Sexual functioning remains the same	Ovaries still produce hormones that influence health
Oophorectomy	Surgical removal of the ovaries	Sexual functioning may be impaired	For a woman of reproductive age, the result is early menopause

Table 2– Male Birth Control Options

Method	Description	Success Rate/ Comments	Side Effects
Natural Methods Abstinence	Refraining from sexual intercourse		
Coitus Interruptus	Also known as the withdrawal method-withdrawing the penis from vagina before ejaculation	Does not protect against sexually transmitted diseases. 60% failure rate	Should not be considered if woman has irregular menstrual cycle
Barriers and intrauterine devices Condom	Sheath that fits over the penis, blocking the sperm from being released into vagina	12% failure rate Good STD protection, especially when containing spermicidal lubricant	Possible allergy to latex or spermicide
Hormonal/ Chemical Depo Provera	Leads to the inability to have an erection, reduction of semen production, and absence of orgasm	All methods need informed consent Used primarily in the treatment of sex offenders, but is used as birth control in individuals who have developmental disabilities	Weight gain and tiredness Diabetes; liver failure; gynecomastia

(table continues)

Method	Description	Success Rate/ Comments	Side Effects
Hormonal/ Chemical Cont'd Anti-Androgen Androcar	Blocks male sexual hormones Lowers the intensity and frequency of sexual drive, but does not change sexual orientation	Used primarily as treatment for sex offenders, but is used as birth control in individuals who have developmental disabilities	Short term side effects include breast development, breast pain; long term side effects are not known. Should not be prescribed for men under the age of 18 or whose bone or testicular development is not complete, which may be the case for males who have a syndrome which interferes with normal sexual development or delayed puberty
Surgical Procedures Vasectomy	Surgical removal of a section of the ductus deferens (duct between testes and penis) to prevent sperm from passing through the ejaculatory ducts.	Does not affect sexual drive Some sperm remain in the man's system after operation, so another method of contraception must be used for at least the first 14 ejaculations Permanent method <1% failure rate	Pain in the testes and nerve endings.
Orchidectomy	Surgical removal of 1 or both testes	Method used for prostate cancer	Causes sterility and impotence

See Tables 1 and 2 for Female and Male Birth Control Options.

The critical need for support in accessing adequate information to assist individuals in making informed healthy decisions is underlined by the complexity of this list.

In family surveys, parents of children with developmental disabilities often admit to confused, ambivalent and anxious attitudes towards the sexuality of their children, acknowledging feelings of inadequacy in providing sexual information. This historically has resulted in parents favouring long-term sterilization or long-term birth control methods for their children. In the 1990's, it has been argued that sterilization without informed consent by the individual should never be done punitively. It has been further argued that sterilization should be offered only after a thorough burden versus benefits analysis identifies this procedure as the least restrictive alternative in allowing individuals increased freedom in the community and interpersonal relationships. Others have argued that the availability of long-term reversible contraceptive methods negates any justification for sterilization based on substitute decision making. If the courts do consider involuntary sterilization for an incapable person, the following due process steps have been recommended:

1. That the individual be represented by an impartial guardian,
2. That a comprehensive medical, psychiatric and social evaluation be reviewed,
3. That the views of the individual be considered,
4. That incapacity is demonstrated,
5. That evidence is given that the person is unlikely to develop sufficiently to make informed decisions in the

future,
6. That the person is shown to be physically capable of procreation and is likely to engage in sexual activity now or in the future,
7. That evidence is given that the person is not capable of caring for a child, even with reasonable assistance,
8. That documentation be provided that less intrusive and more reversible birth control is unacceptable,
9. That evidence is given that appropriate supervision, education and training have been made available.

Finally, recent concerns have been expressed regarding new genetic technologies, noting that they incorporate the eugenic belief that better genes make better people. Spallone (1989) notes "the growth of reproductive technologies is based on an arrogant belief in scientific and social control, a device to assert more social and biological control over women, preparing them to have the perfect baby, ignoring acts of love, bonding and caring". The impact that these technologies will have upon the quality of life of individuals with developmental disability, as well as society's attitudes to this class of individuals, remains to be determined.

Conference Deliberations

Among the group participants were medical professionals, agency support staff, and family members. Discussion developed in respect to the circumstances that arise when birth control or sterilization is being considered for an individual who has a developmental disability. The committee agreed that decisions must always be voluntary and fully informed.

Regardless of established protocols and laws that protect

individuals from involuntary sterilization, the group raised the issue that the value systems of others (caregivers, family) may possibly influence decision-making, noting that these values may or may not be consistent with that of the individual's involved. As well, generally negative attitudes towards the ability of people with developmental disabilities' to parent may influence decision-making. Realistically, participants were in agreement that opinions will vary and decisions are often based on external opinions.

They asked, "What can be done to support the rights of individuals and also consider their well-being?" Consumer education was thought to be a major factor in giving people opportunities to make informed decisions. The group questioned whether people with developmental disabilities are provided with accurate and useful information that is given in a clear and understandable way. If this is not the case, their decisions will often be altered or coerced. Individuals may not be in a position to make an informed choice and may agree to a procedure that may later be regretted. If accurate information is provided in such a way that the individual is able to make a well informed choice, then health practitioners, families and support staff are supporting the rights of the individuals. If the individual makes a decision that is considered to be unsafe or the individual is not able to make a decision based on their cognitive ability, then an advocate such as a substitute decision maker should become involved. This process would not allow for others' value systems to influence the individual's decisions and would also consider health risks or safety issues.

According to the group's experiences, families and support staff at times make decisions on birth control and sterilization based on their fears of the person being sexually abused or becoming sexually active and therefore becoming pregnant or acquiring a sexually transmitted disease. It was noted, however, that sexual abuse is not exclusive to victims that have not been sterilized.

It was agreed that caregivers are likely to attend medical appointments and make requests on behalf of the individual. Finally, the group posed the question, "How can the attitudes of caregivers and family be altered to allow for the individual to be respected in the decision he or she has made?" Education was considered to be a key component in this process. Optimally, there should be a commitment to provide accurate information which could allow for personal, informed decision making. Participants were able to identify that caregivers and families often assume the role of decision-makers in what is believed to be a supportive position. In fact, the group argued that caregivers and family members should only be in an advocating role presenting information, accompanying to medical appointments, and assisting the individual in providing historical information to the physician.

Summary

State of the Art

Despite standards and regulations that have been put into place to protect individuals with developmental disabilities from involuntary sterilization, choices and decisions largely remain in the hands of people most involved in their lives.

Effective medical and non-medical treatment interventions are available for both males and females. Medical options should be discussed with the individual seeking medical intervention. Since we know that caregivers and families are more likely to be included as part of the decision-making process, the need for these individuals to be educated should be the standard, rather than the exception. As well, physicians and surgeons should be updated with the current laws concerning consent and sterilization issues that apply where they are practicing (American Academy of Pediatrics, 1999). Counselling along with sex education should be provided for all people with developmental disabilities who will be considering possible birth control or sterilization procedures.

Fundamental principles and laws have been established to protect individuals with developmental disabilities from being exploited, allowing for voluntary choice. Assuming that an individual lacks capacity or is unable to make a decision is unacceptable. As advocates, we must challenge this premise and assume instead that all people have the ability or capacity to make an informed decision based on education and counselling, until proven otherwise by a professional capacity assessment.

Clinical Implications

In the event that the attending physician or a capacity assessor has determined through careful assessment that the person who has a developmentally disability is unable to consent to treatment, a substitute decision maker is then placed in the role of acting in the best interest of the individual. However, this does not always occur.

Medical practitioners need to consider the following factors to ensure optimum health care:

- the responsibility of familiarizing themselves with the current laws in their jurisdiction,
- the need to address the individual directly, even if a caregiver or family member is in the room,
- the obligation to advocate for the least permanent and intrusive method of birth control for the individual,
- the value of establishing clear communication with local agencies to keep updated on issues,
- the importance of educating caregivers and individuals on available options, and
- the merits of individualizing care according to the ability, needs, and wants of each patient.

Brantlinger (1992) has revealed that attitudes of professionals indicate they continue to require extensive education regarding the legalities, and ethics of sterilization, and in their general approaches to those with disabilities. The factors outlined above to optimize health care will certainly increase positive attitudes if put into practice.

Agency Implications

Agencies have a major responsibility to ensure that each person being supported is given opportunity to attain the necessary information to allow for informed decision making regarding birth control and/or sterilization treatment.

It is understood that people with developmental disabilities often rely on their caregivers, families, and professionals to assist in making decisions; thus, it is incumbent upon this latter group to also become well informed themselves, of all the available options.

It is the responsibility of clinicians to advocate on behalf of individuals and not adhere strictly to the demands or wishes of the family. Sterilization is one particular area where conflict can arise between an individual with a developmental disability and their family. A family may have a strong position where they believe they are acting in the best interest of their child, yet their child is in objection to sterilization. It then becomes the responsibility of the agency to advocate on behalf of that individual in whatever capacity deemed necessary. The agency may offer counselling or education to the family to facilitate a change in attitude or increase their knowledge on the current treatments or laws that are currently in place.

Finally, it is important for agencies to assume a liaison type position to assist the medical practitioner in a) understanding the needs and desires of the individual; b) communicating effectively with the individual; and c) ensuring the individual obtains the treatment they wish.

Most importantly, agencies must have an undivided interest in respecting individual rights to sexual freedom, while providing information to allow for safe and healthy decisions.

What Should Be Done Now

The issues of forced and involuntary birth control and sterilization among individuals who have a developmental disability in today's society has been acknowledged, and to some degree, addressed. Most recently, Dialogues in Contraception (2000) have stated that great strides have been made to enhance a woman's right to reproductive choice and application of reproductive techniques by way of policies and guidelines. Have these frameworks optimally benefited those people with developmental disabilities? Unlikely. Can this change? Yes, but with much additional advocacy.

Protocols should be put into place with local agencies to protect people from unwanted procedures and treatment and ensure the rights of individuals are protected.

Education for all parties is an absolute. This should include information regarding the full range of treatment options currently available. As well as contraception training, education for individuals who have developmental disabilities should include sexual abuse prevention programs and programs discussing aspects of appropriate and healthy sexual relationships, assertiveness training, menstrual hygiene, and sexual transmitted disease protection. Professionals and families should receive further training regarding relevant legislature and ethical decision-making. Brantlinger (1992) states that professionals are influenced by perceptions, attitudes, beliefs, and circumstances. This statement applies to families as well. Through appropriate training, all people advocating for individuals with developmental disabilities could work together in assisting, guiding, and preparing these individuals to make their own personal life choices.

Final Consensus Statement

The American Academy of Pediatrics (1999) has concurred that permanent sterilization becomes increasingly difficult to justify, as more methods of contraception become available options. It can also be said that, while sterilization will usually prevent conception and pregnancy, it is no substitute for safe environments that minimize sexual abuse, nor will it prevent sexually transmitted diseases.

The topic of sterilization has created ethical, moral, political, and legal debate for over a century. Over the years, relevant legislature has evolved considerably. All people, regardless of disability, have the right to being sexual, including the right to bear children. These rights are clearly articulated in the United Nations and Canadian Charters of Rights, and by the United States Civil Rights Commission and the Valencia Declaration. Efforts to uphold these rights have recently intensified. Despite this, we continue to create environments for the individuals with developmental disabilities in which they struggle to exercise their sexual rights.

Much further work is needed to grant each person the right to make intimate and personal decisions free of coercion in respectful and informed contexts.

References

Abramson, P. R., Parker, T., & Weisberg, S. R. .(1988). Sexual expression of mentally retarded people: Educational and legal implications. *American Journal of Mental Retardation, 93(3),* 328-334.

American Academy of Pediatrics (1999). Sterilization of minors with developmental disabilities. *Pediatrics, 104(2),* 337-340.

Brantlinger, E. (1992). Professionals' attitudes toward the sterilization of people with disabilities. *Journal of the Association for People with Special Needs, 17(1),* 4-18.

Buck v. Bell, 274 U.S. (1927).

Contraceptive issues for women with genetic and

developmental disorders. (2000). *Dialogues in Contraception, 6,* 1-2.

E. (Mrs.) v. Eve, 2 S.C. R. at 428 (1986).

Held, K. R. (1992). Ethical aspects of sexuality of persons with mental retardation. In M. Nagler (Ed.), *Perspectives on disability,* pp. 255-260. Palo Alto, CA: Health Markets Research.

Instituto de Sexologia Y Psicoterapia Espill. (1997). Valencia Declaration of Sexual Rights. Valencia, Spain: Author.

Kempton, W. & Kahn, W. (1991). Sexuality and people with intellectual disabilities: A historical perspective. *Sexuality and Disability, 9(2),* 93-111.

Pringle, H. (1997). Alberta Barren. *Saturday Night.* 30-74.

Rioux, M. H. (1990). Sterilization and mental handicap: A rights issues. *Journal of Leisurability, 17(3),* 3-11.

Rowe v. Wade, 410 U.S. 113 (1973).

Sobsey, D. (1995). Enough is enough: There is no excuse for a hundred years of violence against people with disabilities. In D. Sobsey, D. Wells, R. Lucardie, & S. Mansell. (Eds.), *Violence and disability: An annotated bibliography* (pp. ix-xvii). Baltimore, MD: Paul H. Brookes Publishing.

Spallone, P. (1989). Beyond conception. Granby, MA: Bergin & Garvey.

Sullivan, B., & Heng, J. (1994). Ethical issues relating to consent in providing treatment and care. In I. Brown and M. Percy (Eds.), *Developmental disabilities in Ontario* (pp. 83-91). Toronto, ON: Front Porch Publishing.

Sundrum, C. J. & Stavis, P. J. (1999). Sexuality and mental retardation: Unmet challenges. *Mental Retardation, 32 (4),* 255-264.

United Nations. (1998). *Universal declaration on human rights.* New York: Author.

Chapter 7

Parents with Intellectual Disabilities: Impediments and Supports

Maurice A. Feldman

Introduction

It is generally accepted that full social inclusion of people with intellectual disabilities includes sexuality. There is less endorsement for parenting. The current generation of adults with intellectual disabilities is the first in many Western societies to be neither routinely institutionalized nor sterilized. They have grown up internalizing conventional family life values. Not surprisingly, many of these individuals, particularly those with mild intellectual disabilities (IQs between 60 and 80), are expressing interest in doing what the vast majority of adults do - forming loving partnerships and having children.

Conference Deliberations

The members of the parenting group felt that despite the growing realization that people with intellectual disabilities do have the right to parent (and many of them have proven themselves capable), there are numerous obstacles often faced by these adults that make it difficult for them to adequately raise their children. Conversely, there also are conditions that foster success in these families. The group listed and discussed factors that promote or inhibit adequate parenting, and then made several recommendations. Before reviewing impediments and supports that are typically experienced by parents with intellectual disabilities, I will first present an interactional model of parenting that implicitly guided the group's ideas. After the overview of societal and familial factors that may hamper or facilitate positive outcomes, I will highlight recommendations that the group generated regarding assessment, service, and support for parents with intellectual disabilities.

Literature Review

Interactional Model of Parenting

The notion that all of the parenting problems of parents with intellectual disabilities can be blamed on their cognitive limitations is too simplistic. An interactional model of parenting and child outcomes, as elucidated by Belsky (1984) and others (e.g., Sameroff & Chandler, 1975), is probably a more accurate scenario. According to this model, parenting and child outcomes are a function of the accumulating interactions of numerous child, parent, family, and social variables. Similarly, Bronfenbrenner's (1979) ecological model differentiates nested levels of environmental influence: child, parent, and family characteristics (microsystem); the family's community (macrosystem); and society as a whole (exosystem).

Figure 1 presents an interactional model depicting the likely complex relationships between variables that may affect parent and child behaviours and outcomes (examples of some impediments are presented under each variable). At this point, the model is hypothetical, and is based on research with parents who do not have disabilities and what little we know about families with parents who have intellectual disabilities. The directions, paths, and strengths of the relationships between variables still remain to be empirically elucidated (the model shows only unidirectional effects although it is recognized that some relationships are likely bidirectional; the direction chosen is the hypothetical stronger effect). The variables presented in the model are discussed in more detail in the remainder of this chapter.

Figure 1: A Parenting Interactional Model

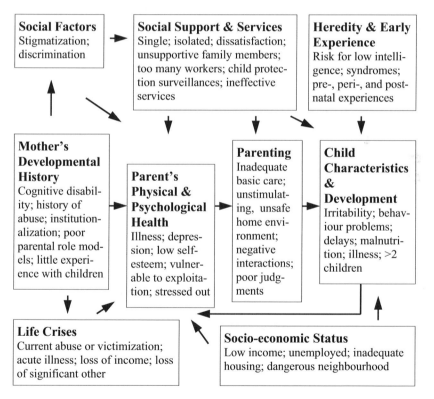

A Parenting Interactional Model. Some possible impediments to effective parenting and child outcomes are listed below each variable. The direction of the arrows are hypothetical and require empirical validation.

The Social Context

The social arena exerts an overarching impact on parents with intellectual disabilities and their children. Society's values toward parents with intellectual disabilities can be reflected in several ways. Governments can pass or rescind laws that make it more or less difficult for people with disabilities to marry, conceive, and raise children. Child protection agencies and the courts can be biased against these parents from the outset or endeavor to try to keep the family together. Media coverage also can be biased or fair.

On the negative side, several research reports have indicated that parents with intellectual disabilities are disproportionately involved in child custody cases (Glaun & Brown, 1999; Schilling, Schinke, Blythe, & Barth, 1982; Seagull & Scheurer, 1986; Taylor et al., 1991).   Typically, the concern is child neglect (primarily due to a lack of parental knowledge and skills), rather than physical or sexual abuse. It is not clear, however, to what extent, this over-representation in custody cases confirms the fact that these parents tend to be less competent or epitomizes the presumption of parental incompetence that leads to closer surveillance and over-reporting of these families. In other words, when it is known that parents have intellectual disabilities, child protection agencies may be more prone to search for, and find evidence of, child neglect, and seek termination of parenting rights than would be the case for unlabeled parents acting in exactly the same manner (Tymchuk, Llewellyn, & Feldman, 1999).

Two examples illustrate this point. Apparently, the state of Washington allegedly had routinely removed children when young parents had IQs less than 70 (Miller, cited in Tymchuk et al., 1999). The second example is from our personal experience. In Canada, we provided child safety training to a couple and we advised them to take their child to the hospital anytime there was an accident with the potential for head injury. Subsequently, they brought their child to emergency after she had fallen down some carpeted stairs in their town home. Although the child was not hurt, when the admitting physician found out that the parents were intellectually disabled, he immediately called child protection which placed the child in foster care on the grounds that the parents were not providing adequate supervision. Do not children of parents without intellectual disabilities fall down stairs? Would the physician and child protection authorities have taken this drastic action if the parents were not intellectually disabled?

Another potentially negative aspect of child custody cases is making decisions "in the best interests of the child" without consideration of other factors. Because most parents with intellectual disabilities are poor, not well-educated, and un- or under-employed, they usually do not have the same material benefits that could be provided by a typical middle-class family seeking adoption. Yet the parent-child bond might be very strong and the parent is providing adequate, although not superior, care. In determining continuation of parenting rights, the question should not solely be what is in the child's best interests from a resource viewpoint, but whether there is evidence of child maltreatment and parental incapacity (i.e., the same criteria that typically is applied to any parent accused of child maltreatment). It is our experience that sometimes child protection agencies are more aggressive in seeking termination of parenting rights of parents with intellectual disabilities when a better endowed family is wanting to adopt that child.

Society's attitudes towards parents with intellectual disabilities are reflected in media portrayals of these families. Over the last decade, media coverage generally has been positive and upbeat, although occasionally a negative slant is presented. There have been a few cases of child murder, accidental death or injury, severe abuse, and neglect where it has been publicly reported that the parents were "mentally retarded". These rare cases unfortunately may reinforce or rekindle the public's inaccurate and negative perceptions that people with intellectual disabilities cannot and should not parent.

On the positive side, discriminatory marriage and sterilization laws have been repealed in many jurisdictions. Although misconceptions about, and bias and discrimination against these families still exist, increasingly court decisions in Canada and the United States are favoring keeping the natural family together and directing the state to provide necessary supports and services (Hayman, 1990, Vogel, 1987). Advocates, self-advocates, civil liberties lawyers, and progressive judges are slowly diminishing the stigma and misconceptions associated with being a parent with intellectual disabilities. Many workers are shifting from a parental incompetence orientation to an empowerment and support model. These attitude changes were associated with more effective early intervention (Espe-Sherwindt & Kerlin, 1990).

The Family Context

<u>The Parents</u>

Parents with intellectual disabilities may have characteristics and experiences that foster or delimit parenting abilities. Unfortunately, our work with hundreds of families, as well as research studies, suggest that many parents with intellectual disabilities face numerous obstacles to being successful parents. The extent to which the parents face these adversities and the countervailing supports and services that they receive determine to a large degree their ability to successfully parent.

Parental Cognitive Limitations

It generally is accepted that low IQ per se, does not predict parenting abilities until it falls below 60 (Tymchuk & Feldman, 1991). Nevertheless, cognitive disabilities tend to impair skills in solving problems, making good judgments and decisions (Tymchuk, Yokota, & Rahbar, 1990), benefitting from didactic instruction (Feldman, 1994), and generalizing new skills (Bakken, Miltenberger, & Schauss, 1993; Feldman, Case, Rincover, Towns, & Betel, 1989).

Stigmatization

Apart from the real impact of cognitive limitations, the parent's attempts to cope with the stigma of being labeled "mentally retarded" may also interfere with effective parenting, or even opportunities to parent. Although stigmatization is a social phenomenon and could be discussed under the social context above, this section will briefly examine how stigmatization affects the parents' beliefs and actions. Indeed, many adults who have been diagnosed with mental retardation do recognize and fear the stigma of that label (Bogdan & Taylor, 1976). Self-advocates now do not hesitate to tell professionals how much they loathe the label, "mentally retarded". To minimize stigmatization, many people with mild and moderate intellectual disabilities may try to deny their limitations, make excuses for failures, and learn to adopt a "cloak of competence" (Edgerton & Bercovici, 1976). That is, they mask their cognitive limitations by acting like they understand and are competent. For example, they may nod their heads and repeat what was just told them. They are reluctant to admit they do not understand or need help. As noted earlier, for parents with intellectual disabilities, stigma may result in a higher probability of having their children taken away than non-labeled parents. Thus, they may endeavor to "wear" a cloak of competence. While this strategy may work for them in other situations, it backfires when they insist that they are perfect parents who do not need any services or help whatsoever, when it is obvious that this is not the case.

Personal History

Many parents with intellectual disabilities have personal life histories that may affect their ability to form close relationships and adequately parent. Many were abused as children, and as adults they continue to have emotional problems; they are vulnerable to exploitation, especially sexually and financially. Some had few opportunities to observe good parental role models, either because they lived in institutions or their home life was chaotic and dysfunctional. Some parents recognize the inadequate care they had received when growing up, and they are eager to participate in parenting programs so they would not make the same mistakes that their own parents made. It has been our experience that those parents who grew up in loving, supportive families (regardless of socioeconomic status) tended to cope better with the parenting role.

Poverty

Virtually all parents with intellectual disabilities are poor

(Fotheringham, 1971). Economic disadvantage is associated with adverse developmental and behavioural outcomes in children (Martin, Ramey & Ramey, 1990; Parker, Greer & Zuckerman, 1988). It is likely that poverty does not directly cause parent and child problems. Rather, events related to low socioeconomic status (SES), such as unemployment; living in substandard, crowded, and unstimulating environments; stress-related illnesses; inferior health care; and malnutrition may have more direct negative impact on parenting and child outcomes (Bee et al., 1982). This view implies that despite these families continuing to live in poverty, the provision of supports, resources, parent training, and early intervention may improve family, parent, and child outcomes (Feldman, Case, & Sparks, 1992; Feldman, Garrick, & Case, 1997; Feldman, Sparks, & Case, 1993; Garber, 1988; Ramey & Ramey, 1992).

Parental Health

Parents with intellectual disabilities often have physical and mental health problems that interfere with parenting. They may suffer from asthma, chronic infections, and other ailments that reflect the effects of inadequate nutrition, smoking, unsanitary living conditions, a sedentary lifestyle, and ongoing high stress. These parents also are at increased risk for mental health problems, as are people with intellectual disabilities in general (Borthwick-Duffy & Eyman, 1990; Eaton & Menolascino, 1982).

Of particular note is the occurrence of depression in mothers with intellectual disabilities (Tymchuk, 1994; Walton-Allen, 1993). Walton-Allen (1993) found that 63% of mothers with intellectual disabilities reported moderate or severe depressive symptoms. This prevalence is considerably higher than the maximum of 40% found in another high risk group - impoverished, young, and single mothers without intellectual disabilities (Wolkind, 1985). Maternal depression may have multiple origins and likely represents the interaction between environmental factors (e.g., poverty, lack of a supportive partner), constitutional characteristics of the mother (e.g., genetic predisposition), parental history (e.g., abuse, ongoing victimization), and child characteristics (e.g., developmental delay, behaviour problems) (Belsky, 1984).

Numerous studies have shown that parental depression is related to dysfunctional parent-child interactions (Hops et al., 1987); insecure attachment (Lyons-Ruth, Connell, Grunebaum, & Botein, 1990), child social and cognitive delays (Lyons-Ruth et al.,1990; Walton-Allen, 1993), childhood depression, oppositional behaviour, conduct disorders, attention deficit, anxiety, and substance abuse (Billings & Moos, 1985; Dumas, Gibson & Albin, 1989; Hammen et al., 1987). Thus, even if parents with intellectual disabilities had no other difficulties, given the high frequency of maternal depression, a considerable number of their children are at risk for developmental, social, and emotional problems.

Parental Stress

Considerable evidence exists that parental stress is related to problems in the parents such as physical and emotional difficulties (Bee, Hammond, Eyres, Barnard & Snyder, 1986; Ilfeld, 1977), parental competency (Weinraub & Wolfe, 1983), mother-infant bonding (Weinraub & Wolfe, 1983), negative and coercive mother-child interactions, and use of corporal punishment (Crnic, Greenberg, Robinson, & Ragozin, 1984; Dumas & Wahler, 1985; Forehand, Lautenschlager, Faust, &

Graziano, 1986;   Panaccione & Wahler, 1986; Webster-Stratton, 1988; Weinraub & Wolfe, 1983).   Parental stress is also associated with developmental and behaviour problems in children (Bee et al., 1986; Feldman, Hancock, Rielly, Minnes, & Cairns, 2000; Garcia-Coll, Vohr, & Hoffman, 1986; Patterson, DeBaryshe, & Ramsey, 1989).

Stress is both a cause of, and affected by, child difficulties. Bee et al. (1986) found that parental stress could precede and predict child problems. Longitudinal data reported by Patterson et al. (1989) indicate that parental stressors exerted an indirect impact on child behaviour problems by increasing negative parenting practices that increased child problem behaviour.   On the other hand, parental stress also may be a reaction to child developmental and behavioural disorders (Benedict, Wulff, & White, 1992; Eyberg, Boggs, & Rodriguez, 1992; Frey, Greenberg, & Fewell, 1989; Mash & Johnston, 1983; Minnes, 1988; Quine & Pahl, 1991).

In general, adults with intellectual disabilities experience many stressors including poverty (Conley, 1973), unemployment (Greenspan & Shoultz, 1981), stigmatization (Edgerton & Bercovici, 1976), and a history of failure experiences (Butterfield & Zigler, 1965).   Studies of parents without intellectual disabilities point to low family income as a major source of stress (Kessler & Cleary, 1980; Quine & Pahl, 1991) and, as stated earlier, virtually all parents with intellectual disabilities are poor. For parents with intellectual disabilities, the constant surveillance and threat of child removal by child protection authorities, as well as numerous workers visiting their home telling them what to do, add other sources of stress not typical of impoverished parents without intellectual disabilities (Hayman, 1990).

A recent study of 82 mothers with intellectual disabilities (living in a large city), who were given the Parenting Stress Index (PSI; Abidin, 1990), found that they indeed experience extremely high (95th percentile) stress levels (Feldman, Léger, & Walton-Allen, 1997). Mothers with school-age children were significantly more stressed than parents of infant/toddler and preschool children. The age of the child and crowded living conditions significantly predicted parenting stress in a multiple regression analysis. The results confirmed that mothers with intellectual disabilities experience extreme stress that, together with other factors, may hinder adequate parenting. Across all three child age groups, scores on the PSI subscales revealed significantly high levels of maternal depression and social isolation, and reduced feelings of attachment to the child and a sense of competency. The mothers felt that their children's behaviour was maladaptive, unacceptable, and unrewarding (to the parent). The high stress levels of the mothers in the above study were not unique to city-dwellers. A follow-up study also found similarly high PSI scores in 30 mothers with intellectual disabilities living in less populated areas (Feldman, Ramsay, & Varghese, 2001).

Social Isolation and Support

Social support involves both emotional and instrumental relationships and can be formal (services) or informal (e.g., family, friends) (Cohen & Hoberman, 1985). In particular, having a warm, nurturing, and intimate relationship (usually with a spouse) is considered the most important form of social support (Crnic et al., 1984; Cutrona & Troutman, 1986; Garcia-Coll et al., 1986). It is widely recognized that social support can buffer the negative affects of stressors in both the parents and children (Dunst, Trivette, & Cross, 1986; Roberts, 1989).

Conversely, a lack of social support is associated with insufficient adaption to life stressors and may partly account for parenting difficulties, dysfunctional parent-child interactions, and nonoptimal child outcomes seen in low SES, adolescent, and poorly educated parents (Bee et al., 1986; Crockenberg, 1987; Kessler & Cleary, 1980; Wahler, 1980).

Many people with intellectual disabilities are socially isolated and this may relate to their increased risk of depression (Reiss & Benson, 1985). The social isolation and lack of social supports of parents with intellectual disabilities also has been widely recognized (Booth & Booth, 1994; Feldman, Léger et al., 1997; Feldman & Walton-Allen, 1997; Llewellyn, 1995; Mattison, 1975; Tymchuk, 1992), and perhaps may partly account for their high levels of depression (Walton-Allen, 1993).

The impact of social support on parents with intellectual disabilities and their children remains unclear. People with few social supports and resources tend to be more stressed out and do not cope well with life's hassles (Lazarus, 1966). In fact, in a recent study we found a negative relationship between social support and parenting stress in parents with intellectual disabilities and that satisfaction with (but not size of) their support networks was associated with more positive parent-child interactions (Feldman et al., 2001). These results are similar to studies of parents without intellectual disabilities (Jennings, Stagg, & Connors, 1985; Weinraub & Wolf, 1983). In another study, maternal social isolation was significantly related to child behaviour problems in families with mothers who had IQs less than 70; this relationship did not obtain in a low income comparison group where the mothers had IQs greater than 85 (Feldman & Walton-Allen, 1997). The support of extended family members may reduce the risk of problems in children of parents with intellectual disabilities (Zetlin, Weisner, & Gallimore, 1985).

Services

We have also examined the parents' impressions of formal supports. In an earlier study (Walton-Allen & Feldman, 1991), we provided a list of services related to child-care, domestic, and personal supports and we asked mothers with intellectual disabilities and their workers (separately) to check off what services they felt the mothers needed and what services were being provided. Both parents and their workers agreed that the parents were not getting all the services that they needed. However, the parents and workers disagreed as to what areas the parents required more support. That is, the workers felt that the parents should be getting more child-care training, but the parents felt that they were being over-serviced in that area, but wanted more services related to personal concerns (e.g., assertiveness training, job training, counselling).

More recently, we again compared the parents' and workers' perceptions of supports. Instead of providing a list of services, we asked mothers with intellectual disabilities and their workers, in separate open-ended interviews, to describe formal and informal sources of family support in several emotional and instrumental domains (e.g., relationship with a confidant, positive feedback, material aid, advice about child-rearing). We again found that parents and their workers disagreed as to the importance of various types of supports. Not surprisingly, the workers invariably listed themselves as significant sources of support to the family. Interestingly, the mothers sometimes neglected to mention services, and instead focused on informal sources of support (sibling, friends, church groups) that oftentimes the workers had not even acknowledged. Thus, as in parents without intellectual disabilities, preliminary evidence suggests that satisfaction with one's (especially informal) social network may moderate the effects of stress in parents with intellectual disabilities and lead to more positive parent-child interactions. More research is needed to determine to what extent social support is related to long-term child outcomes and whether helping socially isolated parents build more satisfactory support networks would result in fewer parenting and child problems.

Effective Interventions

Although our previous studies found disagreements between parents and their workers about family service needs, services that are compassionate, appropriate, coordinated, efficient, and effective can greatly enhance the quality of life of parents with intellectual disabilities and their children. While there are many services that these families want and need, only parent education interventions and specialized preschools have been empirically validated. In a review of published studies of parent education interventions specifically for parents with intellectual disabilities, Feldman (1994) concluded that the most effective programs were skill oriented and used behavioural teaching strategies such as task analysis, prompting, modeling, performance feedback, and positive reinforcement. Not only do parenting skills improve, but also several studies have reported beneficial effects of parent training on the health and development of the children (Feldman et al., 1989; Feldman et al., 1992; Feldman, et al., 1997; Feldman et al., 1993; Slater, 1986), and family preservation (Feldman et al., 1992, 1993). Recent research has demonstrated that a majority of parents with intellectual disabilities can learn child-care skills through self-instruction (Feldman & Case, 1997, 1999; Feldman, Ducharme, & Case, 1999). These latter studies suggest that many families that need parent education may be able to benefit from instruction even when a specialized program is not available.

In addition to parent education programs, placing children of parents with intellectual disabilities in specialized preschools at an early age improves the children's development (Garber, 1988; Martin et al., 1990; Ramey & Ramey, 1992). However, these intensive out-of-home approaches may not be cost effective (Bronfenbrenner, 1974). In the absence of specialized preschool programs, enrolling children of parents with intellectual disabilities in a regular daycare still may have beneficial effects (Ramey & Ramey, 1992). However, out-of-home programs likely do not have much impact on parenting skills and the home environment, thereby leaving the child's health and safety at risk. Two-generation programs that include parenting (and other) education and supports for the parents coupled with specialized preschool placements for the children, may offer the most efficacious and humanitarian alternative to child removal in many cases.

Conversely, ineffective services can be a great detriment to the family. If a program does not offer instructional strategies that have been shown to work with people with intellectual disabilities, it would be logical to attribute failure to the program. However, often it is the parents, not the instructors, who are blamed for a lack of improvement. Parents with intellectual disabilities do not learn well when instruction is primarily didactic or verbal (Bakken et al., 1993; Feldman et al., 1989). Yet, many parent education programs only offer classroom instruction with little opportunity to teach and evaluate parenting skills in vivo. When a parent fails to acquire skills despite concerted (but ineffective) efforts, then the parent may be considered unteachable and/or unmotivated and their parenting rights may be terminated. Before decisions are made to break up the family, a detailed evaluation of the services offered to the family should be undertaken to ensure that state-of-the-art interventions were tried.

Child Factors

The relationship between parent and child factors is complex. The model depicted in Figure 1 hypothesizes that child characteristics not only are affected by parenting styles, but also probably directly or indirectly contribute to inadequate parenting by taxing the parent's abilities and negatively impacting the parent's psychological state (that then directly affects parenting practices).

Child Development

Children of parents with intellectual disabilities are at increased risk for developmental problems, including intellectual disabilities (Feldman, Case, Towns, & Betel, 1985; Reed & Reed, 1965), learning disabilities (Feldman & Walton-Allen, 1997), and cerebral palsy (Nelson & Ellenberg, 1986).

Most studies have reported that children of parents with intellectual disabilities have lower mean IQ scores and more of them have scores less than 70 (the accepted cut-off for a diagnosis of mental retardation) (American Psychiatric Association, 1994) than would be expected from a random, but not necessarily an impoverished, sample of the general population (Baroff, 1974; Bass, 1963; Feldman et al., 1985; Garber, 1988;

Gillberg, & Geijer-Karlsson, 1983; Mickelson, 1947; Reed & Reed, 1965; Scally, 1973; Schilling et al., 1982). For example, Mickleson (1947) estimated that in her sample of 90 children with at least one "feebleminded" parent, 39% would be designated as mentally retarded on the basis of IQ scores. Reed and Reed (1965) studied 7,778 children who were genetically related to 289 probands with IQs less than 69 residing in a Minnesota institution for adults with mental retardation. Reed and Reed found that when both parents had intellectual disabilities, 40% of the children had IQs below 70; 80% had IQs lower than 90 and the mean IQ for this group was 74. When only one parent had intellectual disabilities, 15% of the children scored below 70, and only 54% scored above 90; the mean IQ score was 90. These findings compared to 1% below 70, 91% above 90, and a mean IQ score of 107 for children with two parents without intellectual disabilities. Similar results were obtained in Northern Ireland (Scally, 1973), although in England, Brandon (1957) did not find a higher incidence of developmental delay in the children of parents with intellectual disabilities. In Canada, we found that 42% of a sample of 2-year old children raised by mothers with intellectual disabilities scored at least one standard deviation below the mean on the Mental Developmental Index (MDI) of the Bayley Scales of Infant Development (Bayley, 1969) and the children had significantly lower scores on language compared to nonlanguage MDI items (Feldman et al., 1985). We have also found that (before parent training) young children of mothers with intellectual disabilities vocalized and spoke significantly less than low and middle SES peers who had parents without intellectual disabilities (Feldman et al., 1986; 1993).

Parents without intellectual disabilities raising children with developmental delay report higher stress, depression, and marital disharmony than parents of children without developmental problems (Benedict et al., 1992; Crnic, Friedrich, & Greenberg, 1983; Minnes, 1998). Thus, the high stress and depression reported by mothers with intellectual disabilities discussed earlier, may be related in part to their children also having disabilities. As the child ages and enters school, the impact of the child's developmental delay may become more apparent to the family. This may be one source of the significantly greater stress experienced by parents with intellectual disabilities who were raising school-age children as opposed to preschoolers and infants (Feldman, Léger et al., 1997).

Child Behaviour Problems

Children of parents with intellectual disabilities are also at risk for behavioural and psychiatric problems. O'Neill (1985) reported that 50% of children with average or above average intelligence, who were being raised by parents with intellectual disabilities, had emotional and social problems such as oppositional behaviours and pseudoretardation. In a retrospective study conducted in Sweden, Gillberg and Geijer-Karlsson (1983) found that over 50% of offspring of parents with intellectual disabilities had made use of psychiatric services. Booth and Booth (1997) interviewed 30 adolescent and adult offspring in Great Britain and also reported a high rate of emotional problems. In Canada, Feldman and Walton-Allen (1997) found that children of mothers with intellectual disabilities had significantly more behaviour problems than a low income comparison group of children whose mothers did not have intellectual disabilities. Over 40% of the children (mainly boys) of mothers with intellectual disabilities had conduct disorders compared to 12% of the comparison children. In support of O'Neill's (1985) observations, both Feldman and Walton-

Allen (1997) and Booth and Booth (1997) reported that the offspring who did not have intellectual disabilities had more behavioural, emotional, and social maladjustment than offspring who had below average intelligence.

Child behaviour problems can be a source of stress and parenting difficulties for parents without intellectual disabilities (Eyberg et al., 1992; Mash & Johnston, 1983). Thus, if children of parents with intellectual disabilities are more likely to have behavioural and psychiatric disorders, then this, too, may contribute to the high stress levels and parenting problems seen in these parents (especially those with older and brighter children). Many of these parents who were coping adequately when their children were younger have told us that they can no longer manage their school-age child's behaviour.

Impediment-Support Checklist

This chapter reviewed several of the social, familial, parental, and child factors that interact to make it more or less difficult for a parent with intellectual disabilities to be a competent parent and for the children to optimally develop. The set of variables can be summarized in an Impediment-Support Checklist, which is presented in Table 1 (a similar checklist was devised by Tymchuk & Keltner, 1991). It is important to note that at this point empirical data are not available to confirm that each of these variables actually contributes in either a negative or positive way to parenting and child outcomes in families where parents have intellectual disabilities. Much more research is needed to identify factors that impede or support adequate family functioning. However, the checklist does give researchers, practitioners, child protection workers, lawyers, and judges an appreciation for the interactional, ecological perspective of parenting. Adopting this approach may increase the likelihood that a comprehensive assessment of possible reasons for parenting problems is conducted. Such an assessment should lead to more valid and humane decisions about family continuance, and the provision of appropriate supports and services to help to maintain the child in a safe and nurturing home environment.

Table 1: Impediments/Support Checklist for Parents with Intellectual Disabilities

Parental Development and Demographic Factors

Variable	Impediment	Support
IQ	< 60	>70
Marital Status	Single	Married
Maternal Age at Birth of 1st child	< 21 or > 35 years	Optimal (20-35 years)
Pregnancy	Unplanned; unwanted	Planned
# of Children	3 or more	1
Academic Skills	Illiterate	Reading and Math Skills
Parental Health	Health problems	Excellent health
Family Violence	Victim witness	None
Psychiatric History	Mental Illness	None
Substance Abuse	Yes	No
Life Events	Negative	Positive
Child Protection and Involvement	Previous	Never

Social Factors

Variable	Risk	Opportunity
Stigmatized	yes	no
Discriminated Against	yes	no

Parental Psychological/Personality Factors

Variable	Risk	Opportunity
Mood	Depressed	Content
Self-esteem	Low	High
Parental Attitudes	Punitive; rejecting	Accepting; indulgent
Coping Strategy	Reactive	Proactive
Perceived Stress	High	Low
Motivation	Unwilling	Motivated
Cooperation	Uncooperative	Cooperative
Child Care Experience	None; little	Some

Family Factors

Variable	Risk	Opportunity
Family Income	Below Poverty Level	Middle Class Level
Housing	Unsafe; inadequate; crowded	Safe; adequate
Employment	Unemployment; repeated changes	Stable job
Family Nutrition	Inadequate	Adequate

Social Support Variables

Variable	Risk	Opportunity
Spouse/partner	Not present; unsupportive	Present; supportive
Extended Family	None; few; unsupportive	Many supportive
Quality of Supports	Inhibiting independence	Enhancing Competency
Satisfaction with Supports	Not satisfied	Satisfied
Services	None; few; too many; fragmented; inappropriate; ineffective	Appropriate; effective; coordinated
Workers/ Assessors	Biased; inexperienced	Unbiased; experienced

Child Characteristics

Variable	Risk	Opportunity
Gender	Boy	Girl
Age	School-age	Infant/Toddler
Developmental Status	Developmental Delay	Typical Development
Temperament	Irritable; anxious	Placid
Behaviour	Conduct Disorder; ADHD	Appropriate
Academic Ability	Delays	Grade Equivalent
Emotional State	Depressed	Well adjusted
Separation from Family	Previous; current	None
Health	Sickly	Healthy
Exposure to Family Violence	Witness; victim	None
Abuse	Yes	No

Recommendations

Recommendation 1:
Parents with intellectual disabilities should be judged according to the same criteria as parents without intellectual disabilities and current and future parenting capacity should not be solely determined by tests of cognitive functioning or diagnosis of intellectual disability.

The presumption of parenting incompetence based on having a low IQ and cognitive limitations (e.g., problems in abstract thinking) is not justified or supported by empirical evidence. Just like for other parents, parents with intellectual disabilities should not have their parenting rights terminated in the absence of actual or high potential for child maltreatment (Hayman, 1990; Tymchuk & Feldman, 1991).

Recommendation 2:
Parenting capacity assessments on persons with intellectual disabilities should take into account the impediments and supports for parenting.

The literature shows that parenting ability is affected by a host of variables in addition to cognitive impairment. An adequate and fair assessment should examine parent, child, and family factors that either impede or promote adequate parenting. It also must be recognized that parenting capacity is not a static trait, but can change given different circumstances (e.g., provision of effective services and supports).

Recommendation 3:
Parent capacity assessment should include objective observations of actual parenting skills in the natural environ-

ment.

Feldman, Tymchuk and others have recommended and used ecologically-valid child-care skill observational checklists to evaluate current parenting abilities (as well as the effects of training). In the absence of normative data, however, even these more objective measures need to be carefully interpreted.

Recommendation 4:
Parent education should be considered as an alternative to terminating parenting rights. Child care training should be based on strategies with empirical support.

There is sufficient research to indicate that parents with intellectual disabilities and their children do benefit from home-based behaviourally-oriented parent education (Feldman, 1994, 1997). Furthermore, many parents with intellectual disabilities may improve basic child care skills through self-instruction when the materials are specifically designed for persons with low literacy and cognitive skills (Feldman & Case, 1997, 1999; Feldman et al., 1999).

Recommendation 5:
Services and supports should empower rather than impair, and promote rather than inhibit competence.

Several authors have commented on how services and social supports may or may not foster effective parenting (Espe-Scherwindt & Kerlin, 1990; Tucker & Johnson, 1989). A plethora of uncoordinated services that send in workers who repeatedly tell the parent what to do, could increase the parent's stress and adversely affect the parent's health, current parenting abilities, and receptivity to training. Likewise, persons who tend to be overly critical and take over child-care tasks that the parent is capable of performing may discourage the parents and reduce their self-confidence. Conversely, minimizing and coordinating services and having workers and others providing encouragement, noncritical feedback for errors, and positive reinforcement for improvements may increase the parent's self-esteem, motivation, and success.

Services that are likely to be most effective would be comprehensive and competency-promoting. Components would include parenting education, and other supports for the parents to increase not only their parenting skills, but also their employability, self-esteem, physical and psychological health, and satisfaction with their social support network. In addition, specialized preschool programs should be offered as early as possible in infancy and continue until the child starts grade 1. When specialized preschool programs are not available, then at the very least, parents should be encouraged to place their children in quality daycare (with readily available subsidies).

Recommendation 6:
Community agencies supporting a pregnant woman with intellectual disabilities should consider requesting specialized foster arrangements if the woman wishes to keep her child, but does not have the ability to adequately care for the child on her own.

In Western society, biological parents take complete legal responsibility for the protection, care, and nurturance of the child. Yet in reality, many parents rely on others to help fulfill this commitment. Currently, even if parents with intellectual disabilities can garner sufficient supports to look after the child, if they, themselves, are not deemed capable of eventually caring for the child on their own, then their parenting rights are likely to be terminated. There are few opportunities for long-term foster care that includes not just the child, but also the parents.

Occasionally, a couple or single mother with intellectual disabilities who clearly do not have sufficient parenting skills to safely raise a child on their own, still would like to keep the child and raise him/her to the best of their abilities, with necessary supports. Under these (currently rare) circumstances, perhaps the child protection agency and the community service providing residential support to the couple could consider setting up a specialized long-term foster arrangement whereby the entire family would live with foster parents (perhaps staff from the community service). Under these arrangements, the biological parents would be taught to carry out some child-care activities, with guidance and supervision provided as needed by the foster parents. In this manner, even persons who are unlikely to ever acquire all the necessary skills to be able to independently raise the child can still partially fulfill a parenting role to their child.

References

Abidin, R. R. (1990). *Parenting Stress Index - Manual*. Charlottesville, Virginia: Pediatric Psychology Press.

American Psychiatric Association (1994). *Diagnostic and statistical manual of mental disorders*. Fourth Edition. Washington, DC: Author.

Bakken, J., Miltenberger, R. G., & Schauss, S. (1993). Teaching parents with mental retardation: Knowledge vs. skills. *American Journal of Mental Retardation, 97,* 405-417.

Baroff, G. S. (1974). *Mental retardation: Nature, cause, and management.* NY: Wiley.

Bass, M. S. (1963). Marriage, parenthood, and prevention of pregnancy. *American Journal of Mental Deficiency, 68,* 320-335.

Bayley, N. (1969). *Bayley scales of infant development: Birth to two years.* NY: Psychological Corporation.

Bee, H. L., Barnard, K., Eyres, S., Gray, S., Hammond, M., Spietz, A., Snyder, C., & Clark, B. (1982). Prediction of IQ and language skill from perinatal status, child performance, family characteristics and mother-infant interaction. *Child Development, 53,* 1134-1156.

Bee, H. L., Hammond, M., Eyres, S., Barnard, K., & Snyder, C. (1986). The impact of parental life change on the early development of children. *Research in Nursing & Health, 9,* 65-74.

Belsky, J. (1984). The determinants of parenting: A process model. *Child Development, 55,* 83-96.

Benedict, M. I., Wulff, L. M., & White, R. B. (1992). Current parental stress in maltreating and nonmaltreating families of children with multiple disabilities. *Child Abuse & Neglect, 16,* 155-163.

Billings, A. & Moos, R. (1985) Children of parents with unipolar depression: A controlled 1-year follow-up. *Journal of Abnormal Child Psychology, 14,* 149-166.

Bogdan, R., & Taylor, S. J. (1976). The judged, not the judges: An insider's view of mental retardation. *American Psychologist, 31,* 47-52.

Booth, T. & Booth, W. (1994). Working with parents with mental retardation: Lessons from research. *Journal of Developmental and Physical Disabilities, 6,* 23-41.

Booth, T. & Booth, W. (1997). *Exceptional childhoods, unexceptional children. Growing up with parents who have learning difficulties.* London, UK: Family Policies Studies

Centre.

Borthwick-Duffy, S. A. & Eyman, R. K. (1990). Who are the dually diagnosed? *American Journal on Mental Retardation, 94,* 586-595.

Brandon, M. W. G. (1957). The intellectual and social status of children of mental defectives. *Journal of Mental Science, 103,* 710-738.

Bronfenbrenner, U. (1974). Is early intervention effective? *Columbia Teachers College Record, 76,* 279-303.

Bronfenbrenner, U. (1979). Contexts of child rearing: Problems and prospects. *American Psychologist, 34,* 844-850.

Butterfield, E. C., & Zigler, E. (1965). The effects of success and failure on the discrimination learning of normal and retarded children. *Journal of Abnormal Psychology, 70,* 25-31.

Cohen, S. & Hoberman, H. M. (1983). Positive events and social supports as buffers of life change stress. *Journal of Applied Social Psychology, 13,* 99-125.

Conley, R. W. (1973). *The economics of mental retardation.* Baltimore: John Hopkins University Press.

Crnic, K. A., Friedrich, W. N., & Greenberg, M. T. (1983). Adaptation of families with mentally retarded children: A model of stress, coping and family ecology. *American Journal of Mental Deficiency, 88,* 125-138.

Crnic, K., Greenberg, M., Ragozin, A., Robinson, N., & Basham, R. (1983). Effects of stress and social support on mothers and premature and full term infants. *Child Development, 54,* 209-217.

Crnic, K., Greenberg, M., Robinson, N., & Ragozin, A. (1984). Maternal stress and social support: Effects on the mother-infant relationship from birth to eighteen months. *American Journal of Orthopsychiatry, 54,* 224-235.

Crockenberg, S. B. (1987). Predictors and correlates of anger toward and punitive control of toddlers by adolescent mothers. *Child Development, 58,* 964-975.

Cutrona, C. E., & Troutman, B. (1986). Social support, infant temperament and parenting self-efficacy: A mediational model. *Child Development, 57,* 1507-1518.

Dumas, J., Gibson, J., & Albin, J. (1989). Behavioral correlates of maternal depressive symptomatology in conduct-disorder children. *Journal of Consulting and Clinical Psychology, 57,* 516-521.

Dumas, J., & Wahler, R. (1985). Indiscriminate mothering as a contextual factor in aggressive-oppositional child behavior. *Journal of Abnormal Child Psychology, 13,* 1-17.

Dunst, C. J., Trivette, C., & Cross, A. (1986). Mediating influences of social support: Personal, family and child outcomes. *American Journal of Mental Deficiency, 90,* 403-417.

Eaton, L., & Menolascino, F. J. (1982). Psychiatric disorders in the mentally retarded: Types, problems and challenges. *American Journal of Psychiatry, 139,* 1297-1303.

Edgerton, R. B. & Bercovici, S. M. (1976). The cloak of competence: Years later. *American Journal of Mental Deficiency, 80,* 485-497.

Espe-Scherwindt, M., & Kerlin, S. (1990). Early intervention with parents with mental retardation: Do we empower or impair? *Infants and Young Children, 2,* 21-28.

Eyberg, S. M., Boggs, S. R., & Rodriguez, C. M. (1992). Relationships between maternal parenting stress and child disruptive behavior. *Child and Family Behavior Therapy, 14,* 1-9.

Feldman, M. A. (1994). Parenting education for parents with intellectual disabilities: A review of outcome studies. *Research in Developmental Disabilities, 15,* 299-332.

Feldman, M.A. (1997). The effectiveness of early intervention

for children of parents with mental retardation. In M.J. Gu-
ralnick, (Ed.). *The effectiveness of early intervention: Directions for second generation research.* (pp. 171-191).
Baltimore: Paul H. Brookes.

Feldman, M. A. & Case, L. (1997). Effectiveness of self-
instructional audiovisual materials in teaching child-care
skills to parents with intellectual disabilities. *Journal of
Behavioral Education, 7,* 235-257.

Feldman, M. A. & Case, L. (1999). Teaching child-care and
safety skills to parents with intellectual disabilities via self-
learning. *Journal of Intellectual and Developmental Disabilities, 24,* 27-44.

Feldman, M. A., Case, L., Rincover, A., Towns, F., & Betel, J.
(1989). Parent education project III: Increasing affection
and responsivity in developmentally handicapped mothers:
Component analysis, generalization, and effects on child
language. *Journal of Applied Behavior Analysis, 22,* 211-
222.

Feldman, M. A., Case, L., & Sparks, B. (1992). Effectiveness
of a child-care training program for parents at-risk for child
neglect. *Canadian Journal of Behavioural Science, 24,* 14-
28.

Feldman, M. A., Case, L., Towns, F., & Betel, J. (1985) Parent
education project I: Development and nurturance of children of mentally retarded parents. *American Journal of
Mental Deficiency, 90,* 253-258.

Feldman, M. A., Ducharme, J. M., & Case, L. (1999). Using
self-instructional pictorial manuals to teach child-care
skills to mothers with intellectual disabilities. *Behavior
Modification, 23,* 480-497.

Feldman, M. A., Garrick, M., & Case, L. (1997). The effects
of parent training on weight gain of nonorganic-failure-to-
thrive children of parents with intellectual disabilities.

Journal on Developmental Disabilities, 5, 47-61.

Feldman, M. A., Hancock, C. L., Rielly, N., Minnes, P., & Cairns, C. (2000). Behavior problems in young children with or at risk for developmental delay *Journal of Child and Family Studies, 9*, 247-261.

Feldman, M. A., Léger, M., & Walton-Allen, N. (1997). Stress in mothers with intellectual disabilities. *Journal of Child and Family Studies, 6*, 471-485.

Feldman, M. A., Varghese, J., Ramsay, J., & Rajska, D. (2001). Stress and social support in mothers with intellectual disabilities. Manuscript submitted for publication.

Feldman, M. A., Sparks, B., & Case, L. (1993). Effectiveness of home-based early intervention on the language development of children of parents with mental retardation. *Research in Developmental Disabilities, 14*, 387-408.

Feldman, M. A., Towns, F., Betel, J., Case, L., Rincover, A., & Rubino, C.. (1986). Parent Education Project II: Increasing stimulating interactions of developmentally handicapped mothers. *Journal of Applied Behavior Analysis, 19*, 23-37.

Feldman, M. A. & Walton-Allen, N. (1997). Effects of maternal mental retardation and poverty on intellectual, academic, and behavioral status of school-age children. *American Journal on Mental Retardation, 101*, 352-364.

Forehand, R., Lautenschlager, G., Faust, J., & Graziano, W. G. (1986) Parent perceptions and parent-child interactions in clinic referred children: A preliminary investigation of the effects of maternal depressive moods. *Behaviour Research and Therapy, 24*, 73-75.

Fotheringham, J. (1971). The concept of social competence as applied to marriage and child care in those classified as mentally retarded. *Canadian Medical Association Journal, 104*, 813-816.

Frey, K. S., Greenberg, M. T., & Fewell, R. R. (1989). Stress and coping among parents of handicapped children: A multidimensional approach. *American Journal of Mental Retardation, 94,* 240-249.

Garber, H.L. (1988). *The Milwaukee Project. Preventing mental retardation in children at risk.* Washington, DC: American Association on Mental Retardation.

Garcia-Coll, C., Vohr, B., & Hoffman, J. (1986). Maternal and environmental factors affecting developmental outcome of infant of adolescent mothers. *Developmental Behavioral Pediatrics, 7,* 230-236.

Gillberg, C. & Geijer-Karlsson, M. (1983). Children born to mentally retarded women: a 1-21 year follow-up study of 41 cases. *Psychological Medicine, 13,* 891-894.

Glaun, D. E. & Brown, P. F. (1999). Motherhood, intellectual disability and child protection: Characteristics of a court sample. *Journal of Intellectual and Developmental Disabilities, 24,* 95-105.

Greenspan, S. & Schoultz, B. (1981). Why mentally retarded adults lose their jobs: social competence as a factor in work adjustment. *Applied Research in Mental Retardation, 2,* 23-38.

Hammen, C., Adrian, C., Gordon, D., Burge, D., Jaenicke, C., & Hiroto, D. (1987) Children of depressed mothers: Maternal strain and symptom predictors of dysfunction. *Journal of Abnormal Psychology, 96,* 190-198.

Hayman, R. L. (1990). Presumptions of justice: Law, politics and the mentally retarded parent. *Harvard Law Review, 103,* 1201-1274.

Hops, H., Biglan, A., Sherman, L., Arthur, J., Friedman, L., & Osteen, L. (1987). Home observations of family interactions of depressed women. *Journal of Consulting and Clinical Psychology, 55,* 341-346.

Ilfeld, F. W. (1977). Current social stressors and symptoms of depression. *American Journal of Psychiatry, 134,* 161-166.

Jennings, K. D., Stagg, V., & Connors, R. (1985, Apr.). Social support and mothers' interactions with their preschool children. Paper presented at the biennial meeting of the Society for Research in Child Development, Toronto.

Kessler, R. C. & Cleary, P. (1980). Social class and psychological distress. *American Sociological Review, 45,* 463-478.

Lazarus, R. (1966). *Psychological stress and the coping process.* New York: McGraw-Hill.

Llewellyn, G. (1995). Relationships and social support: Views of parents with mental retardation/intellectual disability. *Mental Retardation, 33,* 349-363.

Lyons-Ruth, K., Connell, D. B., & Zoll, D. (1989). Patterns of maternal behavior among infants at risk for abuse: relations with infant attachment at 12 months of age. In: D. Cicchetti & V. Carlson (Eds.), *Child maltreatment: Theory and research on the causes and consequences of child abuse and neglect.* (pp. 464-493). Cambridge: Cambridge University Press.

Lyons-Ruth, K., Connell, D., Grunebaum, H., & Botein, S. (1990) Infants at social risk: Maternal depression and family support services as mediators of infant development and security of attachment. *Child Development, 61,* 85-98.

Martin, S., Ramey, C., & Ramey, S. (1990) The prevention of intellectual impairment in children of impoverished families: Findings of a randomized trial of educational day care. *American Journal of Public Health, 80,* 844-847.

Mash, E. J. & Johnston, C. (1983). Parental perceptions of child behavior problems, parenting self-esteem, and mother's reported stress in younger and older hyperactive and normal children. *Journal of Consulting and Clinical Psychology, 51*, 86-99.

Mattison, J. (1975). *Marriage and handicap.* (2nd edition). London, UK: Tavistock Institute.

Mickelson, P. (1947). The feebleminded parent: A study of 90 family cases. *American Journal of Mental Deficiency, 51*, 644-653.

Minnes, P. (1988). Family stress and resources associated with a mentally retarded child. *American Journal on Mental Retardation, 93*, 184-192.

Minnes, P. M. (1998). Mental retardation: The impact upon the family. In J. A. Burack, R. M. Hodapp &. E. Zigler, (Eds.). *Handbook of mental retardation and development.* (pp. 693-712). NY: Cambridge University Press.

Nelson, K. B. & Ellenberg, J. H. (1986). Antecedents of cerebral palsy: Multivariate analysis of risk. *New England Journal of Medicine, 315*, 81-86.

O'Neill, A. M. (1985). Normal and bright children of mentally retarded parents: The Huck Finn Syndrome. *Child Psychiatry and Human Development, 15*, 255-268.

Panaccione, V. F. & Wahler, R. (1986). Child behavior, maternal depression and social coercion as factors in the quality of child care. *Journal of Abnormal Child Psychology, 14*, 263-278.

Parker, S., Greer, S., & Zuckerman, B. (1988) Double jeopardy: The impact of poverty on early child development. *The Pediatric Clinics of North America, 35*, 1227-1240.

Patterson, G. R., DeBaryshe, B. D., & Ramsey, E. (1989). A developmental perspective on antisocial behavior. *American Psychologist, 44*, 329-335.

Quine, L., & Pahl, J. (1991). Stress and coping in mothers caring for a child with severe learning difficulties: A test of Lazarus' transactional model of coping. *Journal of Community and Applied Social Psychology, 1*, 57-70.

Ramey, C. T. & Ramey, S. L. (1992). Effective early intervention. *Mental Retardation, 30*, 337-345.

Reed, E. W. & Reed, S. C. (1965). *Mental retardation: A family study*. Philadelphia: Saunders.

Reiss, S. & Benson, B. A. (1985). Psychosocial correlates of depression in mentally retarded adults I. Minimal social support and stigmatization. *American Journal of Mental Deficiency, 89*, 331-337.

Roberts, W. L. (1989). Parents' stressful life events and social networks: Relations with parenting and children's *competence.* Canadian Journal of Behavioural Science, 21, 132-146.

Sameroff, A. J., & Chandler, M. (1975). Reproductive risk and the continuum of caretaking causality. In: F. Horowitz (Ed.) *Review of child development research* (Vol. 4, pp. 157-243). Chicago: University of Chicago Press.

Scally, B. G. (1973). Marriage and mental handicap: Some observations in Northern Ireland. In F. F. de la Cruz and G. D. La Veck (Eds.) *Human sexuality and the mentally retarded* (pp. 186-194). New York: Brunner/Mazel.

Schilling, R., Schinke, S,. Blythe, B., & Barth, R. (1982). Child maltreatment and mentally retarded parents: Is there a relationship? *Mental Retardation, 20*, 201-209.

Seagull, E. & Scheurer, S. (1986). Neglected and abused children of mentally retarded parents. *Child Abuse & Neglect, 10*, 493-500.

Slater, M. A. (1986). Modification of mother-child interaction processes in families with children at-risk for mental retardation. *American Journal of Mental Deficiency, 91*, 257-267.

Taylor, C. G., Norman, D., Murphy, J., Jellinek, M., Quinn, D., Poitrast, F., & Goshko, M. (1991). Diagnosed intellectual and emotional impairment among parents who seriously mistreat their children: Prevalence, type, and outcome in a court sample. *Child Abuse & Neglect, 15*, 389-401.

Tucker, M. B. & Johnson, O. (1989). Competence promoting versus competence inhibiting social support for mentally retarded mothers. *Human Organization, 48*, 95-107.

Tymchuk, A. J. (1992). Predicting adequacy of parenting by people with mental retardation. *Child Abuse & Neglect*, 16, 165-178.

Tymchuk, A. J. (1994). Depression symptomatology in mothers with mild intellectual disability: An exploratory study. *Australia and New Zealand Journal of Developmental Disabilities, 19*, 111-119.

Tymchuk, A. & Feldman, M. A. (1991). Parents with mental retardation and their children: Review of research relevant to professional practice. *Canadian Psychology, 32*, 486-494.

Tymchuk, A. J. & Keltner, B. (1991). Advantage profiles: A tool for health care professionals working with parents with mental retardation. *Pediatric Nursing, 14*, 155-161.

Tymchuk, A. J., Llewellyn, G., & Feldman, M. A. (1999). Parenting by persons with intellectual disabilities: A timely international perspective. *Journal of Intellectual and Developmental Disabilities, 24*, 3-6.

Tymchuk, A. J., Yokota, A., & Rahbar, B. (1990). Decision-making abilities of mothers with mental retardation. *Research in Developmental Disabilities, 11*, 97-109.

Vogel, P. (1987). The right to parent. *Entourage, 2*, 33-39.

Wahler, R. G. (1980). The insular mother: Her problems in parent-child treatment. *Journal of Applied Behavior Analysis, 13*, 207-219.

Walton-Allen, N. (1993). Psychological distress and parenting by mothers with mental retardation. Unpublished doctoral dissertation, University of Toronto.

Walton-Allen, N. & Feldman, M. A. (1991). Perception of service needs by parents with mental retardation and their workers. *Comprehensive Mental Health Care, 1*, 137-147.

Webster-Stratton, C. (1988). Mothers' and fathers' perceptions of child deviance: Roles of parent and child adjustment and child deviance. *Journal of Consulting and Clinical Psychology, 56*, 909-915.

Weinraub, M. & Wolf, B. (1983). Effects of stress and social supports on mother-child interactions in single- and two-parent families. *Child Development, 54*, 1297-1311.

Wolkind, S. (1985). The first years: Pre-school children and their families in the inner city. In J. E. Stevenson (Ed.) *Recent research in developmental psychopathology. Journal of Child Psychology & Psychiatry*, Supplement, No. 4.

Zetlin, A., Weisner, T., & Gallimore, R. (1985). Diversity, shared functioning and the role of benefactors: A study of parenting by retarded persons. In S. K. Thurman (Ed.), *Children of handicapped parents: Research and clinical perspectives.* (pp. 69-94). New York: Academic Press.

Chapter 8

Sexual Assault against Individuals who have a Developmental Disability

Diane Cox-Lindenbaum and Shelley L. Watson

Introduction

Regardless of age, individuals who have a developmental disability appear to be more vulnerable to abuse than individuals who do not have a disability (Goldman, 1994). Sobsey (1988) cites similar findings, stating that individuals who have all types of disability are at a much higher risk of sexual assault, sexual abuse, and sexual exploitation. In a survey of 85 women who had a disability, 70% indicated that they have been violated sexually (Goldman, 1994). Although the exact degree of risk varies from study to study, it appears to be at least 150 % of that for individuals of the same sex and similar age who do not have disabilities (Sobsey, 1994).

There are a number of factors that render individuals who have a developmental disability particularly vulnerable to sexual abuse. One such factor is the false and illogical assumptions that many people make about individuals who have developmental disabilities. These assumptions include the beliefs that no one would take advantage of an individuals who has a disability, that any form of sexual contact is enjoyed by individuals who have disabilities as they are more stimulated sexually than other people, and that individuals who have disabilities have impaired sexuality (Carmody, 1991).

The increased vulnerability for abuse of individuals who have a developmental disability is not related directly to the nature of the individual's disability (Griffiths, 1999; Muccigrosso, 1991; Sobsey, 1994; Sobsey & Varnhagen, 1991; Ticoll & Panitch, 1993). Rather, it has been suggested that abuse is more likely to occur because of the way society treats individuals who have a developmental disability and views their sexuality (Griffiths, 1999; Griffiths et al., 1995; Sobsey, 1994). "Sexual abuse is not just a sexual act - it is an expression of power" (Griffiths, 1999, p. 449).

The following chapter will look at the issue of sexual assault/ abuse of individuals who have a developmental disability. Abuse prevalence as well as agency responsibilities and obligations will be discussed. Treatment and prevention will also be addressed, suggesting possible preventions and solutions to this problem, as demonstrated in the following case studies.

Case Examples

Example 1

Justin, a 26 year-old man with Autism, has been living in a group home for seven years. He does not speak, but communicates with the use of picture symbols that must be interpreted by a "facilitated communicator". Over the years, he has developed strong and meaningful relationships with staff. Although he has a history of extreme aggression, bizarre behaviours, and Obsessive-Compulsive Disorder, he had reached a period of stabilization. However, after a scheduled vacation with staff, Justin returned fearful, paranoid, withdrawn, aggressive, and disoriented. Through his facilitated communicator, he stated that three of his staff had sexually abused him while on vacation. He demonstrated post-traumatic stress symptomatology, but no one would believe that these "treasured" friends had betrayed him in such an aggressive and inhumane way. Given his controversial method of communication, charges were not pursued.

Example 2

Mary, a 30 year-old woman with a developmental disability and psychotic disorder, was found in her room, "beneath a young man who was partially naked". The young man was not a resident of the home, but was utilizing the group home as respite for the weekend.

Staff had heard a "No! No!" coming from her room. As staff entered, they found the young man with his pants down, on top of Mary, who appeared to be in a dazed, catatonic-like state. As they approached, the young man was verbally re-directed from the room. The incident was charted as two people engaging in sexually illegal, but "voluntary" interaction.

After the incident, Mary deteriorated emotionally and psychologically. Her functioning in both vocational and social relationships became dysfunctional. The woman's change in symptomatology was not attributed to her sexual assault because she "already had mental health problems".

Example 3

An early intervention pre-school had noted an extreme change in the behaviour of a 4-year-old boy, Todd, who had delayed speech and a severe communication disorder. He was initially seen as shy and withdrawn, however, he became increasingly hostile, aggressive toward peers, and even bit a male teacher. During a toileting program, the child's undergarments were seen to be bloodied. The case was reported to the Child Abuse Hotline and the staff brought the child to a local emergency room at the hospital. The child was examined and found to have some rectal abrasions. Because of the child's overall delayed development (speech, communication disorder, and ambulatory delays), the rectal tearing was deemed to be "self-imposed" and the child seen as "incapable of giving a normal sexual abuse interview". In spite of the clinical symptomatology, physical evidence, and findings of a high-risk parental/family environment, the child was still not deemed to be considered at high risk for sexual abuse. The clinical and physical symptomatology was assumed to be the result of his developmental disability.

Literature Review

According to Carmody (1991), accurate statistics concerning the prevalence and incidence of sexual assault among people who are intellectually disabled are difficult to obtain. This is largely because the majority of cases of sexual abuse are likely never reported. Using FBI statistics and data collected by the Seattle Rape Relief Disabilities Project, Ryerson (cited in Sobsey & Varnhagen, 1991) estimates that only 20 percent of the cases of sexual abuse involving people with disabilities are ever reported to the police, community service agencies, or other authorities. Consequently, it is very difficult to compile accurate statistics concerning the incidence of sexual abuse among the disabled population.

Carmody (1991) states that individuals who have a developmental disability are particularly vulnerable to being sexually assaulted and that the systems designed to assist them are failing to recognize or address their specific needs. Conway (1994) asserts that a further complication is that many professionals and support providers find it difficult to recognize the subtle symptoms of abuse. The following literature review will examine the vulnerabilities to abuse of individuals who have developmental disabilities, including power inequities, characteristics of the disability, gender differences, and isolation, as well as abuse by caregivers.

Power inequities

Abuse, whether it be individuals who have a disability or not, is characterized by inequities in power (Doe, 1990). Sobsey (1995) supports this and states that individuals who have disabilities have been vulnerable to abuse because of power inequities. While some of the power inequities experienced by individuals who have disabilities are the direct effects of impairments (e.g., a person who uses a wheelchair is less likely to be able to carry out effective self-defense or to escape a violent confrontation), most of these inequities result from disempowerment. Sobsey (1995) goes on to state that the liberties and rights of people with disabilities have often been severely restricted, leaving them vulnerable to violence and exploitation.

He suggests that as individuals who have disabilities empower themselves individually and collectively, some of these power imbalances are restored. The central issues of power and sexuality must therefore be integrated into the understanding of abuse (Doe, 1990). Power inequities are nowhere more evident than in caregiving relationships, as will be discussed in the next section.

Caregiving relationships

Doe (1990) clearly asserts that the nature of abuse is a complex combination of aggression and sexuality in the form of abuse of power. She further elaborates that within the dynamic of offender and victim is an understanding, or coercion, that the abuse will not be disclosed. With offenders who are caregivers or close relatives, threats and psychological abuse can be used to maintain secrecy.

Less than 10% of offenders have disabilities themselves, yet more than half of the perpetrators, have 'caregiving' relationships with their victims (Doe, 1990). The term "caregiver" or "support provider" is a wider category that is used to include natural family, step-family, generic service providers, and specialized caregivers such as personal care attendants, psychiatrists, residential care staff, and foster families. In their caregiving roles, these people have power over the service consumer both through social and physical means (Doe, 1990).

While individuals who have developmental disabilities are often negatively stereotyped, caregivers are typically viewed as patient, dedicated, quasi-religious figures that are beyond reproach. "Consequently, we may have difficulty believing that the same man who was honored by his international religious and fraternal organizations for his dedication in adopting handicapped children from the third world countries, is now charged with sexually abusing these children" (Sobsey & Mansell, 1993, p 288). However, we cannot afford to dismiss suspicious events or behaviour simply because we believe some individuals are beyond censure (Sobsey & Mansell, 1993).

A Canadian nationwide survey of victims of sexual abuse who had disabilities revealed that in 96% of cases, the identities of offenders were generally known to the victims and/or their caregivers (Sobsey, 1988). Sobsey (1988) also found that offenders came into contact with their victims as a result of exposure to disability-based services in 29% of the cases reported. Levine Powers, Mooney, and Nunno (1990), Rindfleisch and Bean (1988), as well as Rindfleisch and Rabb (1984) all discuss the abuse of children in institutions, presenting staggering incidences of abuse by caregivers.

Although the high incidence of abuse by service providers is disheartening, Sobsey and Doe (1991) assert that it should not be interpreted to mean that most caregivers are abusive. It is important to remember that a single abusive caregiver may abuse a large number of victims. The average sex offender is believed to have about 70 victims before being apprehended and this number may be much higher in isolated group living environments (Sobsey & Doe, 1991). Furthermore, children and adults who have disabilities may be exposed to many more individuals. For example, Lakin, Bruininks, Hill, and Hauber (1982) found an average annual staff turnover rate of 32.8% in public residential facilities and 54.2% in private residential facilities. Moreover, around-the-clock staffing requires at least five staff for each one on duty at any given time, and staff are often rotated from unit to unit. Consequently, most individuals living in institutional settings come in contact with hundreds of caregivers in contrast to a much smaller number encountered in natural families (Sobsey and Varnhagen, 1991). Individuals removed from their homes are often moved through a number of settings, each with a number of caregivers. Assuming the same risk from each caregiver, the greater the number of caregivers with whom an individual has contact, the greater the risk for sexual abuse.

The system continues to "self-select" offenders (Sobsey & Doe, 1991). Many agencies continue to hire with little or no attempt to screen out people with histories of abuse or assault. Furthermore, many agencies seek physically powerful and assertive staff because they believe that these individuals will exert better control over service consumers. In these cases, people with previous convictions and fugitives on charges of sexual offenses were hired as caregivers and committed further offenses (Sobsey & Doe, 1991). Caregivers who report abuse are often harassed or threatened by their coworkers and employers, sometimes forcing them to resign, while no action was taken against the reported abuser (Sobsey & Doe, 1991).

Sobsey and Varnhagen (1991) developed a survey to investigate services provided to victims of sexual abuse who had a disability. There were four major concerns addressed by the survey. These included (1) characteristics of the victims, offender, and offense; (2) whether and how the victim's disability contributed to the victim's vulnerability to sexual abuse; (3) whether the offender was charged and/or convicted of the offense and, if the offender was not charged, whether the victim's disability was a contributing factor; and (4) the nature of and satisfaction with any community services obtained to treat and/or support the victim. The researchers found that 47% of the victims of sexual abuse were 18 years of age and over and that victims were predominantly female (85%). Offenders were most frequently members of the victim's natural family or disability-based service providers (20% for each group). This was followed by family friends (13%), strangers (12%), and other individuals who had disabilities receiving services in the same settings as the victim (11%). Child victims were most often sexually abused by relatives (44%), followed by support providers (19%). Adolescent victims were generally abused by either support providers (25%) or neighbours/family friends. Adult victims were most often abused by support providers or co-disability support recipients (Sobsey & Varnhagen, 1991).

There were 70 responses to the questions dealing with whether the victim's disability might have contributed to being at greater risk for sexual abuse. The predominant comments, comprising 35% of the responses, had to do with the victim not having enough knowledge about appropriate sexual behaviour and/ or having poor judgment. Twenty four percent of respondents also cited "overcompliance" as a factor contributing to abuse, suggesting that the current focus of compliance training in special education may be harmful to students and a greater focus on assertiveness may be needed (Sobsey & Varnhagen, 1991).

In spite of the large incidence of abuse by caregivers, many instances of sexual abuse are never reported to authorities. Sobsey and Mansell (1992) conducted a validation study where they asked experts to rank priorities and concerns with regards to the sexual abuse of individuals who have a developmental disability. Experts ranked the requirement to report abuse of all vulnerable people and complainant protection legislation as important in providing protection to persons reporting incidences of abuse (Sobsey & Mansell, 1992). Nevertheless, in a sample of abuse in caregiving facilities, charges were laid by law enforcement agencies in only 22% of cases (Sobsey, 1988). In a study of child welfare institutions, Rindfleisch and Rabb (1984) also reported that only one out of five suspected abuse situations were reported to child protection agencies. Failure to report abuse to authorities is due in large part to over reliance on caregivers and disability factors (Muccigrosso, 1991; Sobsey & Mansell, 1992). This topic will be further discussed in Chapter 12 on Sexual Offenses and the Legal System.

Disability increases probability of sexual abuse

A number of risk factors link disabilities to sexual abuse. These include society's de-sexualized image of people with disabilities, society's myths about individuals who have a developmental disability, the severity of the disability, and communication factors. Sobsey and Varnhagen (1991) contend that in considering the ways in which disability may lead to sexual abuse, it is important to recognize that it is often not the disability that appears to increase risk; it may be society's treatment of that disability. Changing these beliefs may prove to be significant in detecting and reducing the abuse of individuals who have disabilities. However, our underlying cultural beliefs that often devalue people with disabilities and support the use of power and aggression against others may prove among the most difficult factors to modify (Sobsey & Doe, 1991).

Sobsey and Mansell (1993) cite several myths that may contribute to the increased sexual assault of individuals who have a developmental disability. The first of these myths is the *dehumanization myth*: the individual is seen as less than human and the offender sees himself or herself as more human and therefore, more important than the victim. Consequently, the offender sees nothing wrong with exploiting the less valued individual to meet his or her own needs. The second myth is the *damaged merchandise myth*, which provides the offender with a rationalization not only for the choice of victim, but also may alleviate any guilt of inhibition about exploiting an individual who has a developmental disability. The third myth described by Sobsey and Mansell (1993) is the *feeling no pain myth*: some victims may not fully understand what is happening to them, so they may suffer less from abuse. They therefore rationalize their crime by contending that the victim was not really hurt. The fourth myth is the *disabled menace myth*, which portrays individuals who have developmental disabilities as menaces to society who are both dangerous and unpredictable. The offender therefore blames the victim for the abuse, perhaps citing aggressive behaviour on the part of the victim. The final myth is the *helplessness myth*: the perception of vulnerability of the individual who has a developmental disability affects the selection of victims by sex offenders (Sobsey & Mansell, 1993).

Society's de-sexualized image of people with disabilities often results in our failure to recognize the possibility of sexual abuse of children and adults with disabilities (Sobsey & Mansell, 1993). For example, if a physician finds that an adolescent girl is not sleeping well, having difficulties in school, seems fearful of people, and resists physical examination, the physician and caregivers should begin to wonder about the possibility that she is being abused. However, if that child has a diagnosis of mental or emotional disability, the physician may be likely to attribute the symptoms to her disability and therefore be less likely to detect abuse (Sobsey & Mansell, 1993).

Goldman (1994) contends that individuals who have a developmental disability are at risk for abuse because they may be less able to articulate the fact of abuse. They may be unable to differentiate between appropriate and inappropriate physical contact, whether it is sexual or violent. He goes on to declare that they are frequently more dependent on others for care or assistance and therefore more trusting since dependency and trust often translate into compliance and passivity. Individuals who have disabilities may be more reluctant to report instances of abuse for fear of losing vital ties to major care providers. As well, they are likely to be considered less credible than individuals who do not have disabilities when and if they report abuse (Goldman, 1994). This will be further discussed in the chapter on Sexual Offenses and the Legal System.

Zirpoli, Snell, and Loyd (1987) found that the severity of disability and the extent of maladaptive behaviour contributed significantly to risk of abuse among residents of state training centers who had developmental disabilities. This suggests that the degree, as well as the nature, of the impairment may be an important factor in the incidence of abuse (Sobsey & Varnhagen, 1991). Marchetti and McCartney (1990) state that individuals living in institutions and those with higher IQ scores or more adaptive behaviour appear to be at somewhat greater risk for abuse than those with lower IQ scores and less adaptive behaviour. However, this is inconsistent with Rusch, Hall, and Griffin (1986), who found that clients who were abused had lower social quotients than clients who were not abused.

Another major factor in the increased vulnerability of individuals who have developmental disabilities to sexual abuse is impaired communication. Many individuals who have developmental disabilities often lack the ability or opportunity to protest effectively. Deficits in communication among adolescents who have developmental disabilities, children who have physical disabilities, children who have multiple disabilities, and children who have hearing impairments not only reduce the amount of communication, but also heavily influence the content and circumstances of communication (Sobsey & Varnhagen, 1991). All individuals who experience significant communication deficits show very low rates of initiation and often communicate only when responding to others. These individuals would be unlikely to report abuse, particularly if not explicitly asked.

Sobsey (1988) contends that impaired communication skills may lead to greater risk of sexual abuse in two ways. First, individuals who have disabilities and those who have poor communication skills may be simply unable to report an occurrence of sexual abuse. Second, even when abuse is reported and the victim has a disability, it is often not investigated, generally because of the legal issues concerning the acceptability of the testimony of an individual who has a developmental disability. Sobsey (1988) concludes that all of this makes individuals who have developmental disabilities easy marks for offenders. Doe (1990) supports this and states that it is not likely that anyone says "yes" to abuse. It is more likely that someone could not or did not say "no". But it is equally likely that the victim did protest and was still abused. An ability to physically defend oneself may also be a factor. Physical, sensory, and intellectual impairments are all likely to interfere with the individual's abilities to escape or resist abuse (Sobsey

& Varnhagen, 1991).

Some argue that certain characteristics of persons within institutionalized settings provoke abuse by staff (Conway, 1994).
This is called the dependency-stress model of abuse (Sobsey,
1994). In a study of residents in American institutions for people with intellectual disability, Rusch et al. (1986) found that
aggressive residents caused staff to attack back. Ambulatory
residents were more likely to be abused because less mobile
residents were restricted and therefore less likely to rebel.
Younger residents were more likely to challenge staff because
they often had more challenging behaviours than older, more
sedate residents. More dependent residents were found to provoke frustration in staff who were consequently more likely to
abuse them. Finally, self-injurious residents were more likely
to provoke staff abuse in an effort to stop the behaviours. The
solution in part was to ensure that staff had respite time from
residents, together with better training to meet residents' needs
(Rusch et al., 1986). Although this study was about physical
abuse by caregivers, many of these attitudes come into play
when discussing sexual abuse.

In the dependency-stress model of abuse (Sobsey, 1994), the
disability of the individual is thought to increase his or her dependency on caregivers beyond their limited resources for coping with these demands. However, the dependency-stress
model is subject to several important criticisms. First, it can
be viewed as blaming the victims for the actions of the people
who offend against them. Second, this model is not consistent
with many of the empirical findings regarding abuse of individuals who have developmental disabilities. For example, as
described above, placement in settings with multiple caregivers has been found to increase risk rather than reduce it

(Levine Powers et al., 1990; Rindfleisch & Bean, 1988; Rindfleisch & Rabb, 1984). Finally, research connecting disability, dependency, stress, and abuse does not provide a clear demonstration of these relationships (Sobsey, 1994). Consequently, the dependency-stress model of abuse and the findings posited by Rusch et al. (1986) must be considered to be unsupported as a model for identifying abuse of individuals who have a developmental disability.

Gender differences

Sobsey, Randall, and Parrila (1997) found that gender and age differences are apparent for some categories of abuse. The same total numbers of girls and boys are victims of abuse. However, research suggests that boys are more likely to experience more severe forms of physical abuse while girls are more likely to be sexually abused (Sobsey et al., 1997). However, when it comes to the population of individuals who have disabilities, Sobsey et al. (1997) found that twice as many boys who had disabilities were victims of sexual abuse than boys without disabilities. Nevertheless, even among children who have disabilities, girls were more frequently victims of substantiated sexual abuse, whereas all other categories of abuse had more boys than girls as victims. In sum, Sobsey et al. (1997) concluded that female gender is clearly associated with increased risk for sexual abuse. Disability status, in turn, seems to interact with gender and is associated with increased risk for all types of abuse for boys with disabilities (Sobsey et al., 1997).

Researchers have reported a difference in abuse rates in adolescent data as compared to the other age groups (Sobsey et al., 1997). While girls and boys were about equally represented in the younger groups of nondisabled children, adolescent girls were more likely to be victims of substantiated abuse than adolescent boys. In the group who had disabilities, the number of boys also dropped, resulting in about equal distribution of boys and girls in the adolescent sample. However, boys who had disabilities were again over-represented as victims of sexual abuse in relation to their non-disabled peers (Sobsey et al., 1997).

Isolation

The increased vulnerability of individuals who have disabilities has been postulated to be due to the isolation faced by many of these individuals. Doe (1990) asserts that in group homes or institutions where similarly disabled people, including abusive and vulnerable individuals, are placed in relative isolation, abuse between individuals who have disabilities is more likely to occur. Rindfleisch and Bean (1988) support this and state that the risk of being sexually abused within an institutional setting is two to four times as high as for being sexually abused in the community. Therefore, serving more people with disabilities within the community and fewer in institutions may be a powerful prevention strategy. Sobsey and Mansell (1993) contend that for individuals who continue to be served in institutional settings, reducing the isolation of this service delivery system may have similar preventive effects.

Prevention

In a study conducted by Sobsey and Mansell (1992), experts ranked "teaching persons who have disabilities and their service providers the signs of abuse" to be the most important component of abuse detection. However, Sobsey and Varnhagen (1991) assert that it is time for researchers and clinicians to switch their focus from documenting the existence of this problem to developing the appropriate prevention and treatment services for people with disabilities.

An understanding of sexual behaviour is a crucial requirement in ensuring that people with an intellectual disability are protected from sexual assault (Carmody, 1991). While sexual assault is primarily a crime of violence, the sexual component of the assault distinguishes it from other forms of assault. If individuals who have a developmental disability are not made aware of healthy sexuality and their right to choose their own sexual partners and behaviours, the possibility of sexual exploitation is increased. A lack of sex education and opportunities to develop a sexual identity result in confusion and uncertainty about what is acceptable behaviour from other people. Carmody (1991) contends that it is not possible to protect people from sexual assault unless they have an understanding of their own bodies and human anatomy. Any discussion of sexual assault is most useful within a discussion of the range of appropriate sexual behaviours.

Denying individuals who have disabilities access to sex education may produce several related consequences (Sobsey & Mansell, 1993). It may increase the vulnerability of people with disabilities to possible pregnancy and venereal diseases, but also to potential abuse by those who will exploit their lack of knowledge about sexuality. These researchers found cases where sexual abuse was rationalized by offenders as a form of sex education for the victim.

Although the positive aspects of sexuality are integral to sex education, Fifield (1986) contends that there is an ethical responsibility to bring up less positive topics like abuse, harassment, and assault. He feels that omission of such topics neglects the concerns and experiences of the audience and suggests that the facilitator is only concerned with positive sexuality. He goes on to state that little can be done to facilitate disclosure of sexual abuse by individuals who have developmental disabilities if the topic of sexual assault is not raised. Fifield (1986) asserts that sex education is best done within a balanced presentation of the positive and negative aspects of sexuality.

Sobsey (1994) supports this and states that training should be provided to help students understand when to comply and when to refuse the demands of others. They should be taught that no one has a right to hurt or abuse them. Noncompliance with unreasonable requests should be rewarded not punished, and mixed messages should be avoided. Sobsey (1994) goes on to state that because abuse occurs most often in the context of power inequities, empowering vulnerable individuals is a logical approach to abuse prevention. Both treatment and prevention programs must integrate this issue for increased effectiveness (Doe, 1990; Muccigrosso, 1991).

Researchers suggest that prevention training programs may also produce several unwanted side effects (Sobsey & Mansell, 1993). Placing the exclusive responsibility for abuse prevention on those individuals who are likely to be victimized by requiring them to learn to resist abuse, ignores the responsibility for prevention of the remainder of society. It also has the danger of implying that the potential victims are themselves solely responsible for their own victimization. That is, if potential victims fail to prevent sexually abusive or assaultive situations, they may be held responsible for the incident.

Ironically, prevention training programs that intend to help potential victims protect themselves may ultimately contribute to victim blaming (Sobsey & Mansell, 1993).

Training potential victims to avoid or resist abuse has been the standard approach to sexual abuse prevention for some time. Nevertheless, it is unrealistic to expect that any program that places sole responsibility for abuse prevention on potential victims will adequately protect or serve the needs of the disabled (Sobsey & Mansell, 1993). Sobsey (1994) cautions that training can and does help to prevent abuse, but it is important to recognize that many abused people with disabilities, as with other victims of abuse, face extreme power inequities that no amount of individual training can overcome. Therefore, training individuals to resist abuse must be accompanied by efforts to change the administrative, legal, social, and cultural conditions that foster abuse. Program developers need to be aware that training in the area of sexuality will produce little change in the incidence of sexual abuse, or reporting of sexual abuse, so long as no effort is made to address the power imbalance within the setting (Conway, 1994).

Conference Deliberations

The group initially focused on the high incidence of abuse among people who have developmental disabilities in residential settings. The group raised the issue of definition of sexual abuse/assault and how its definition is often compromised when dealing with sexual abuse of persons who have developmental disabilities.

At times, there was confusion about what constitutes abuse and neglect for a person with a disability, merely based upon the attitudes of society on individuals who have disabilities. The ethical challenge that is raised is: Does the person, agency and family apply a different set of values regarding abuse/assault when a person has a disability? And if so, why? How can agencies be advocates for the protection of persons with developmental disabilities? The group discussion involved the following four topics.

1. It was concluded that there is a need to advocate for the recognition of the symptoms of abuse, including "masked symptomatology" in any person with a disabling condition. This information should be available to participants of all ages - children, adolescents, and adults who have disabilities. This population should not be expected to tolerate a higher level of pain, both physical and emotional, than the general population. In addition, we must raise the awareness of the general public, including police, hospitals, and courts, included within the systems that serve and care for them, such as Early Intervention Programs, schools, families, pre-vocational, vocational, and residential settings.

2. It was also agreed that along with the definition of sexual abuse and the importance of providing information to all the key system components, the individual with the disability should be the central person to receive this information. This is the case whether the individual is a child, adolescent, or adult. Issues and rights of privacy, personal boundaries, respect, confidentiality, individual rights, and choices must be integrated into all aspects of the person's education. This attitude should begin at birth and continue through the entire life cycle of the individual.

3. It was the consensus of the group that all components of the health system, whether it be families, schools, or agencies receiving any government funding, must be provided with information regarding abuse and abuse prevention specifically designed for people who have disabilities. This information should be detailed as far as developmental level and age. Each agency therefore has an obligation to provide proactive, self-advocacy, and abuse prevention programs to the individuals that they support.

4. The group also felt that agencies have an obligation to be knowledgeable about crisis intervention and sexual assault sequelae. Therefore, agencies should provide state-of-the-art crisis, long- and short-term treatment to participants who are suspected of having been abused. All persons have a right to treatment and there should be a centralized government Office of Protection and Advocacy that thoroughly investigates the sexual abuse of children and persons with developmental disabilities. This government bureau should also make recommendations for a safe environment and there should be coordination within that bureau amongst all community agencies.

Individuals who have developmental disabilities were the first members in our group to state that they did not have clear information about what constitutes sexual abuse during their early development as a child, adolescence, or as adults. They also felt that they were poorly informed about how to express concerns about sexual mistreatment and how to avoid it. They described their major gaps in knowledge, education, and respect for personal and interpersonal boundaries and privacy. They also stated that issues and attitudes of compliance superseded any accepted internalized concept of entitlement to respect, privacy, personal choice, appropriate boundaries. By late adolescence and early adulthood, most had already experienced some level of abuse or inappropriate behaviours that could have been avoided.

This brings us to recommendations for what can be done to minimize or prevent the sexual abuse of individuals who have a developmental disability. An ecological model of abuse will be presented, as well as recommendations for clinicians and agencies. Abuse can only be understood within a context of power inequities, and attempts must be made to change the legal, administrative, social, and cultural conditions that foster abuse.

Summary

State of the Art

The interactions between offender and victim are characterized by an inequity of power, but this inequity can only be understood by considering the environment in which they interact and the cultural milieu in which they exist (Sobsey & Doe, 1991). Sobsey (1994) presents an integrated ecological model of abuse that examines physical and psychological aspects of the interacting individuals within the context of environmental and cultural factors. It examines power inequity at multiple levels and provides a structural framework for understanding the abuse of individuals who have disabilities.

Sobsey (1994) states that the individual characteristics of victims and offenders must be considered when a developing a model of abuse. These include limited social skills, learned helplessness, and dependency. Abuser characteristics are also integral to the ecological model, but few details are known about those who abuse people who have disabilities due to the low number of convictions and charges against these individuals. However, some trends include the need to exercise control, exposure to abusive models, devaluing attitudes, and impulsive behaviour (Sobsey, 1994).

Perhaps the most important aspect of Sobsey's (1994) model is the interactions and relationships between the abuser and the victim. Individuals who have disabilities who are victimized are often compliant and disempowered (Sobsey, 1994). The asymmetrical nature contributes to the abuse. Environmental factors must also be considered since they can bring people who are likely to be offenders together with people who are likely to be victims.

As stated by Goldman (1994), while the eradication of all abusive behaviour is the ultimate goal, the problem is likely to persist. Nevertheless, educators and support providers can and must take a proactive position to protect vulnerable individuals. Recognition that individuals who have developmental disabilities are particularly vulnerable to abuse places additional responsibility for ensuring protection. An understanding of Sobsey's (1994) integrated ecological model will serve as a basis for the prevention strategies, clinical, and agency implications that follow.

Clinical Implications

While sexually abused individuals who have disabilities suffer from the same feelings, trauma and psychic and physical pain as those who do not have disabilities, the ways in which this suffering presents itself may be different than in the general population. Symptoms of abuse and suspicions of abuse must be widely recognized by individuals, families, system providers, courts, and legislative bodies. These symptoms must be separated from the disability and seen in and of themselves. In all three examples presented earlier in the chapter, the people by ordinary standards displayed symptoms or behaviour that suggested abuse. The assessment and therefore treatment process was not initiated immediately because different standards of care were applied to the individuals who had a developmental disability. There was blatant denial, rationalization, and probably fear of liability for the abuse that superseded the emotional and physical traumas that were so apparent in these individuals. Only when systems integrate knowledge of suspected abuse with established protocols for assessment and treatment, can healing occur.

Sexual abuse can be accompanied by terror, fear, and a feeling of total helplessness (Cohen, 1993). Individuals often report difficulties with sleep, recurrent nightmares, intrusive thoughts, and an inability to feel emotions of any type, especially those associated with intimacy, tenderness, and sexuality. These are all symptoms of Post Traumatic Stress Disorder, which is a very relevant issue for individuals who have a developmental disability. However, the disorder is seldom diagnosed in or treated for victims who have disabilities (Cohen, 1993).

In her work in medical management of Post Traumatic Stress Disorder of individuals who have a developmental disability, Ryan (1992) stresses that treatment of this disorder involves a multi-disciplinary approach. She stresses that goals of treatment include a subjective sense of healing and improvement, reduction and remission of problematic symptoms, desired levels of social functioning, best possible cognitive functioning and best possible physical health. Her five-point protocol includes:

1. Careful use of medications
2. Identification of medical problems
3. Reduction of iatrogenic factors
4. Appropriate psychotherapy
5. Habitation changes (identification of and reduction of triggers of disassociation)

Treatment programs for offenders are also important, since many offenders will repeat their offenses without effective treatment. Treatment for victims is also an important prevention strategy since a significant proportion of victims will become future offenders in the absence of successful treatment. Programs should have the aim of preventing all members of society from becoming offenders, emphasizing social adjustment and attitudes consistent with support rather than exploitation of others (Sobsey & Doe, 1991).

Agency Implications

Traditionally, offenses against individuals who have developmental disabilities have been viewed as isolated occurrences beyond the control of the agencies that are responsible for the services provided (Sobsey & Doe, 1991). However, as more is known regarding the patterns of these offenses, questions of agency responsibility must be addressed. For example, if an agency fails to screen employees for history of abuse, can the agency be held responsible for future abuse committed by that person while in their employ? If an agency clusters known offenders with vulnerable individuals without providing adequate safeguard against assaults, is the agency responsible for the abuse that results? Questions such as these are being considered by courts across North America and agencies are increasingly being held responsible. A further discussion of this topic can be found in Chapters 2 and 3: Sexual Policies in Agencies Supporting Persons who have Developmental Disabilities.

Sobsey and Doe (1991) assert that no agency or institution can be expected to provide an absolutely risk free environment, but every agency must be expected to provide at least the same level of safety available within the community. Failure to provide reasonable safeguards represents carelessness on the part of these agencies and a violation of the rights of the individuals that these agencies serve. Agencies at all levels of functioning - administration, professional, and direct care, have a responsibility to be involved in proactive prevention programs. This can be accomplished through both client and staff training, thorough staff screening procedures, provision of a safe, risk free environment, and agency protocols that require mandatory reporting of sexual assault.

a) Education for Individuals who have Developmental Disabilities

Agencies must provide a philosophical, programmatic, and methodological approach to abuse prevention programs. Environmental constructs must be considered with a view towards creating healthy functioning and a healthy environment. Agencies must also have a sense of responsibility in creating new and efficient methods of proactive intervention and curriculums. Such methods of empowering individuals against vulnerabilities to abuse are essential to adequate program development.

We must then, through proactive prevention programs, intervene so that the vulnerabilities of individuals who have developmental disabilities are reversed and/or reduced substantially. This programmatic exercise can only be created through a holistic approach (a whole person approach). The education and training regarding healthy sexuality and how it is defined for people with disabilities must be a life-long process. It is only through healthy concepts of body image, emotional well-being, appropriate communication, and interpersonal socialization that we can be begin to overcome abuse. Through acknowledgment of the concepts of individualization, love, consent to sexuality, sexual appropriateness, sexual knowledge and use of body parts, building relationships, friendships, safety, freedom from intrusion, and gender identity, we can arrive at definitions of abuse, coercion, force, and inappropriate sexual interaction. As stated by Sobsey and Doe (1991), "The belief that keeping sex a secret from people with disabilities somehow protects them is as unrealistic as it is distasteful" (p. 255). It is through responsible wellness, principles of sex education, and training in all aspects of human development, that we can develop education and training concepts regarding abuse and trauma.

As children who have disabilities grow into young adults, they must learn age-appropriate behaviour (Sobsey, 1994). Many people who have developmental disabilities are subtly encouraged to act in more inappropriate ways than are appropriate for younger children. They may display affection in ways that are inappropriate to their social relationships. For example, it is typically acceptable for a young woman to give her brother a casual goodbye hug, but it is typically unacceptable for her to give the same kind of hugs to her teacher. Often this kind of mildly inappropriate behaviour will be tolerated in individuals who have developmental disabilities and by those who may pass it off as harmless social ignorance. However, this kind of conduct is not harmless because it increases the individual's risk of victimization by others who see the behaviour as a sign of vulnerability or who interpret any show of affection as "sexual seduction" (Sobsey, 1994).

Individuals who have developmental disabilities should also be taught to identify appropriate occasions for compliance and for assertiveness. They should not be taught generalized compliance with everyone for all things. As with victims who do not have disabilities, saying "no" is not always enough. Prevention programs should clearly teach this.

Education plays a key role in risk reduction, but it will only produce significant risk reduction when other interventions are applied concurrently to help equalize the power imbalances between individuals who have disabilities and those who interact with them. Prevention programs are only as good as the sense of empowerment they impart.

b) Staff Education and Training

The importance of education and training applies not only to persons with disabilities but to staff, programs, and agencies at large. Staff members who are providing educational, vocational, residential, and other related services will also benefit from training. It is important for staff to have an early introduction to a clear policy regarding abuse and sexual behaviour. The mere definition of sexual abuse and how it applies to persons with disabilities must be a concept learned and understood by all of the key components of the system. Staff should be trained to recognize and respond appropriately to early signs of abuse, and to their own feelings of aggression or sexual attraction that may arise (Sobsey & Mansell, 1993).

As a resourceful community, agencies must acknowledge high risk factors and vulnerabilities and provide all personnel with knowledge in these areas of concern. Proactively, the social community of friends, family, and the key components of the provider systems must ensure sex education and training for healthy functioning, as well as provide abuse awareness training and education programs. Key systems must recognize that persons with disabilities at all functioning levels and all developmental stages can be taught concepts of loving and learning to be loved in a respectful, appropriate manner. Agencies have a responsibility to utilize available current curricula and to create individual, group, and family training in these areas.

c) Provision of a Risk-Free Environment

Once staff and agencies become educated about sexual abuse and assault of individuals who have developmental disabilities, they may begin to understand how they can provide a safe environment for the individuals they support. Many institutional settings cluster potentially sexually aggressive and vulnerable individuals together with little attention to the prevention of violence. Institutionalization of dangerous individuals may improve safety in the community, but without adequate safeguards to protect vulnerable individuals living in institutional settings. Certainly, violence among residents is rarely tolerated and typically some attempt is made to maintain order, but agencies have failed to recognize their legal obligation to maintain a level of personal safety for the individuals they claim to support (Sobsey & Mansell, 1993).

Environments can bring together people who are likely to be offenders with victims and can create power inequities. Agencies have a responsibility to evaluate and carefully monitor settings that increase limits of high risk and dangerousness as to their security. As well, peers of persons with disabilities with histories of high risk behaviours should be afforded their own training and treatment and should not be provided with opportunities environmentally or personally that would jeopardize the safety of others.

Agencies must also take responsibility for contract staff (Sobsey & Mansell, 1993). For example, many agencies contract for transportation services for their clients. However, Sobsey and Mansell (1992; 1993) have found many cases of these transportation providers sexually assaulting individuals who have a developmental disability. Agencies have an obligation to acknowledge this risk and a responsibility to control it.

Reducing the isolation of individuals in group home settings is another preventative measure that agencies should endorse. The privacy of individuals living in institutions and group homes is a significant concern (Sobsey & Mansell, 1993), but research indicates that isolation from society increases risk and inclusion in society decreases it (Sobsey, 1994). Agencies cannot entirely eliminate risk for the individuals they support, but they do have an obligation to provide a level of safety that is similar to the level provided for individuals who do not have disabilities (Sobsey & Mansell, 1993). Agencies and staff have a responsibility to take reasonable precautions to reduce the risk of abuse for the individuals they support.

d) Thorough Staff Screening Procedures

Perhaps the best way of ensuring a safe environment is through the implementation of strict staff screening and hiring procedures. Support providers working with persons who have disabilities should be carefully and routinely screened concerning their professionalism and trustworthiness. Yet, Sobsey and Mansell (1993) have found that in a number of cases, sex offenders have been known to take jobs providing personal care to individuals who have disabilities in institutions, group homes, and private residences. Although the number of applicants who are sex offenders is small, the number of potential victims per offender allowed into the system is large, posited at likely 100 or more (Sobsey & Mansell, 1993). Therefore, careful and thorough reference and police checks are essential to a screening process. Employers in the service delivery system need to be both sensitive to the problems produced by sexual abuse of people with disabilities and conscientious about screening staff in order to prevent it.

Sobsey and Mansell (1993) go on to state that in the past, many abusers have been allowed to resign from an agency rather than face charges for their offenses. Unfortunately, many of these individuals move on to another service delivery setting and continue to abuse the individuals in their care. It is therefore imperative that whenever possible, charges are laid and convictions are obtained. This will prevent the possibility of abusers moving from agency to agency. When employees leave an agency because of concerns over the nature of their interactions with service consumers, it is imperative that this concern be included in any reference information provided to prospective future employers.

e) Mandatory Reporting of Sexual Assault

All agencies should have a protocol for suspected abuse and treatment of the abuse. This protocol should be guided by state-of-the-art assessment and treatment programs. There should be a state or federal agency that provides a comprehensive protocol for suspicion of abuse. This protocol should have mandated policies and procedures regarding reporting, as well as a protocol for providing safety for the person whom is suspected of being abused.

Along with this protocol, there should be a written and practical set of guidelines for crisis intervention, sexual assault counselling, and clinical and therapeutic procedures for intervention. Each agency should have an in-house Sociosexual Committee that mandates procedures and policies for investigation, assessment and treatment, as well as follow-up. Agencies may develop an investigating committee that is composed of professionals and/or administrative personnel who are not directly involved with the program. Some agencies may follow a protocol that involves community and outside governmental agencies and supports which would provide on-site technical assistance to crisis intervention, assessment, and treatment.

The most important aspect of an agency's responsibility is to remove the victim from harm's way and provide intervention that will yield a comprehensive assessment and treatment plan that will ensure safety and appropriate intervention. This protocol must be utilized in a manner that involves state-of-the art knowledge and adaptation for persons with disabilities and their family. If there is no existing mandate, each agency has a current obligation to create policies and procedures that integrate the accumulation of the best available knowledge in the field. Part of licensure and accreditation of the agency should be dependent upon the adequate development of such a protocol, and the comprehensive and responsible operation of its articles and procedures. Failure to provide such a protocol with a viable committee to exercise its principles should result in the agency's suspension of licensure or accreditation. There will be further discussion of the need for agency protocol for reporting sexual assault in the chapter on Sexual Offenses and the Legal System.

What Should Be Done Now

Lowering risk factors and empowering individuals through prevention, education, training, assessment, and treatment, if sexual abuse does occur, can be successfully accomplished. Implementing known options that are available, such as educational component assessment and treatments, as well as how they can be adapted to current trends of treatment can be utilized. On-going support services to individuals, families, educators, and agencies must be coordinated according to general standards of care. Following through of guidelines regarding the standards of care must be mandated through a Central Office of Protection and Advocacy to disperse, recommend state-of-the-art prevention assessment and treatment. These concepts can only attempt to minimize the impact of abuse.

Training is effective in reducing and preventing abuse; however it must be recognized that many abused individuals who have disabilities, as with other victims of abuse, face power inequities that no amount of individual training can change (Sobsey, 1994). Moreover, placing the exclusive responsibility for abuse prevention on those individuals who are likely to be victimized by requiring them to learn to resist abuse disregards the accountability of the rest of society for the problem. It also implies that potential victims are themselves solely responsible for their own victimization (Sobsey, 1994). Therefore, training individuals to resist abuse must be accompanied by efforts to change the administrative, legal, social, and cultural conditions that foster abuse.

Final Consensus Statement

Prevention of sexual assault requires early and pragmatic intervention . It involves systemic, programmatic, and personal cooperation and collaboration. Preventative measures include individual, group, family, administrative, and legal review. Individuals who have developmental disabilities and who are victims of sexual assault must be consulted and involved in the development and delivery of services. It is vital that services be accessible to all, appropriate, flexible, and integrated with services for consumers without disabilities (Sobsey & Doe, 1991).

References

Carmody, M. (1991). Invisible victims: Sexual assault of people with an intellectual disability. *Australia and New Zealand Journal of Developmental Disabilities, 17(2),* 229-236.

Cohen, M. V. (1993). Sexual abuse and post-traumatic stress disorder. *Sexuality and Disability, 11(4),* 255-257.

Conway, R. N. F. (1994). Abuse and intellectual disability: A potential link or an inescapable reality. *Australia and New Zealand Journal of Developmental Disabilities, 19(3),* 165-171.

Doe, T. (1990). Towards an understanding: An ecological model of abuse. *Developmental Disabilities Bulletin, 18* (2), 13-20.

Fifield, B. B. (1986). Ethical issues related to sexual abuse of disabled persons. *Sexuality & Disability, 7(3/4)*, 102-109.

Goldman, R. L. (1994). Children and youth with intellectual disabilities: Targets for sexual abuse. *International Journal of Disability, Development, and Education, 41(2)*, 89-102.

Griffiths, D. (1999). Sexuality and people with developmental disabilities: Mythconceptions and facts. In I. Brown & M. Percy (Eds.), *Developmental disabilities in Ontario* (pp. 443-451). Toronto, ON: Front Porch Publishing.

Griffiths, D., Baxter, J., Haslam, T., Richards, D., Stranges, S., & Vyrostko, B. (1995). *Building healthy boundaries project*. Unpublished manuscript.

Lakin, K. C., Bruininks, R. H., Hill, B. K., & Hauber, F. A. (1982). Turnover rate of direct-care staff in a national sample of residential facilities for mentally retarded people. *American Journal of Mental Deficiency, 87,* 64-72.

Levine Powers, J., Mooney, A., & Nunno, M. (1990). Institutional abuse: A review of the literature. *Journal of Child and Youth Care, 4(6)*, 81-95.

Marchetti, A. G. & McCartney, J. R. (1990). Abuse of persons with mental retardation: Characteristics of the abused, the abusers, and the informers. *Mental Retardation, 6,* 367-371.

Muccigrosso, L. (1991). Sexual abuse prevention strategies and programs for persons with developmental disabilities. *Sexuality and Disability, 9(3)*, 261-271.

Rindfleisch, N. & Bean, G. J. (1988). Willingness to report abuse and neglect in residential facilities. *Child Abuse and Neglect, 12,* 509-520.

Rindfleisch, N. & Rabb, J. (1984). How much of a problem is resident maltreatment in child welfare institutions? *Child Abuse and Neglect, 8,* 36-38.

Rusch, R. G., Fall, J. C., & Griffin, H. C. (1986). Abuse-provoking characteristics of institutionalized mentally retarded individuals. *American Journal of Mental Deficiency, 90(6),* 618-624.

Ryan, R. (1992, December). Post traumatic stress syndrome: Assessing and treating the aftermath of sexual assault. *National Association for Dual Diagnosis conference proceedings.* (pp. 8-11). New York: National Association for Dual Diagnosis.

Sobsey, D. (1988). Sexual victimization of people with disabilities: Professional and social responsibilities. *Alberta Psychology, 17(6)* 8-9.

Sobsey, D. (1994). *Violence and abuse in the lives of people with disabilities: The end of silent acceptance?* Baltimore, MD: Paul H. Brookes Publishing Co.

Sobsey, D. (1995). Enough is enough: There is no excuse for a hundred years of violence against people with disabilities. In D. Sobsey, D. Wells, R. Lucardie, & S. Mansell (Eds.), *Violence and disability: An annotated bibliography.* (pp. ix- xvii). Baltimore, MD: Paul H. Brookes Publishing Co.

Sobsey, D. & Doe, T. (1991). Patterns of sexual abuse and assault. *Sexuality & Disability, 9(3),* 243-259.

Sobsey, D. & Mansell, S. (1992). The prevention of sexual abuse of people with developmental disabilities. *Network, 2(3),* 8-17.

Sobsey, D. & Mansell, S. (1993). The prevention of sexual abuse of people with developmental disability. In M. Nagler (Ed.), *Perspectives on disability* (pp. 283-292). Palo Alto, CA: Health Marketing Research.

Sobsey, D. Randall, W., & Parrila, R. K. (1997). Gender differences in abused children with and without disabilities. *Child Abuse & Neglect, 21(8)*, 707-719.

Sobsey, D. & Varnhagen, C. (1991). Sexual abuse, assault, and exploitation of Canadians with disabilities. In C. Bagley, R. J. Thomlinson (Eds.), *Child sexual abuse: Critical perspectives on prevention, intervention, and treatment* (pp. 203-216). Toronto, ON: Wall and Emerson.

Ticoll, M. & Panitch, M. (1993). Opening the doors: Addressing the sexual abuse of women with an intellectual disability. *Canadian Woman Studies, 13(4)*, 84-87.

Zirpoli, T. J., Snell, M. E., & Loyd, B. H. (1987). Characteristics of persons with mental retardation who have been abused by caregivers. *The Journal of Special Education, 21(2)*, 31-41.

Chapter 9

Inappropriate Sexual Behaviour: Inherent or Taught?

Marc Goldman and Orson Morrison

Introduction

Inappropriate behaviour has historically implied that a problem exists within the individual. When someone who has a developmental delay is described as "a behaviour problem", he or she is often subject to a myriad of treatments and restrictions. Habilitation may focus on elimination of misbehaviour at the expense of maximizing strengths, social skills, and independence. When the inappropriate behaviour is of a sexual nature these problems are often multiplied.

This chapter will survey some of the ethical issues concerning inappropriate sexual behaviour. The task group was asked to reach consensus on several controversial issues involving sexual misbehaviour. One challenge was to determine why sexual misbehaviour appears to be over represented in the population of people with developmental disabilities. Is this over representation due to characteristics inherent in developmental delay, characteristics of the support system, characteristics of the treatment system, or a combination of factors?

Case Examples

1. Two individuals living in a large community agency are discovered having consensual sexual relations. The facility has a clear policy that prohibits such activity. The support workers request that behaviour programs be written to address the behavior.
2. A male, when introduced to a female peer, places his hand on her breast.
3. A male resident of a group home is sent home from his job because he reported for work wearing women's clothing.
4. Two residents of a group home are discovered having sexual relations in a public park.
5. The administrator of a thirty bed co-ed institution for individuals who have developmental delay, mental health needs and criminal charges is informed that "safeguards" must be built into the program designed to discourage consensual sexual activity.
6. A woman with developmental delay is frequently observed masturbating in public.
7. A group home resident is found viewing a pornographic video in the home.

Discussion was facilitated through the presentation of the following scenarios.

Literature Review

Three years prior to becoming president of The American Association for The Study of the Feeble Minded, Henry Hubert

Goddard published "proof" that "feebleminded women" were a threat to society. Goddard (1912) claimed to have scrutinized two lineages of offspring fathered by Martin Kallikak Sr.; 480 descendents of a union between Martin and a woman believed to have developmental delay compared to descendants of his marriage with an individual of normal mental abilities (Goddard, 1912). Goddard (1912) claimed that descendants of the legitimate family were all of good character: "Indeed, in this family and its collateral branches, we find nothing but good representative citizenship." Of the descendants between Mr. Kallikak Sr. and the woman believed to have developmental delay, Goddard submitted dramatic findings, claiming that many were "feebleminded." He observed that many were prostitutes, criminals, perverts, paupers, horse thieves, and whorehouse madams (Perske, 1995). Henry Hubert Goddard warned, "There are Kallikak families all about us. They are multiplying at twice the rate of the general population, and not until we recognize this fact, and work on this basis, will we begin to solve these social problems." Goddard went on to propose a systematic solution; he submitted that any individual who threatened the better "human stock" should be separated from society and barred from reproduction (Smith, 1985.)

In 1924, a leader of the Eugenic Records Office, Harry Laughlin, shaped a sterilization law for the state of Virginia. The first individual designated for sterilization under the new law was Carrie Buck. She challenged constitutional support for the state's intrusion of a citizen's procreation pursuits. The case progressed to the Supreme Court, which upheld the right of state government to forbid reproduction of those determined to be defective in some way.

The majority opinion, delivered by Justice Oliver Wendell Holmes, set the stage for the sterilization of 50,000 people in the United States (Perske, 1995). He said: "It is better for all the world, if instead of waiting to execute degenerate offspring for crime, or to let them starve for their imbecility, society can prevent those who are manifestly unfit from continuing their kind. The principles that sustain compulsory vaccination is broad enough to cover cutting the Fallopian tubes...Three generations of imbeciles are enough."

The predominate twentieth century perception of sexuality of individuals having developmental delay as perilous to society appears to have remnants of influence. As the trend moved from control through institutionalization to one of treatment for inappropriate sexual conduct, behaviour modification procedures were all but exclusively utilized until the late 1960's. The goal of these "treatments" was often the elimination of sexual behaviour through aversive methods. Researchers published case studies demonstrating success at eliminating undesirable behaviour through a variety of punishments. Despite knowledge within the field of behavioural learning that teaching and rewarding functional replacement behaviour were most effective, such an approach was rarely followed (Griffiths, Quinsey, & Hingsburger, 1989). It appeared that behavioural control was the accepted practice. Treatment designed to result in permanent, adaptive change, was not considered when dealing with aberrant behaviours of a sexual nature.

Opportunity for people with developmental disabilities to reside in normal community settings has resulted in considerable growth potential for individuals and communities. While people are demonstrating that they have capabilities that far exceed prior expectations, the deinstitutionalization process has also illuminated social deficiencies among some people with developmental delay (Kempton, 1998). Communities hold citizens accountable for their actions in ways quite different than institutions supporting individuals with developmental delay. In addition to being "treated" for misbehaviours with behaviour plans and medications, the individual residing in the community risks serious legal sanctions when they violate community standards.

Barbaree and Marshall (1998) organized treatment of individuals who have committed sexual crimes into three categories. *Organic treatments* usually involve administration of drugs that lower male hormone levels. This approach attempts to control deviant sexual behaviour through reduction of sexual urges (Bradford, 1985). The effectiveness of this approach remains uncertain. There are problematic side effects and drop out rates are high (Barbaree & Marshall, 1998). *Nonbehavioural Psychotherapy* includes divergent orientations and procedures. These include psychodynamic, individual, and group treatment as well as treatments that focus on social competency. Barbaree and Marshall (1998) note that there appears to be a shift away from application of nonbehavioural psychotherapy techniques to the exclusion of alternative approaches. *Comprehensive Cognitive-Behavioural Therapy* assumes that sexual crimes are the result of multiple influences. These influences must all be addressed in order to reduce risk of recidivism. Cognitive, physiological, socioeconomic, behavioural, social, as well as historical variables, are all included in this approach.

Authors in the field of developmental disabilities have emphasized the need to evaluate the multiple factors that influence aberrant behaviour. In their treatment manual for self-injurious behaviour, Gardner and Sovner (1994) emphasized that the first task in designing treatment interventions is development of interrelated formulations that consider the influence of bio-medical, social, and psychological variables. A clinical manual by Griffiths, Gardner, and Nugent (1998) described an inte-grated approach to challenging behaviour that investigates the potential interactions of biomedical, psychological, and social/environmental influences. Gardner, Graeber, and Machkovitz (1988) stressed that treatment programs for individuals having developmental delay and criminal behaviours should focus on the numerous personal characteristics and skill deficits. The multiple factor approach described by the above authors closely parallels the cognitive-behavioural approach to treat-ment of sex offenders - that sexual crimes are the result of multiple influences. All influences must be addressed in order to reduce the risk of recidivism.

Haaven, Little, and Petre-Miller (1990) described a residential treatment program for sex offenders having developmental dis-abilities. Underlying assumptions included that all behaviour in the program environment is relevant for treatment and that every resident was capable of taking responsibility for, and understanding, their own behaviour. The program imple-mented modified cognitive-behavioural techniques used with offenders without intellectual impairment as well as addressing habilitative needs. They maintained that clinical elements of such treatment should include a "multidiagnostic, holistic ap-proach" that empowers clients to participate in their own treat-ment. Teaching and treatment were carried out in an environ-ment that enriched learning. They concluded that specialized treatment impacted criminal activity and that recidivism was inversely related to length of time in treatment.

Individuals with developmental disabilities appear to be over represented within the population of sex offenders (Day, 1993). Although the overwhelming majority of people with developmental delay do not engage in sexual offenses, over representation might be attributed to multiple influences. Influences such as impaired mental abilities and adaptive skills (Day, 1997) are inherent in individuals with developmental delay. Additional variables, which potentially contribute to aberrant sexual behaviour, can be attributed to systems responsible for the support and treatment of such individuals.

Griffiths et al. (1989) argued that a lack of appropriate sexual development might be the result of multiple systemic influences. Absence of a normal learning environment, segregation from the community, restrictive and punitive sexual policies, lack of privacy, lack of sexual education and responsibility training, poor partner selection, and societal attitudes, all contribute to lagging development of sexuality. They maintained that modification of sexual misbehaviour can generally occur through implementation of positive teaching and counselling techniques but they noted that individuals engaging in paraphilic behaviours would require additional interventions.

Furey and Niesen (1994) submitted that "institutional abuse" results from practices that prevent residents from appropriate learning about, and/or expression of sexuality. Such practices included prohibition of sexual expression, segregation by gender, absence of sex education, and sexual abuse by staff and peers. They suggested that such abuse was not limited to those residing in institutions.

The restriction of sexual freedom has been one of the major areas of historical infringement of rights and freedoms of individuals with developmental delay. These restrictions have resulted in significant emotional and behavioural problems (Mayer & Poindexter, 1997). Mayer and Poindexter (1997) encouraged discontinuation of the imposition of "super human" standards of sexual restriction on people with developmental delay, stating that "artificial environments tend to produce artificial behaviour."

In 1991, Hingsburger, Griffiths, and Quinsey submitted that sexually offensive behaviours, regardless of the level of intrusiveness, do not always result from deviant arousal. They suggested that in some cases sexual misbehaviour is the only type of sexual behaviour in the individual's repertoire. They coined the term "counterfeit deviance" to describe behaviours that appear deviant upon initial observation but can be attributed to factors other than deviant arousal upon closer analysis. Although safety of community members remains a constant priority, selection of treatment modalities will vary greatly, dependent on whether the behaviour is due to deviant arousal or other variables. They discouraged clinicians from making assumptions about an individual, based solely on the "look" of the offensive behaviour. They concluded that incidents of counterfeit deviance would continue until the service system provided living situations that promoted normal sexual expression.

Dementral (1993) presented an Ecological Assessment Inventory designed to assist in determining if an individual's inappropriate sexual behaviour was attributable to counterfeit deviance. Through a series of inquiries, the assessment attempts to determine if the aberrant behaviour results from the individual's interaction between one or more systems in the environment. Treatment strategy is designed to impact the individual's "system" as well as the individual. Treatment is developed after all the potential sources of "counterfeit deviance" have been investigated.

The World Health Organization (1975) conceptualizes sexual health as, "...freedom from fear, shame, guilt, false beliefs and other psychological factors inhibiting sexual response and impairing sexual relationships." People with developmental delay often live in systems that have considerable power over individual behaviour. If such systems fail to develop comprehensive sexuality policies, decision making power falls into the hands of staff who must make decisions on a case by case basis (Hingsburger, 1994). In such situations sexual health, as defined by the World Health Organization cannot be achieved. The Association for Community Living (1994) developed a policy handbook on sexuality concerning people having developmental disabilities. The handbook emphasizes training of support staff and consumers. Policies clearly describe responsibilities of consumers and staff on a variety of subjects related to sexuality. An underlying assumption of the handbook is that sexual expression is a guaranteed right as well as a matter of personal choice. The authors contend that agencies providing residential supports should offer education opportunities concerning sexual issues to the same degree that opportunities for personal development are offered in other areas of growth.

Conference Deliberations

The task group discussed each scenario outlined at the beginning of the chapter. This was done individually and the group arrived at consensus on several issues.

In some situations, inappropriate behaviour is defined by agency policy rather than by law, violation of social norms, or victimization. Just as juveniles can be found guilty of crimes based on their age (i.e., consuming alcohol), people with developmental delay are vulnerable to status offenses. That is, a behaviour is considered inappropriate simply because the individual has a developmental disability or lives in an environment in which the behaviour cannot be coined out in private.

Many agencies and institutions have policies that prohibit sexual activity between consenting adults. These policies are created for a variety of reasons including the false belief that people with developmental delay are eternal children incapable of understanding what they are doing. Such prohibitive policies are also established based on the equally false assumption that individuals who have a developmentally disability are sexually dangerous. Some prohibitive policies are based on issues of liability and/or parental pressure.

Although one group member argued that an agency/facility is a subculture that may establish rules defining any sexual activity as inappropriate, the majority maintained that consensual sex between two adults in a private setting is not inappropriate regardless of agency/facility policy.

Several group members noted that their experience had been that whenever an agency had policies prohibiting consensual sexual activity, "inappropriate" sexual activity occurred. When privacy was not provided or allowed, sexual activity took place in areas that society prohibits (i.e., parks, stairwells, parking lots, etc.). Thus, illegal or inappropriate sexual activity in public places may occur, at least in some cases, due to policy rather than characteristics inherent in individuals with developmental delay. This is an example of how the system providing supports paradoxically encourages "counterfeit" deviant behaviour in individuals.

The consensus was that sexuality is a basic human right that agencies/facilities should not prohibit. Some participants suggested that agencies that prohibit sexual behaviour between consenting adults could be legally challenged as violating basic human rights. Although consensus on pursuing litigation in such cases was not reached, it was agreed that agencies were in need of education and challenge of their prohibitory practices.

Regardless of policy, an individual engaging in consensual sex should never be described as someone who engages in inappropriate sexual behaviour and in need of a behaviour management plan. Comprehensive assessment of sexual behaviour considered problematic should occur in order to determine the multiple factors influencing the behaviour. Agency policy and other environmental factors influencing such behaviour should be addressed, as well as personal characteristics of the individual.

Some group members were aware of agencies that tend to overlook sexual behaviour rather than deal with the many ramifications of acknowledging such behaviour. These agencies were described as being particularly motivated to avoid parental concerns. When a parent discovered that their adult child had engaged in consensual sex, the consumers were frequently separated by the agency in an attempt to "appease" the parent. One danger inherent in overlooking sexual behaviour rather than following clear guidelines is that non-consensual sexual behaviour (sexual offending) is not identified. The victim of non-consensual activity might continue to experience abuse while the offender is "overlooked." The offender may learn that his behaviour is acceptable or that the only consequence is a move to another residential setting with new opportunities to victimize others.

The group agreed that considerably more effort should be directed toward the education of parents. This effort should not simply be directed at sexual issues but also toward helping parents to understand that the individual is an adult with specific rights, needs, and responsibilities. Bluntly informing parents that they have no right to influence the sexual behaviour of their adult child can result in alienation from the treatment team and jeopardize treatment. The group agreed that this education process should be done with sensitivity and respect. Such education should not be dependent on the individual expressing interest in sex but should be incorporated into general information given to parents when they begin to learn about developmental delay and should continue throughout their relationship with service providers. Such an approach would encourage teaching concepts such as privacy and consent as well as providing opportunities for the individual to develop additional sociosexual skills.

The group agreed that an individual with developmental delay has the right to express sexuality according to his or her sexual orientation. Policies concerning sexuality of individuals with developmental delay should respect sexual preference.

After reaching consensus on the issue of expression of sexual behaviour as a basic human right that should not be labeled as inappropriate, the group discussed behaviours that society labels deviant. They acknowledged that some individuals with developmental delay engage in dangerous predatory behaviours that necessitate confinement. Other individuals who engage in sexual misbehaviour are not predators. They engage in such behaviours due to a variety of factors. Regardless of behaviour dynamics, a thorough assessment of risk should be completed to determine the least restrictive setting in which the individual can safely reside. Care should be taken not to mistake someone who has skill and/or knowledge deficits with an anti-social predator who has deviant arousal.

It is not uncommon for professionals in both the human services and criminal justice fields to regard anyone who has engaged in sexual misbehaviour as untreatable and in need of permanent incapacitation. An individual with developmental delay who engages in inappropriate sexual behaviour may require close supervision in order to protect the community. This does not imply, however; that the individual is incapable of ever learning socially acceptable sexual behaviour. Upon successful completion of treatment, many may be capable of safely living in the community in a less restrictive setting.

The group believed that a significant number of individuals with developmental delay engage in sexual misbehaviours in response to characteristics of their environments rather than inherent factors. While acknowledging legal reporting responsibilities, they were reluctant to recommend immediate legal action or punitive behavioural interventions . The group's proposed alternatives to the aforementioned "knee-jerk" response was a comprehensive assessment of the individual. The assessment should include, but not be limited to, the following:

Review of agency policy

Restrictive rules that might have influenced sexual behaviour should be considered. Although it is hoped that restrictive policies be reconsidered, understanding how such external environmental factors influenced aberrant sexual behaviour should be the focus of the review. This of course assumes that the behaviour violated norms. It is possible that the behaviour was influenced by policies from previously involved agencies.

Review of historical information

A thorough understanding of the individual is crucial to development and application of effective treatment interventions. It is often beneficial to investigate historical as well as current social and environmental conditions. After carefully reviewing all available records, effort should focus on resolving significant contradictory information, filling lapses of time, and obtaining as much additional detail as possible. Detailed information should be obtained from the individual of interest as well as people who were involved with the individual in the past. Specific reasons for termination from community activities, jobs, schools, and/or residential settings warrant investigation. Past and/or current psychological, physical, and/or sexual abuse should be investigated. The individual's recollection of his or her early sexual experiences is often of significant value. The person's reaction, as well as the environment's reaction (i.e., family, teachers, staff, etc.) to those experiences should be determined.

Context in which the behaviour occurred

Police reports are useful. Additional information should always be obtained from multiple sources including the individual and staff present at the time of the behaviour. One author is familiar with a case where a man having moderate mental retardation was detained in jail for ten months as a result of criminal charges of attempted rape. Close investigation, including confirmation from a staff member from his previous residential setting, revealed that he was attempting to "fuel the fires" in his sexual partner of twenty years. She was recovering from a fall and cerebral accident. The "offender" was enrolled in a treatment group comprised of sex offenders of normal intelligence.

Destabilizers that influenced the behaviour

Influences on the behaviour such as drugs, alcohol, mental illness, mood dysphoria, and environmental conditions should be assessed.

Personal characteristics

Numerous person specific characteristics can influence aberrant sexual behaviour. Some individuals lack understanding of community standards and expectations. For others, lack of sociosexual skills, education, and/or experience are contributory factors. Behavioural learning and maintenance, impulse control, and possible medical influences should be included in the review. If deviant arousal is under consideration or established, an offense-specific evaluation should be completed by a qualified professional familiar with people having intellectual impairment.

The group noted that in many cases, there are two victims when an incident of sexual misbehaviour occurs. Not only is the recipient of the abuse in need of support and treatment, but the perpetrator may also need help. The consensus was that the individual who engaged in the inappropriate behaviour towards another could be a victim of the systems designed to support him or her. It was the belief of the group that the traditional repressive attitude and lack of education of sexuality for people with developmental delay often results in such victimization.

The group acknowledged a lack of treatment resources and an urgent need for them. They agreed that the treatment team is responsible for providing appropriate treatment, and needs to acknowledge "ownership" of their responsibility to treat sexual misbehaviour. They concluded that treatment teams must develop their own expertise and design treatment and prevention programs, rather than waiting for additional resources that are currently in short supply. Advances in treatment will require that professionals familiar with working with individuals having developmental disabilities design, implement, and evaluate sex offense specific treatment.

The group predicted resistance from their own agencies and the community if they became more active in treating inappropriate sexual behaviour. At least two group members, one working in a community residential facility in Canada and the other previously employed in a state hospital in the United States, had been told by their supervisors that any treatment of sexual misbehaviour would have to be carried out discreetly. Both were informed that the mandate for clandestine treatment was based on administrative concerns that the agency/facility would come to be known as a resource for the treatment of individuals who engaged in inappropriate sexual behaviour. Such a reputation was perceived by the administrators as undesirable. The group adamantly maintained that treatment teams must insist on providing such treatment and oppose the policy of incarceration of all offenders in lieu of treatment.

In discussing the issue of public masturbation, the group again declined repressive behavioural management techniques. There was consensus that the treatment team must take responsibility for treatment. The first step in providing such treatment would, once again, be a comprehensive assessment. The group suggested considering the following variables:

The group's attention was directed toward medical issues, specifically how adaptation could be mistaken for maladaptive behaviour. The individual could possibly be suffering from a vaginal ailment and attempting to alleviate discomfort. The group agreed medical issues should always be ruled out prior to considering other hypotheses. It was noted that obtaining thorough medical evaluations was difficult in some settings but that the treatment team is responsible for assuring that they are performed.

The last scenario reviewed by the group concerned a man with developmental delay, residing in a group home, who was sent home from work because he wore female attire. As with previous scenarios, the group agreed that a behaviour plan was not required. It was felt that the residential agency and staff had several responsibilities in this situation:

1. Protect the individual's right to dress as he sees fit (within legal parameters).
2. Assure that the individual understands the possible conse-

quences of his behaviour.

3. Educate the workplace and the community concerning individual rights and choice.

4. Train staff on issues of rights, choice, and non-judgmental intervention.

5. Develop fair and humane policies and guidelines concerning issues of sexual behaviour.

Summary

The State of the Art

The consensus group considering inappropriate sexual behaviour, with representatives from Canada and the United States, suggested that current practices are disturbing and often contribute to sexual misbehaviour. Many, but not all, agencies and facilities lack policies on sexual behaviour that promote sexual health. Prohibiting or ignoring sexual behaviour will often result in inappropriate behaviour, as defined by the agency and/or society.

Some agencies are reluctant to provide any treatment for individuals who engage in sexual misbehaviour or to publicly acknowledge that they do so. Underreporting aberrant sexual behaviour permits continued predatory behaviour and prevents both the victim and the offender from receiving treatment.

Some professionals in the field who acknowledge the need for treatment of individuals who engage in inappropriate sexual behaviour are reluctant to advocate for such service due to their employers' preference to avoid involvement in that aspect of habilitation and treatment.

There appears to be a reluctance to educate parents concerning sexuality of individuals with developmental delay until their loved one expresses interest in sex.

With rare exceptions, research aimed at promoting sexual health of people with developmental disability is nonexistent.

Clinical Implications

It is significant to note that the group suggested that treatment teams should initially attempt to assess and treat clients who engage in sexual misbehaviour without clinical consultation. The reasons for this tendency to avoid clinical expertise can only be speculated upon, as the question was not brought before the group. It may simply be due to the difficulty treatment providers encounter when they attempt to locate clinicians willing to deal with such challenges. Another possibility could be that team members have been disappointed in the clinical services that they have experienced. The historical tendency toward repression and punitive practices may also be a factor. There is a need for clinicians to investigate and remediate this issue. They will have to inform service providers about how they can assist in managing sexual misbehaviour and assist individuals with developmental delay from living in increasingly restrictive settings.

The authors do not condone the group's avoidance of clinical support. Clinicians experienced in sexuality as well as individuals having developmental disabilities are essential to assessment and development of intervention strategies.

Clinicians also have an important role in educating agencies, facilities, and parents. This information should include general issues of sexuality, for people with developmental delay, multi-factor explanations of sexual misbehaviour, and the ramifications of repressive and punitive approaches to sexuality. Such training should be done with respect to the sensitivity of the issues.

Clinicians who take on this challenge can expect to meet with resistance from all systems. The process of changing the current mindset concerning the sexuality of people with developmental delay will be slow, but necessary, if gains are to be made in the reduction of sexual misbehaviour.

Agency Implications

Some agencies respect the rights of people with developmental disability to appropriately express their sexuality and have policies that promote sexual health. Unfortunately, many agencies continue to prohibit sexual expression or ignore it. Prohibiting sexual expression will continue to result in individuals engaging in sexual behaviour in secret, dangerous, and maladaptive ways. Telling an individual that feelings of sexuality are "wrong" will result in lower self-esteem. Such agencies are at risk of being held accountable for human rights violations. Ignoring sexual behaviour puts individuals at risk of maladaptive learning and victimization.

What Should Be Done Now

Effort should be directed at education of all people supporting individuals with developmental delay. This education should emphasize the need to eliminate repressive and punitive approaches concerning sexuality directed toward people with developmental delay.

Research efforts should be directed toward establishing education curricula that are effective in reducing sexual misbehaviour and in refining assessment techniques that distinguish individuals who engage in counterfeit deviance from sexual predators. Incentives should be made available to encourage systematic assessment of treatment efficacy.

Agencies should develop policies and procedures that promote the sexual health of individuals with developmental disability. Agencies that modify current restrictive practices can expect resistance from parents, staff and community members. Concerns must be treated with respect, keeping in mind that issues of sexuality are often laden with emotion. Legal consultation should be sought to clarify issues of liability.

Criminal justice system personnel should be given information that will assist them to understand that many individuals with developmental delay who engage in sexual misbehaviour, although in need of treatment and possibly restricted freedom, are not all predators requiring incarceration. When courts order treatment, such treatment should be mandated to make reasonable accommodations for the individual having intellectual impairment. Collaborative efforts with the criminal justice system should develop a consistent approach to addressing aberrant sexual behaviour in the community. The courts should obtain evaluations of offenders by clinicians experienced in sexuality and disability. Such evaluations should include security needs as well as suggestions for effective treatment interventions. Careful court monitoring of individuals released on probation with Probation Officers sensitive to the issues should occur when warranted.

Clinicians should focus on assisting residential settings to design environments and policies that promote sexual health rather than inappropriate behaviour. The clinician providing treatment for individuals who have engaged in sexual misbehaviour should work closely with support staff. Treatment should extend beyond what transpires in the clinician's office. Support staff should implement techniques designed to enhance and generalize what is discussed in treatment sessions. Learning will be facilitated if the individual reviews subject matter through multiple modalities. For instance, the client in treatment might make posters at home illustrating the consequences of aberrant behaviour. The client in latter stages of treatment might regularly discuss with support staff his/her plan for avoiding high-risk situations. Such strategies will only occur when agencies acknowledge the seriousness of the behaviour and the importance of treatment.

Final Consensus Statement

Inappropriate sexual behaviour is often arbitrarily defined by treatment providers and others interested in the well being of people with developmental delay. Policies designed to prohibit and/or punish consensual sex result in sexual misbehaviour, victimization, and undermines self-esteem. Parents of individuals with developmental disabilities, residential agency and facility administrators and staff, and criminal justice personnel need to understand the complex issues of sexuality and people with developmental delay. Prior to labeling an individual as sexually deviant, a comprehensive assessment of medical, psychiatric, psychological, social, and environmental factors should be completed to determine their contribution to the behaviour. Interventions should address internal characteristics as well as environmental influences.

References

Barbaree, H. E., & Marshall W. L. (1998). Treatment of the sexual offender. In R. M. Wettstein (Ed.), *Treatment of offenders with mental disorders* (pp. 265-328). New York: The Guilford Press.

Bradford, J. M. W. (1985). Organic treatments for the male sex offender. *Behavioral Sciences and the Law*, 3, 355-375.

Day, D. (1997). Clinical features and offense behavior of mentally retarded sex offenders: A review of research. *The NADD Newsletter*, 6, 86-90

Day, D. (1993). Crime and mental retardation: A review. In K Howells & C. R. Holland (Eds.), *Clinical approaches to the mentally disordered offender* (pp. 111-144). Chichester: John Wylie & Sons, Ltd.

Dementral, D. (1993). Assessing counterfeit deviance in persons with developmental disabilities: A ecological assessment inventory. *The Habilitative Mental Healthcare Newsletter*, 1, 1-7.

Furey, E., M. & Niesen, J., J. (1994). Sexual *abuse of adults with mental retardation by other consumers. Sexuality and Disability, (4),* 173-180

Gardner, W. I., Graeber, J. L., & Machkovitz, S. J. (1998). Treatment of offenders with mental retardation. In R.M. Wettstein (Ed.), *Treatment of offenders with mental disorders* (pp. 329-364). New York: The Guilford Press.

Gardner, W. I., & Sovner, R. (1994). *Self-injurious behavior: Diagnosis and treatment.* Pennsylvania: Vida Publishing.

Goddard, H. H. (1912). *The Kallikak family.* New York: The MacMillan Company.

Griffiths, D. M., Gardner, W. I., & Nugent, J. A. (1998). *Behavioral supports: Individual centered interventions. A multimodal functional approach.* Kingston, NY: NADD Press.

Griffiths, D., Quinsey, V. L.. & Hingsburger, D. (1989*).* *Changing inappropriate sexual behavior: A community based approach for persons with developmental disabilities.* Baltimore, MD: Paul H. Brookes.

Haaven, J., Little, R. & Petre-Miller, D. (1990). *Treating intellectually disabled sex offenders: A model residential program.* Orwell, VT: Safer Society Press.

Hingsburger, D. (1994). Sexuality update: Developing a sexuality policy for residential agencies. *The Habilitative Mental Healthcare Newsletter,* 4, 69-70.

Hingsburger, D., Griffiths, D. & Quinsey, V. (1991). Detecting counterfeit deviance: Differentiating sexual deviance from sexual inappropriateness. *The Habilitative Mental Healthcare Newsletter,* 9, 51-54.

Kempton, W. (1988). *Sex education for persons with disabilities that hinder learning: A teacher's guide.* Santa Barbara, CA: James Stanfield Company.

Mayer, M. & Poindexter, A. (1997). *Self instruction program series on mental and behavioral disorders in people who have mental retardation.* Durham, NC: TheraEd.

Perske, R. (1995). *Deadly innocence?* Nashville, TN: Abingdon Press.

The Association for Community Living. (1994). *Human sexuality handbook: Guiding people toward positive expressions of sexuality.* Springfield, MA: The Association for Community Living.

World Health Organization. (1975). *Education and treatment in human sexuality: The training of health professionals. Report of a WHO meeting.* Geneva: World Health Organization. WHO Technical Report No.572

Chapter 10

Consent to Treatment Issues in Sex Offenders with Developmental Delay

Paul Fedoroff, Beverley Fedoroff, and Cheryl Peever

Introduction

Few topics in clinical practice raise more controversy than the question of how to best manage sex offenders (cf. Fedoroff & Moran, 1997). Frequently, when the individual to be treated (or not) has a developmental disability, the complexity of the ethical and management issues increases exponentially (cf. Fedoroff, Fedoroff, & Ilic, 1999; Mikkelsen & Stelk, 1999). Among the many important issues that arise in the assessment of any alleged sex offender are the following questions:

> Did he or she do it?
> Why did they do it?
> What are the diagnoses?
> What are the treatment alternatives?
> What is the prognosis?
> What are the risks?
> What are the consent to treatment issues?

The purpose of this chapter is to review the last question in the list above.

"Consent to treatment issues" were considered in detail at a recent consensus conference convened to review the ethical issues involved in the treatment of sex offenders with developmental delay (Fedoroff, 1998). While there is extensive literature on consent to treatment (cf. Bloom & Bay, 1996; Hoge, 1994; Simon, 1987; Grisso & Appelbaum, 1998), very little has been written on the topic for sex offenders who have developmental delay. In addition, most papers about consent to treatment focus almost exclusively on the issue of consent to pharmacologic treatment. This is unfortunate since it isolates a single aspect of treatment options from the context in which it is administered. As a result, debates about the ethical issues involved frequently conflate theoretical, socio-political, religious, moral, and clinical issues (e.g., Szasz, 1982).

In an attempt to partially address the problem, this paper will deal with the relevant topics in the context of a fictitious, though typical case presentation, beginning well before the issue of treatment arises. In this way, it is hoped a more realistic picture of the complexities of management and methods to resolve or avoid ethical quandaries will emerge.

Case Examples

The presentation of the case of Alex

Alex is a 34 year old man with "Trisomy 21" (Down Syndrome). His parents are elderly. He has mild mental retardation. He is always cheerful, very sociable, and easily befriends everyone he meets. He is athletic and loves sports. Although he has never lived independently, he is comfortable in the community, and regularly uses public transportation primarily to attend sports events. He has never been employed, and has never been in a romantic relationship. He has no alcohol or substance abuse problems. There is no history of conduct disorder or criminal activity.

One day the police arrive on his parents' doorstep with news that their son has been identified as the offender in a sexual assault. A woman says Alex touched her breast as she was getting off a subway car. Alex's parents are understandably shocked and horrified by these events and immediately seek treatment for their son at a community treatment agency responsible for assessing people with developmental delay.

This case poses many issues which will be explored in the following sections: legal proceedings, the assessment, and course of treatment.

Nature of the treatment team

The first task for the treatment team is to establish for whom it is working. There are several interested parties: Alex, his parents, the victim, the police, the transit authority which manages the subway, the agency for which it works, and the community. In addition, different members of the treatment team may have current or past allegiances (official and non-official) to each of the interested parties. Further, the relationship between the treatment team and the other parties may change as the case progresses.

For example, if the police elect to charge Alex, it is probable that the prosecution (Crown) will be interested in what Alex told his treatment team about the events in question. Since the expectations of the criminal justice system are different from the expectations of the mental health system, most facilities that specialize in the treatment of sex offenders decline to become involved until the criminal proceedings are completed. The ability of the treating agency to ethically manage an individual in Alex's predicament depends on how well it navigates the initial contact. This is particularly important if the agency has assumed responsibility for Alex's care prior to the incident in question, since the agency's role as a treatment provider is different from its role in a pre-trial assessment.

The legal proceedings: Part 1

Alex is charged with "sexual interference". On the advice of the treatment agency, Alex's parents retain a lawyer. His lawyer asks for a "pre-trial" report from a forensic psychiatrist. This assessment indicates that Alex is "fit to stand trial", and that a defense of "not criminally responsible on account of mental illness" is not justified. In court, Alex enters a plea of guilty.

Identifying the immediate problem

Contrary to his parents' analysis of the situation, at the time of presentation, Alex's main problem was his arrest (that is why his parents came to the treatment team). The team correctly identified the problem and referred him to a lawyer. It should be noted that this decision is independent of whether or not Alex is guilty. While treatment teams are often tempted to "investigate" the case prior to the court proceedings, this is often a mistake. Not only does this confuse the role of the treatment team, it can also interfere with the work of the true experts in this area: police detectives, lawyers, and the judiciary.

Fitness to stand trial and criminal responsibility

The forensic psychiatrist's first report, prepared prior to the trial proper, considers the issues of "fitness to stand trial" and whether Alex is suitable for a defense of "not criminally responsible of account of mental illness". Fitness to stand trial proceedings deal with the question of whether the accused is able to understand the meaning of the charges, the legal process, and most importantly, whether he can aid his attorney in his own defense. In Canada, the criteria for "fitness to stand trial" have been intentionally set low, and in practice, most people with moderate mental retardation will easily meet the fitness to stand trial criteria, and all accused are assumed to be fit to stand trial until proven otherwise (Canada Criminal Code, 1999a).

The question of whether the accused is "not criminally responsible on account of mental illness" (NCR) deals with the issue of whether mental illness caused the accused to fail to appreciate the nature and consequences of his actions at the time of the events in question (Canada Criminal Code, 1999b). This is a major topic in the field of forensic psychiatry and far beyond the scope of this chapter (cf. Miller, 1994; for review). Nevertheless, it is important to acknowledge that sexual deviations (paraphilias) generally do not meet the criteria for successful NCR defenses (e.g., Williams, 1996).

The legal proceedings: Part 2

The court next requests a "pre-sentence report", and the forensic psychiatrist proceeds to conduct a second evaluation for the purposes of sentencing. This assessment includes phallometric testing that shows Alex has primary sexual responses to adult females. Psychiatric examination reveals signs of major depression that "may have preceded the event in question." He is assessed as being "impulsive with poor concentration". Treatment for depression and frotteurism (touching and rubbing against non-consenting persons) is recommended. The forensic psychiatrist's report concludes that "sex drive reducing medication may be indicated".

The judge gives Alex a conditional sentence that includes an order that he seek treatment for his psychiatric disorders, and complies with the recommendations of the psychiatrist, including treatment with sex-drive reducing medication.

Forensic pre-sentence reports

The forensic psychiatrist's pre-sentence report includes the results of phallometric testing. Phallometry or penile plethysmography is a test in which change in penis size is measured while the subject is presented with a variety of visual and/or auditory stimuli. The test assumes that greater changes in penis size are correlated with sexual arousal directed toward the presented stimuli. While useful for research and for treatment, it is not an appropriate test for the determination of guilt or innocence (Fedoroff & Moran, 1997). The finding that Alex shows sexual responses to adult women in the lab says little about his ability to behave normally with women in the real world. Nor does it rule out the possibility that he may act sexually with males or children in other contexts.

The report identifies several areas of psychiatric concern: depression, impulsivity, poor concentration, and "frotteurism". However, the nature of a forensic assessment is different from a standard clinical assessment since Alex would have been informed that any information obtained during the forensic assessment could be reported to the court. Although defense lawyers can, in theory, elect not to disclose expert reports that are unhelpful to their clients, in practice, this is difficult to do in the case of pre-sentence reports.

The limitations on conditional sentences

The judge in this case elected not to incarcerate Alex. Instead, a decision was made to impose a "conditional" sentence requiring Alex to satisfy specific expectations or face additional sanctions. The wording of the treatment condition is important. Alex is required to seek psychiatric treatment, but the treatment team is not required to treat Alex. This is not only because judges ordinarily have no authority to direct the activities of treatment agencies, but also because the treatment team may come to the conclusion that treatment is not indicated.

That is, while Alex may be required to comply with the treatment recommendations of the treatment team, the judge is not allowed to specify what the psychiatric treatment recommendations are. The forensic psychiatrist and judge have both suggested the use of "sex drive reducing medications", but neither can ethically order the use of medication, since the forensic psychiatrist is not the treating psychiatrist, and the judge is not a physician.

The assessment

Alex and his parents return to the treatment team's clinic with Alex's conditional sentence papers in hand. "The doctor says Alex needs chemical castration," his parents report. They also say that Alex's probation officer would like a copy of the treatment team's assessment and proof that he is taking his medication.

Consent forms allowing the treatment team to obtain the forensic psychiatrist's pre-sentence report and the probation officer's pre-sentence report, including the prosecution (Crown's) brief, are obtained from Alex. The clinic's duties to report are carefully explained to Alex before any assessment is undertaken. He voluntarily undergoes a full assessment by the treatment team.

He is discovered to be severely depressed with poor sleep, poor appetite, and some suicidal ideation. His cognitive abilities are now below what they were prior to the offence. His parents disclose they have discovered some notes in Alex's bedroom that involve sadistic themes about sexually torturing women. They are frightened. They are "too old to look after him any longer", and want him institutionalized. They want to know what the treatment team is going to do.

Changing perspectives

At this point, things do not appear to be going well. This is hardly unusual. Much of the current "problem" is due to the fact that Alex's status has undergone several dramatic shifts in a short time: from "child" in his parents' eyes; to "prisoner" in the view of the police; to "accused" in the view of his lawyer and forensic psychiatrist; to "convicted sex offender" in the view of the court and probation officer; to "patient/client" in the view of his treatment team. While each party is correct within its own perspective, the potential confusion experienced by the official parties pales in comparison to the confusion experienced by Alex's parents and by Alex himself.

An independent treatment assessment

Again, the most important task for the treatment team at this moment is to be clear about its role. At this stage, the treatment team must satisfy itself that it is the most appropriate agency to help Alex. In order to do this, it must conduct its own independent assessment.

As with every evaluation, before it begins, Alex has the right to know what will be done with the information obtained. The degree of disclosure is negotiable. Some offenders are happy to waive all rights to keep information private from their probation officer and parents. Others are more circumspect. Alex should be encouraged to discuss his decision with his lawyer and anyone else he trusts.

However, he also must be informed that the treatment team is required by law to report any known or suspected sexual offenses against identifiable minors. The specific details of reporting laws vary between jurisdictions, and therefore, will not be reviewed in detail here.

Disposition

Once the initial assessment is completed, the treatment team must decide whether it can accept responsibility for Alex's care. It may be that it does not have sufficient resources or support to do so. Alex may require admission to hospital if his current psychiatric state is sufficiently severe to represent a danger to himself or others. If so, then he can be "certified" without his or his parent's consent under the Mental Health Act (Ontario Government Statute, 1990). If this option is entertained, it is important to remember that the Mental Health Act only permits the receiving hospital to detain him. It does not permit the involuntary administration of medication, and it does not permit indefinite hospitalization. Again, the specific requirements of the Mental Health Act will vary from jurisdiction to jurisdiction; so these details will not be reviewed here. In general, most experts agree that the diagnosis of a paraphilic disorder alone is insufficient grounds for certification under the Mental Health Act since paraphilias are life-long disorders, and do not by themselves signify immediate danger to self or others.

Since Alex is not "certifiable" even though he is under a conditional sentence that requires him to seek treatment, he retains the right to decide if he will accept it. This fact is often forgotten by offenders, their parents, clinicians, and other interested parties such as probation and parole officers, particularly in the case of offenders with developmental delay.
Assuming the agency accepts Alex for treatment, its duties are clearly defined. The treatment team must act in a fiduciary relationship with Alex. This means it must act at all times in his best interest. While the treatment team can and should work in cooperation with Alex's probation officer, it is not an

arm of the criminal justice system. It cannot disclose information obtained during its assessment or treatment without Alex's written consent.

Forensic reports

The forensic psychiatrist's report is unique in that it belongs to the lawyer who commissioned it. The treatment team should request a copy of the report from the lawyer, not the forensic psychiatrist. Alternatively, if the report was presented in court, the probation officer usually can obtain it easily. The forensic psychiatrist's report should not be viewed by the treatment team as the ultimate authority or final word on the case. The forensic psychiatrist will have produced the report in order to answer only the questions posed by the lawyer who retained him or her. The time spent on the assessment will have been necessarily limited by the time restraints of the court, and by the ability of the lawyer to pay for the time spent on the case. In addition, the information obtained pre-sentence may be different from the information available once the legal consequences of disclosure have been removed (i.e., post-sentence).

Finally, although the police, forensic psychiatrist, prosecution, judge, and probation officer may all genuinely believe that treatment of Alex with sex drive reducing medication is a good idea, there is no authority for the treating psychiatrist to prescribe it before fulfilling a series of requirements as outlined in Figure 1.

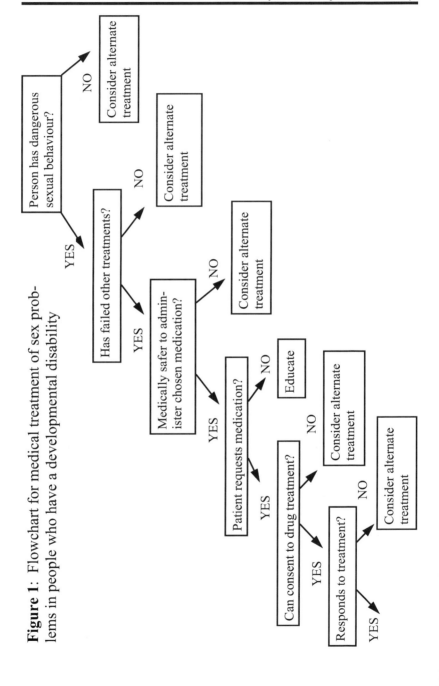

Figure 1: Flowchart for medical treatment of sex problems in people who have a developmental disability

Course of Treatment: Part 1

Alex does not want to be admitted to hospital and he does not meet criteria for involuntary certification under the Mental Health Act. He is accepted for outpatient treatment in the clinic. The clinic's duties to report are again carefully explained to all the parties involved. Treatment options for his depression are explained. Due to the severity of his depression and because of the evidence suggesting possible paraphilic disorders (unconventional or "kinky": sexual interests), "specific serotonergic re-uptake inhibitor" (SSRI) medications are discussed with Alex. The risks and benefits of several types of SSRI's are explained. He is told that SSRI's may alter his sexual interests, but they are not "chemical castration medications," and their effects are reversible. Antiandrogen medications are also discussed, including possible risks and benefits of each one.

He is clearly informed that the decision to take medication is one that he and his treating psychiatrist will make together and that ultimately, it is Alex's decision alone. Alex agrees to try an SSRI, and it is prescribed. A psychotherapy program is devised for Alex, and measures to monitor his progress are agreed upon by Alex, his parents, the treatment team, and his probation officer.

After six weeks, Alex's mood has improved dramatically. However, he continues to sleep poorly and frequently falls asleep during the day. His parents are increasingly worried by his forgetfulness and distractibility. He seems increasingly irritable. They have read about the high incidence of Alzheimer dementia in people with Down Syndrome and again wonder if he should be institutionalized. They have also found more sadistic writings in his room that they have secretly photocopied to show the treatment team.

Alex is referred for a sleep study that reveals he has sleep apnea syndrome. Continuous positive airway pressure (CPAP) is prescribed with Alex's consent. He is questioned carefully about possible sadistic sexual interests. He admits to this on condition that the team not tell his parents. He asks if there is any medication that can help him control these interests.

Duty to report/duty to caution

The treatment phase begins with a reminder of the duty to report dangerous or criminal behaviours. This is important because the experience of being in treatment is very different from the experience of being assessed. Individuals in treatment often develop very open and trusting feelings toward their therapists. They deserve to be protected from misperceiving the limitations of the confidentiality of the relationship. At the same time, it is vital that the team feels free to communicate with each other and with the necessary authorities if treatment is not proceeding successfully. By clearly establishing the limits of confidentiality at the start of treatment, the team will avoid ever appearing to betray its word, if disclosure to the appropriate authorities later becomes necessary.

Consent to treatment

Treatment of psychiatric disorders such as depression follows the same rules in sex offenders with developmental delay as it does in any other patients. All treatment options (pharmacologic and non-pharmacologic), as well as the risk and benefits of both accepting or refusing treatments, must be reviewed with the patient in terms that he/she can understand. Often, they need to be reviewed more than once. With Alex's permission, his parents should also be informed, since the treatment is unlikely to be successful if they do not agree with the plan. However, the decision to accept the treatment plan ultimately rests with Alex, not only because of the ethical implications, but also because the treatment is certain to fail if he does not accept it wholeheartedly.

Unmasking co-morbid disorders

This case demonstrates three other principles of treatment. First, the successful treatment of one disorder sometimes will uncover other problems that were previously masked. In Alex's case, treatment of his depression unmasked a sleep disorder that was previously attributed to his depression. People with developmental disabilities often have facial dysmorphia that increases their likelihood of having obstructive sleep apnea. Sleep apnea is a treatable condition that can have dramatic effects on mental status. Symptoms may be altered in people with developmental delay.

Second, people with developmental delay often have exaggerated responses to disease. Sleep deprivation caused by sleep apnea syndrome is associated with decreased concentration, cognitive impairment, and irritability in all populations, but particularly in the case of people with pre-morbid cognitive impairment. Accurate diagnosis and appropriate treatment of medical and psychiatric disorders is crucial in this population. Co-morbid medical problems are common and important.

Third, there is a tendency to attribute problems to a single disorder, particularly in the case of people with developmental delay. This is unfortunate, since it is precisely this group which is prone to having multiple psychiatric and medical disorders. It is easy to explain away irritability, depression, cognitive impairment, and impulsivity in people with developmental delay. Treatment teams who care for these people should be constantly vigilant for alternative explanations for the symptoms they observe.

At this point, Alex has learned that the treatment team is trustworthy and working to help him. He has discovered he can talk about private sexual issues without being ridiculed or punished by the staff. Therefore, it is not surprising he decided to disclose having sadistic sexual fantasies.

Keeping secrets

The difficulty for staff is the fact that they have been included in deceptive behaviour by Alex's parents who have been surreptitiously searching his bedroom. Problems like this are unavoidable, but can be minimized by following two rules. First, treatment staff must never engage in deceptive behaviour or encourage it. Not only is deception ethically indefensible, but the act of engaging in or condoning deceit, models precisely the mode of conduct that the team wishes to eliminate from Alex's behaviour. Individuals with developmental delay may have cognitive impairments, but they are not stupid. If Alex had thought he was being "tricked" or not included in the treatment plan, he would not have disclosed his private sadistic fantasies. This fact is often overlooked as is demonstrated by the sex offender literature that frequently refers to "cognitive distortions" that on closer inspection amount to "distortions" designed to keep the therapists from getting angry (Laws, 1989; Wright & Schneider, 1997).

Likelihood of disclosure

The initial phase of treatment ends with Alex requesting medication to control his sadistic interests. Is this request likely? Surprisingly, not only is it likely, providing certain conditions are met, it is almost inevitable. First, an honest, respectful, confidential, and hopeful treatment atmosphere must be established. The treatment team cannot lie, make false promises, or encourage any deceitful behaviour. Convincing Alex that the team can be trusted and is working in his best interest is crucial, and should be a top priority in any treatment plan. Diligent adherence to the principle of giving Alex control of what happens to him is the key to the success of his treatment.

Second, the team must be respectful. While the actions of a convicted sex offender are always reprehensible, the courage of any offender who actively engages in treatment for the purpose of preventing relapse (as opposed to avoiding further punishment) is always laudable. Alex has changed overnight from being an "innocent" 34 year old "child" to a convicted, sadistic sex offender. His parents want to institutionalize him, and are spying on him. His probation officer does not believe him. The treatment team is his last refuge. If the team achieves what it says it will do (i.e., cure his depression, fix his insomnia, listen to what he has to say, and help him with his sexual problems), and treats him respectfully, not only when decisions about treatment are necessary, but also in its day to day interactions with him, treatment success will increase.

Limits of confidentiality

A common misconception is that treatment requires absolute confidentiality. The fact is that successful treatment of sex offenders with developmental delay requires a clear exposition of the limits of confidentiality. Alex knew that within the limits of the statutory reporting laws, what he disclosed would be kept confidential within the treatment team and those individuals outside the team that he, and he alone, designated. On this point, parents and "significant others" are often confused. It is important to explain that while within the statutory limits of the law, there is an ethical limitation which forbids members of the treatment team from disclosing information from therapy or assessment without consent, there is nothing that forbids the team from gathering information from any source.

Therefore, parents should be told that while the team cannot discuss information without the patient/client's consent, nothing forbids them from providing information to the treatment team (on the understanding that the team will share the information amongst itself).

Finally, the team must be realistic but hopeful. If the treatment team is pessimistic about the treatment outcome, the patient/client will quickly learn this, and intentionally or unintentionally work to fulfill the team's expectations (Fedoroff & Moran, 1997; Frank & Frank, 1991; Nolley, Muccigrosso, & Zigman, 1996; Shapiro & Shapiro, 1997).

Course of Treatment:- Part 2.

Alex's motivations for seeking further treatment were carefully explored. He indicated an abhorrence of recurrent sadistic fantasies that he knew were criminal. He said although he was worried about acting on these fantasies, he would contact a member of the treatment team before acting on the fantasies. No specific victim was identified and his parents were never included in these fantasies. Alex indicated that he would be more comfortable if his sex drive was lower and his sadistic fantasies disappeared. He again asked if there was anything that could help him.

Anti-androgen medications were discussed with him again. After the risks and benefits of anti-androgen medications were discussed, he chose oral medroxyprogesterone. After being given a 24-hour number to call if he needed to talk with a member of the treatment team, he was encouraged to discuss his decision with his parents. He was also given a copy of the progesterone consent form to review. He was told to obtain the appropriate lab tests (with assistance of the treatment team), and was given a follow-up appointment. At the follow-up appointment, he signed the consent form, and was given a prescription for medroxy-progesterone acetate. Alex's parents, with his permission, were invited to this session and encouraged to ask questions about the treatment plan. They were also provided with the name of an independent therapist who could assist them during this difficult time.

At follow-up and after increasing the oral dosage of me-droxy-progesterone to 500 mg daily, Alex continued to report troublesome sadistic fantasies. He was reminded about the option of medroxy-progesterone weekly injec-tions or leuprolide monthly injections. He was also told about the unique risks and benefits of leuprolide treat-ment (particularly anaphylactic shock and osteoporosis). He was given a copy of a leuprolide consent form and again encouraged to consult with the people he trusted about what he should do.

Alex elected to try monthly leuprolide injections. After completing the necessary medical investigations, he signed the consent form and began treatment with this medication. Notably, he was also encouraged to con-tinue participating in all the other aspects of his treat-ment program, including individual and family psycho-therapy; vocational training; group sex offender therapy; and relapse prevention therapy for depression.

A month after beginning treatment with leuprolide, Alex reported he felt "free" for the first time he could remem-ber. His mood was normal. His concentration was nor-mal. His sleep was normal. His energy had returned. His sadistic fantasies had disappeared. He was participating actively in his vocational training program and his re-lapse prevention group. His parents reported that they felt they had "gotten our own son back". Alex summed it up when he said, "I am sorry for what I did when I was arrested, but I am glad because I got the help I needed. I feel normal now and I'm happy."

After some progress, treatment has uncovered a new set of problems. Some would regard this as a setback or even a relapse. Nothing could be further from the truth. Treatment teams should be much more worried about the problems they do not hear about. New problems reported by the patient/client before they have been acted upon are not only a sign that a productive therapeutic relationship has been established, but also an indication that therapeutic progress is being made.

Antiandrogen treatment

On learning about Alex's continued preoccupation with sadistic fantasies, the staff appropriately first assessed the risk of immediate danger. The therapeutic context in which Alex has learned to trust the team not only makes disclosure of problems more likely, but also makes it easier to assess risk. At this point, it is Alex who is requesting antiandrogen treatment rather than the team insisting on it. Antiandrogen treatment of sex offenders is a long-established tradition, but antiandrogens have never been approved for this purpose in North America.

Therefore, unlike the case with more common psychotropic medications, a signed consent form is required. Various medical tests are also indicated that are beyond the scope of this chapter. Importantly, while Alex is clearly the central figure in any treatment decision, attempts should be made to include those he trusts such as his parents.

It is also extremely important to be clear about the purpose of therapy which is to alter or control the patient's criminal sexual urges. The truth is that while antiandrogens lower testosterone, they are not reliable contraceptives and their effects are reversible. Therefore, aside from reducing testosterone, treatment with antiandrogen bears no relationship to surgical castration, and the antiquated term "chemical castration" should be abandoned. Further, given that antiandrogens remain experimental, most would argue that they should never be prescribed without voluntary consent, particularly in the case of people with developmental delay.

In this case, Alex found that medroxy-progesterone acetate was not sufficiently effective. Some experts believe that medroxy-progesterone acetate administered by weekly intramuscular injection is more effective than by oral administration, but there are no studies on this issue. If intra-muscular medications are considered, patients usually choose leuprolide that can be given by once monthly intramuscular injections. A new formulation of this medication is available which allows injections every three months. While the "three-monthly" formulation may be more convenient, it is expensive and begs the question of whether anyone who is so seriously ill as to need injectable antiandrogens should be seen by a psychiatrist only once ever three months. Further information about the rationale for pharmacologic treatment of sex offenders is available elsewhere (Bradford, 1996; Bradford, 1997; Bradford & Greenberg, 1996; Bradford & Pawlak, 1993; Clarke, 1989; Cooper, 1995; Dickey, 1992; Fedoroff, 1988; Fedoroff, 1994; Fedoroff, 1995; Fedoroff, Wisner-Carlson, Dean, & Berlin, 1992; Gijs & Gooren, 1996; Gotestein & Schubert, 1993; Hucker, Langevin, & Bain, 1988; Kellett, 1993; Land, 1995; Laschet & Lachet, 1971; Money, 1970; Money, 1987; Rosler & Witztum, 1998).

Conference Deliberations

At the start of its deliberations, conference members expected there would be a great deal of disagreement about consent to treatment issues in sex offenders with developmental delay. However, it quickly became clear that expert's apprehensions could be allayed by reframing pre-conference perceptions.

The major themes of the consensus meeting are summarized in Table 1.

Table 1- Conference Themes

Pre-conference Perception	Consensus	Recommendation(s)
Treatment is involuntary	Sex offender treatment must always be voluntary	Education re: patient rights, consent, treatment options
Treatment is medical	Treatment is multidisciplinary	Fuller integration of modern medical investigations and interventions into the full treatment plan
Medical treatment is irreversible	Pharmacologic treatment is reversible	Sex offenders should be offered a full range of treatments, including pharmacologic, if indicated

It was agreed that sex offender treatment of people with developmental delay must always be voluntary and fully informed. While it is conceivable that some sex offenders with developmental delay will require apprehension by police, this should not be confused with treatment. The committee recommended that treatment providers be educated about not only the full range of treatment options for sex offenders with developmental delay, but also about the rights that people with developmental delay retain even after being accused or convicted of a sexual offense.

The committee agreed that medical interventions are but one of many treatment options for sex offenders with developmental delay. It was agreed that medical interventions should be considered only as part of a fully developed treatment plan that should also include psychological, social, and family/caretaker interventions. However, the committee also agreed that individuals seeking treatment should always be presented with a full explanation of all the treatment options available so that they can make voluntary, independent and informed choices.

The committee also agreed that only reversible medical interventions should be considered. Individuals seeking treatment need to be fully informed of the potential risk and benefits of both accepting and refusing medical interventions (as well as other treatment options).

The committee unanimously agreed upon these opinions and recommendations. The committee deferred on the more complicated issues of situations in which substitute consent is required, or in which the individual's parents or guardians are opposed to a treatment option that the individual with developmental delay has chosen. However, the committee expressed the opinion that rare situations like these are best dealt within the spirit of open disclosure and respect for the wishes of the individual with developmental delay.

Summary

The State Of The Art

Effective pharmacologic and non-pharmacologic treatment interventions are available for the treatment of sex offenders with and without developmental delay. Treatment interventions must never be confused with investigative procedures undertaken for third parties. All treatment interventions should be fully discussed with the person seeking treatment before treatment is begun. In addition, opportunities for independent assessment ("second opinions") should be available and encouraged. Any treatment should be consented to by the individual seeking treatment and the option to withdraw consent should always be available. Any specific treatment that is undertaken should be integrated into a comprehensive treatment plan. In addition, verifiable treatment objectives should be identified at the start of treatment, and progress should be measured at regular intervals. If progress is not being made, the entire treatment program should be re-evaluated and changed as necessary. However, no alterations in the treatment plan should be made without the informed consent of the individual being treated. Finally, limits of confidentiality as well as the rights and responsibilities of both the individual being treated and the members of the treatment team should be made explicit before treatment is undertaken. Further research into optimal assessment techniques, treatment options, assessment of response to treatment, and alternative interventions in this population is needed.

Clinical Implications

While it was the committee's belief that the recommendations listed above are applicable to all people with developmental delay, the committee also acknowledges that every person with developmental delay is a unique individual with unique strengths and vulnerabilities. The same can be said about any treatment team. "Cookie-cutter" treatment programs are unlikely to be optimal for any specific person, and need to be adapted to the situation. They will also need to be modified as treatment progresses. Nevertheless, the importance of honesty, respect, responsibility, autonomy, and realistic optimism cannot be overemphasized. Agreed upon standards of treatment adhering to these principles have been published and are widely accepted by the treatment community (cf. Coleman et al., 1996).

Agency Implications

This paper has focused primarily on the responsibilities of the treatment team. However, in the case of sex offenders, there are always other stakeholders including the victim(s), the community, and the agency in which the treatment team works. Agency directors have their own concerns. A single sex offense "relapse" by an individual receiving treatment under the auspices of an agency may endanger the entire agency. Treatment teams need to bear this in mind, and should regularly consult with agency administrators about what they are doing. This does not mean they should disclose confidential clinical material to non-clinicians, but by the same token, it is unfair to expect agency administrators to tolerate being "left in the dark" about the types of problems with which the treatment team is dealing. It was the committee's hope that its recommendations would be compatible with most agency's terms of reference.

However, the committee felt it important to emphasize that not all agencies can treat all sex offenders. The establishment of agreed upon criteria for the acceptance of sex offenders for treatment is important and should be periodically reviewed. Finally, some agency administrators will be more "tolerant" than others will. The committee felt strongly that agencies are ethically obliged to disclose their policies regarding the treatment of sex offenders so that individuals seeking treatment can make informed decisions about whether a particular agency is right for them.

What Should Be Done Now

As noted above, the committee's recommendations are summarized in Table 1. The committee's recommendations concerning the steps necessary prior to commencing pharmacologic therapy of sex offenders with developmental delay are summarized in Figure 1. Specific advice about likely treatment decisions is highlighted in the text above. These recommendations are based on consensus about what is currently known concerning the treatment of sex offenders. However, the committee acknowledges that advances in research into the humane treatment of this population are likely to uncover new and increasingly effective treatment interventions. Nevertheless, the underlying principles of treatment as outlined in this paper are unlikely to change.

Final Consensus Statement

Convicted sex offenders with developmental delay have the right to full disclosure of the limits of confidentiality prior to entering therapy. They have the right to be informed of the findings of the treatment team, and the treatment team's recommendations for treatment. They also have the right to hear about all possible treatment options both pharmacologic and non-pharmacologic, including those that the agency in question may not be qualified to administer. They have a right to know what specific treatments the team is prepared to offer, and of all the treatment agency's policies concerning their management, prior to treatment. Within the statutory obligations of the treatment agency, the treatment team has the right to decline to accept responsibility for the care of any individual who is unable or unwilling to provide informed, voluntary consent to a mutually agreed upon treatment plan. Once treatment is commenced, the individual seeking treatment has the right to humane, respectful care, and to be fully informed of any changes in the treatment plan to which he/she voluntarily consents.

References

Bloom, H. & Bay, M. (1996). *A practical guide to mental health, capacity, and consent law of Ontario.* Toronto: Carswell.

Bradford, J. (1996). The role of serotonin in the future of forensic psychiatry. *Bulletin of the American Academy of Psychiatry and Law, 24,* 57-72.

Bradford, J. (1997). Medical interventions in sexual deviance. In D. R. Laws, & W. O'Donohue (Eds.), *Sexual deviance: Theory, assessment and treatment* (pp. 449-464). New York: Guilford Press.

Bradford, J. M. W. & Greenberg, D. M. (1996). Pharmocological treatment of deviant sexual behaviour. *Annual Review of Sex Research, 7,* 283-306.

Bradford, J. M. W. & Pawlak, A. (1993). Double-blind placebo crossover study of cyproterone acetate in the treatment of the paraphilias. *Archives of Sexual Behavior, 2,* 383-402.

Canada Criminal Code (1999a). Section 672.72 Fitness to stand trial. In E. L. Greenspan, & M. Rosenberg (Eds.), *Martin's Annual Criminal Code of Canada* (pp. 1058-1061). Aurora: Canada Law Book Inc.

Canada Criminal Code (1999b). Section 16. Defense of mental disorder. In E. L. Greenspan, & M. Rosenberg (Eds.), *Martin's annual Criminal Code of Canada* (pp. 47-53). Aurora: Canada Law Book Inc.

Clarke, D. J. (1989). Anti-libidinal drugs and mental retardation: a review. *Medical Science and the Law, 29,* 136-146.

Coleman, E., Dwyer, S. M., Abel, G., Berner, W., Breiling, J., Hindman, J., Knopp, F. H., Langevin, R., & Pfafflin, F. (1996). Standards of care for treatment of adult sex offenders. In E. Coleman, S. M. Dwyer, & N. J. Pallone (Eds.), *Sex offender treatment. Biological dysfunction, intrapsychic conflict, interpersonal violence* (pp. 5-11). New York: Haworth Press.

Cooper, A. J. (1995). Review of the role of two anti-libidinal drugs in the treatment of sex offenders with mental retardation. *Mental Retardation, 33,* 42-48.

Dickey, R. (1992). The management of a case of treatment-resistant paraphilia with a long-acting LHRH agonist. *Canadian Journal of Psychiatry, 37,* 567-569.

Fedoroff, J. P. (1988). Buspirone hydrochloride in the treatment of transvestic fetishism. *Journal of Clinical Psychiatry, 49,* 408-409.

Fedoroff, J. P. (1994). Serotonergic drug treatment of deviant sexual interests. *Annals of Sex research, 6,* 105-107.

Fedoroff, J. P. (1995). Antiandrogens vs. serotonergic medications in the treatment of sex offenders: A preliminary compliance study. *The Canadian Journal of Human Sexu-*

ality, 4, 111-122.

Fedoroff, J. P. (1998). *Consent to treatment*, Sexuality and ethical dilemmas in people with developmental delay: Welland District Association for Community Living: 3rd Annual Sexuality Conference. Niagara Falls Ontario.

Fedoroff, J. P., Fedoroff, B. I., & Ilic, K. (1999). Sexual disorders, developmental disorders, developmental delay and co-morbid disorders. *NADD Proceedings, 16*, 90-96.

Fedoroff, J. P. & Moran, B. (1997). Myths and misconceptions about sex offenders. *The Canadian Journal of Human Sexuality, 6*, 263-276.

Fedoroff, J. P., Wisner-Carlson, R., Dean, S., & Berlin, F. S. (1992). Medroxy-progesterone acetate in the treatment of paraphilic sexual disorders: Rate of relapse in paraphilic men treated in psychotherapy for at least five years with or without medroxyprogesterone acetate. *Journal of Offender Rehabilitation, 18*, 109-123.

Frank, J. C. & Frank, J. B. (1991). *Persuasion and healing*. Baltimore, MD: Johns Hopkins University Press.

Gijs, L. & Gooren, L. (1996). Hormonal and psychopharmacological interventions in the treatment of paraphilias: An update. *The Journal of Sex Research, 33*, 273-290.

Gotestein, H. G. & Schubert, D. S. P. (1993). Low-dose medroxy progesterone acetate in the management of paraphilias. *Journal of Clinical Psychiatry, 54*, 182-188.

Grisso, T., & Appelbaum, P. S. (1998). *Assessing competence to consent to treatment: A guide for physicians and other health professionals*. Oxford: Oxford University Press.

Hoge, S. K. (1994). Treatment refusal in psychiatric practice. In R. Rosner (Ed.), *Principles and practice of forensic psychiatry* (pp. 127-132). New York: Chapman & Hall.

Hucker, S. J., Langevin, R., & Bain, J. (1988). A double blind trial of sex drive reducing medication in pedophiles. *An-*

nals of Sex Research, 1, 227-242.

Kellett, J. (1993). The nature of human sexual desire and its modification by drugs. In A. J. Riley, M. Peet, & C. Wilson (Eds.), *Sexual pharmacology* (pp. 130-145). Oxford: Clarendon Press.

Land, W. B. (1995). Psychopharmacological options for sex offenders. In B. K. Schwartz, & H. R. Cellini (Eds.), *The sex offender: Corrections, treatment and legal practice* (pp. 18-1 to 18-7). Kingston, NJ: Civic Research Institute.

Laschet, U. & Lachet, L. (1971). Psychopharmacotherapy of sex offenders with cyproterone acetate. *Pharmackopsychiatrie Neuropsychopharmakologic, 4,* 99-104.

Laws, D. R. (1989). *Relapse prevention with sex offenders.* New York: Guilford Press.

Mikkelsen, E. J. & Stelk, W. J. (1999). *Criminal offenders with mental retardation: Risk assessment and the continuum of community-based treatment programs.* New York: NADD Press.

Miller, R. D. (1994). Criminal responsibility. In R. Rosner (Ed.), *Principles and practice of forensic psychiatry* (pp. 198-215). New York: Chapman & Hill.

Money, J. (1970). Use of an androgen-depleting hormone in the treatment of male sex offenders. *Journal of Sex Research, 6,* 165-72.

Money, J. (1987). Treatment guidelines: Antiandrogen and counseling of paraphilic offenders. *Journal of Sex and Marital Therapy, 13,* 219-223.

Nolley, D., Muccigrosso, L., & Zigman, E. (1996). Treatment successes with mentally retarded sex offenders. In E. Coleman, S. M. Dwyer, & N. J. Pallone (Eds.), *Sex offender treatment. Biological dysfunction, intrapsychic conflict, interpersonal violence* (pp. 125-141). New York: Haworth Press.

Ontario Government Statutes (1990). *Form 1: application by physician for psychiatric assessment.* Ontario: Mental Health Act Queens Press.

Rosler, A. & Witztum, E. (1998). Treatment of men with paraphilia with a long-acting analogue of gonadotropin-releasing hormone. *New England Journal of Medicine, 338,* 416-422.

Szasz, T. S. (1982). The myth of mental illness. In R. B. Edwards (Ed.), *Psychiatry and Ethics* (pp. 19-28). Buffalo, NY: Prometheus Books.

Shapiro, A. K. & Shapiro, E. (1997). *The powerful placebo.* Baltimore, MD: Johns Hopkins University Press.

Simon, R. I. (1987). The right to refuse treatment and the therapeutic alliance. In R.I. Simon (Ed.), *Clinical psychiatry and the law* (pp. 78-99). Washington DC: American Psychiatric Association.

Williams, S. (1996). *Invisible darkness: The horrifying case of Paul Bernardo and Karla Homolka.* Toronto: Little Brown and Company.

Wright, R. C. & Schneider, S. L. (1997). Deviant sexual fantasies as motivated self-deception. In B. K. Schwartz, & H. R. Cellini (Eds.), *The sex offender: New insights, treatment Innovations and legal developments* (pp. 1-14). New Jersey: Civic Research Institute.

Chapter 11

Assessment and Treatment of Sex Offenders who have a Developmental Disability

Ron Langevin and Suzanne Curnoe

Introduction

When individuals who have a developmental disability are accused, charged, and/or convicted of a sexual offense, a major issue has been whether they should be treated like any other sex offender and whether the same assessment procedures and treatments apply. "Special considerations" may lead to a violation of civil liberties of individuals who have a developmental disability, as in the case of Mr. A.

The Case of Mr. A

When he was 14 years of age, he engaged a 6 year old girl in non-violent sex play and was caught. It was decided "in his better interests and that of the community" to institutionalize him. When he was seen at age 23 he had received no treatment and there had been no trial. A 14 year old who was not developmentally delayed and was charged with the same offense in Canada would not be sentenced to 9 years in institution and most likely would have been ordered into treatment as part of a probation order.

In some cases a full sexological and forensic assessment of a sex offender who has a developmental disability may only be requested when there is concern about aggressiveness or danger. Consider Mr. B, a 26 year old high functioning youth with a developmental disability from a dysfunctional family.

The Case of Mr. B

He was institutionalized but with privileges to leave the facility and so had a girlfriend with a developmental disability in the community. Her case worker was concerned that she had black eyes and bruises at times. Apparently her boyfriend, Mr. B, was 'very rough' when they had intercourse. Although there were no charges, there was concern that his aggressiveness was escalating and he was sent for phallometric assessment. Results showed the presence of a courtship disorder with a predominant interest in sexual aggression and sadism. Should he be charged? What is his risk to harm other women and the community in general? What treatments should be used, if any? What are the ethical responsibilities of case workers and mental health professionals?

The literature on the sex offender who has a developmental disability is remarkably silent in addressing such ethical issues surrounding risk, treatment, and assessment.

Literature Review

Guidelines such as those of the Canadian Psychological Association's (cf. Sinclair, 1998) offer general principles that are broad and include respect for the dignity of persons, responsible caring, integrity in relationships, and responsibility to society, but do not offer specific guidelines about assessing and treating sex offenders or individuals who have a developmental disability. Two organizations have developed guidelines for the assessment and treatment of sex offenders generally, the Association for the Treatment of Sexual Abusers (ATSA, 2001) and the International Association for the Treatment of Sexual Offenders (IATSO) (Coleman et al., 1995). These guidelines are also broad and attempt to deal with sex offenders in general rather than deal specifically with the sex offender who has a developmental disability. The older of the two organizations, ATSA, has attempted to develop guidelines for training of professionals dealing with sex offenders again, generally without specific focus on the sex offender who has a developmental disability. IATSO is stricter in its guidelines and indicates that a minimum requirement of treatment providers is a master's degree or equivalent in a clinical field from an accredited institution. They also recommend that therapists be licensed by a certification body, such as government agencies, medical board, etc. as well as having special training in the areas of counselling and assessing paraphilics and sexual offenders. Typically this has not been the case so that "sex therapists" abound who have no credentials and are not restricted by licensing boards. Paradoxically, a therapist cannot advertise themselves as "psychologist" without a license.   Possible criminal charges may be laid if they do. However, currently anyone can call themselves a "sex therapist". Moreover, the College of Psychologists of Ontario would only require that a psychologist wishing to work with sex offenders read on the subject, attend meetings and workshops, or have some home-study accreditation (see Quinsey & Lalumiere, 1996, for example). Thus, one can see why administrators may be reluctant to provide extensive programs for sex offenders who have developmental disabilities. Harvey Stancer of the Clarke Institute of Psychiatry established a rule for evaluating research studies in mental health generally that can be applied to assessment and treatment. "For a research study to be ethically sound, it must have a valid research design and method." The principle can be extended to research on individuals who have a developmental disability. An ethically sound assessment should include reliable and valid instruments that examine all major relevant factors pertinent to the case at hand. Treatment should include contemporary knowledge of effective treatment, it should be beneficial and not harmful, and should have an evaluative component to determine its effectiveness for the individual being treated. These issues will be addressed again later.

There are many problems in the contemporary assessment and treatment of sex offenders in general that are only amplified when dealing with individuals who have a developmental disability. For one, reporting laws have been enacted to protect children in the community so that any revelation by a client about a child at risk for sexual or physical abuse must be reported to the Children's Aid Society or police under penalty of loss of license and possible incarceration. Some individuals have approached clergy, psychiatrists, psychologists, or social workers, with the intention of having treatment for their sexually deviant behaviour and found themselves facing criminal charges. It behooves the mental health professional to warn new clients about this reporting law so the role of therapist and law enforcer are clearly distinct. However, some naive individuals who have a developmental disability may still tell their worker/therapist about encounters with children or other sexual behaviour that constitutes a criminal offense. A patient's advocate may serve a useful role in addressing this problem. Thompson-Cooper, Fugere, and Cormier (1993) noted that the reporting laws have changed the focus of child protection workers from helping families to investigating cases for abuse and reporting it to the police which may lead to lengthy court processes and to incarceration rather than to appropriate intervention by mental health professionals. They suggest a system such as the 'confidential doctor' used in the Netherlands, whereby the police are informed of abuse only if the family and accused are not cooperating with the helping professionals.

Another contemporary issue faced by therapists are lawsuits by victims of sexual assault. When a therapist treats a sex offender who is released to the community and commits another crime, accusations are made that the therapist, who released this person prematurely, did not perform the appropriate therapy, or did not do the suitable therapy appropriately. One therefore can expect some reticence on the part of mental health professionals to engage in therapy at this juncture in history, especially in cases that are considered dangerous or difficult to treat. Victim impact has become a more prominent issue and when dealing with any sex offender, danger to the community, robustness of treatment, and general risk should be addressed.

Assessment Issues

The guidelines offered by ATSA and IATSO are attempting to ensure that a proper assessment is done and appropriate treatment administered. As indicated earlier, an ethically sound assessment should evaluate all major relevant factors to the case at hand and the best available reliable and valid instruments and methods should be used. Langevin and Watson (1996) have outlined the pertinent factors that should be assessed in any sex offender: sexual history and preference, substance abuse, mental illness and personality, history of crime and violence, neuropsychological functioning, and other biological factors that may influence sexual behaviour and cognitive functioning, especially endocrine disorders such as sex hormone abnormalities. These factors will be considered in turn.

Sexual History and Preference

The most significant motivation for sexual offenses is the presence of a sexual disorder, that is, a sexual preference that is unconventional and may involve nonconsenting partners, e.g., children, or rape of an adult. Langevin and Watson (1996) found that 80% or more of offenders have an identifiable sexual disorder. While the exact incidence of sexual disorders among individuals who have a developmental disability is unknown, Langevin, Marentette, and Rosati (1996) found that individuals with WAIS IQ scores in the "retarded or borderline retarded range" and "neuropsychological impairment" were over-represented among known sex offenders. These results indicate a greater need for the training of professionals working with individuals who have a developmental disability who likely would be the first to identify sexual disorders in this population. Moreover, it is not known what the incidence is of sex offenders who have developmental disabilities may be who are not sexually deviant, but are expressing loneliness, or curiosity, or lack the appropriate social skills to approach their age peer adult female. A survey and literature review by Tudiver, Broekstra, Josselyn, and Barbaree (1997) reported that sex offenders who have developmental disabilities displayed more social skill deficits, were sexually naive, and lacked interpersonal skills resulting in more difficulties interacting with the opposite sex. The psychological and psychiatric literature on sex offenders in the 1960's through to the early 1980's emphasized the poor social skills and lack of sex education among sex offenders generally and did not always subdivide men with sexual disorders from those without deviant sexual interests. Those who are not sexually deviant may be much more amenable to intervention and placement in the community than individuals with a true sexual disorder that may be very resistant to change. It is important to determine whether a true sexual disorder exists in a given client, but many sex offenders seen currently are reluctant either to tell the mental health professional, or to admit it to themselves (cf. Langevin, 1988).

Offenders who have a developmental disability are no exception. While some may attempt to conceal their sexual preferences from the examiner, others are unable to verbally report their sexual behaviours and preferences. In contrast, some will be eager to please the examiner and, as a result, may reveal a sexual disorder that does not in fact exist.

The Case of Mr. C

Mr. C, a 28 year old male with a developmental disability, was eager to be accepted by the males in his small town. At their urging he went into a washroom and touched the genitals of a 6 year old boy. He was immediately apprehended. When questioned by the police about other similar incidents he 'acknowledged' them. When asked for the names of the boys he gave them many names of boys who did not exist in order to please the police. There were no other verified incidents of child sexual abuse by this man.

External sources of past sexual history and previous treatment and assessment information on sex offenders are important to ascertain, but especially so in individuals with developmental disabilities who, without malice, may not tell the whole *story* or the correct *story* of their lives or of their sexual behaviour in particular.

It is not unusual for many sex offenders in general to be unable to tell an examiner exactly what their sexual preferences may be. If they experience an attraction to adults and children, and they find different features attractive about the two age groups, they may not be able to specify an exact preference for children. This distinction may be particularly difficult for people with developmental disabilities. The authors believe that phallometric testing is invaluable in all cases of sexual offenders and paraphilics to help resolve questions of sexual preferences and to further define treatment goals and risk to the community. In this testing, penile erection is measured while the male views pictures of males and females, adults and children, and hears taped stories about sexual interactions.

The Freund Test (Freund, McKnight, Langevin, & Cibiri, 1972; Freund & Watson, 1991) is the best documented and validated and offers up to 90% sensitivity in identifying pedophiles. Other sexual disorders, such as a preference for sexual aggression over consenting sexual relations, are also identifiable, but with less sensitivity (cf. Lalumiere & Quinsey, 1993). There are two classes of measuring devices, circumference and volumetric. The volumetric is more sensitive than the circumference device which may misdiagnose in 10%-to-15% of cases, so the former is recommended (cf. Kuban, Barbaree, & Blanchard, 1999). Phallometric testing is especially valuable in assessing individuals with a developmental disability who are having sex with children. When audio tapes are used there must be an additional assessment to assure that individuals who have a developmental disability are able to understand the narrative. Although some workers legitimately worry that their client may be "labeled for life" because of phallometric test results, the clinician, as a result of such testing and other results, may enact more effective treatment plans, including degree of supervision required. In addition, the community may be protected from dangerous sex offenders.

Alcohol and Drug Abuse

Alcohol abuse and alcohol dependency are common among all sex offenders in general. Langevin and Lang (1990) indicated that between one third and one half of various sex offender groups were alcoholics and over half had tried some street drug, although only a small fraction had a drug abuse problem. About half of all sex crimes are carried out under the influence of alcohol, making it the single most important disinhibiting factor to evaluate. Moreover, the more violent the crime, the more likely alcohol was involved (cf. Rada, 1975).

Sex offenders who have a developmental disability in institutions may be closely supervised and not have access to alcohol, but those living in community settings are among a population in which 85% of males drink alcohol. There may be pressures to drink. Therefore, it is an important aspect of assessing the sex offender who has a developmental disability to determine his use and dependence on alcohol, if any, and its role in his particular crimes. Consider the case of Mr. D.

The Case of Mr. D

Mr. D told us that he did not drink at all, whereas his case worker noted that he "drank a lot" and was forced to leave his previous placement because of drunk and disorderly behavior. He and his cousin, who appeared to be an alcoholic, drank at every opportunity. Mr. D would become loud and aggressive while drinking and during one drinking bout, he committed a sexual assault and was arrested. His case worker reported that he was not allowed to drink as part of his probation order. He told her that he was not drinking, but she met him by chance on the street and he smelled of alcohol.

Tudiver et al. (1997) found that alcohol and drugs play a role in less than 4% of the sex crimes committed by individuals who have a developmental disability, indicating that it has a less frequent role in their crimes. However, the disinhibiting role of alcohol may be more pronounced in individuals who have a developmental disability, especially when traumatic brain injury is a factor. Although there is no definitive information, it is believed that alcohol will have a more profound effect on individuals who have a developmental disability or brain injury, controlling for confounding factors such as amount consumed and body size variables, etc. Alcoholics generally may fail to report the amount of alcohol they consume or may minimize the extent of the problem they have. Some alcoholics display sexually deviant behaviour that appears only when they are drinking. Others may show pathological intoxication, a peculiar disposition to become aggressive and psychotic under the influence of even small amounts of alcohol. It also is not known if these problems are more common among sex offenders who have developmental disabilities, but, at the very least, alcohol and drug abuse should be given the same consideration as it is for its role in sex offenders in general.

Crime, Violence, Personality, and Mental Illness

Mr. D, noted earlier, illustrated the next significant factors to assess; antisocial behaviour and personality. He was the product of a very dysfunctional and aggressive family which was a source of antisocial values for him. Tudiver et al. (1997), in their survey, noted that sex offenders who have developmental disabilities have a higher incidence of family psychopathology, psychosocial deprivation, school maladjustment, behavioural problems, and criminal behaviour, compared to non-delayed adult sex offenders. Individuals with antisocial behaviour patterns and personality disorders (ASPD) are over-represented in the criminal population generally and among sex offenders as well, wherein 20%-to-40% may have an ASPD diagnosis. ASPD adds an additional burden to address in assessing the sex offender and it may be one more factor that convinces administrators and politicians that some sex offenders who have developmental disabilities should just be institutionalized rather than assessed and treated. It is certainly important to distinguish inappropriate behaviour driven by ignorance of appropriate behaviour versus that which has a long history and is driven by ASPD. A full assessment of family background and parental behaviour, client's institutional behaviour, physical and/or sexual abuse as a child, criminal acts (whether they resulted in court proceedings or not), and history of lying, stealing, and aggression will offer the treatment provider the information that may be the difference in convincing administrators that treatment is an acceptable alternative to institutionalization.

Major mental illnesses, such as schizophrenia, in which there is a loss of touch with reality, are observed in less than 10% of sex offenders in general. However, Tudiver et al. (1997) reported a high incidence of psychiatric illness in the sex offender who has a developmental disability, and therefore it too should be assessed as most psychoses are treated with medication today and a specialist in psychoses should be consulted, especially when there may be other medication administered to individuals who have a developmental disability.

Bersoff, Glass, and Blain (1994) have reviewed the difficult legal and ethical issues in dealing with dual diagnoses, i.e., individuals have both a developmental disability and mentally illness. Such individuals may have their constitutional rights violated: the right to marry, have children and determine what shall be done to their own bodies. Bersoff et al. (1994) offer guidelines for individuals working with dual diagnosis cases. They note foremost that such workers must have even more training that the average worker dealing with individuals who have a developmental disability, and heightened awareness of their rights, albeit there is very little in the ethics literature that gives psychologists explicit guidelines in serving and studying individuals with multiple handicaps. They further suggest that, although one may be acting benevolently, it is important to ensure that the desire to help these people does not unduly overshadow the obligation to respect their self-determination, autonomy, and rights. Such knowledge not only helps the client, but protects the practitioners and researchers against liability. They further recommend that in criminal cases, expert sources should be consulted to learn more about procedures and about psychometrically sound instruments that should be used in assessment. They conclude that the loyalty of the worker to the client, legal system, the public, or institution is a debatable issue, but they believe the most important is that of fidelity of the worker to the client.

Biological Factors

Although all of the foregoing factors are important, biologically based factors are often especially pertinent to individuals who have a developmental disability for whom biological factors and brain injury may be at the root of the developmental disability, and/or interact with it in significant ways. Frequently, biological variables are ignored in the assessment of sex offenders in general, although Langevin and Watson (1996) found that up to 60% of sex offenders generally show neuropsychological impairment. Neuropsychological test batteries are available and may be used in conjunction with vocational test batteries to determine the client's strengths and weaknesses that may have a bearing on therapy and his potential future in the community. Although lower IQ is typically linked to a general impairment on neuropsychological tests, some individuals may show specific deficits.

The Case of Mr. E

Mr. E was described as "slow" by his probation officer and indeed his IQ score was in the borderline to developmentally delayed range. However, standard neuropsychological testing showed he suffered from aphasia and was creating his own language as he encountered novel situations. What was taken for lack of cooperation was really a lack of understanding which could be circumvented by a therapist who knew what the underlying problem was.

Reports over the years indicate that sex hormone abnormalities may appear in certain cases (see Langevin, 1992, for a review). Testosterone, for example, may be associated with increased libido and aggressiveness in sex offenders. There appear to be no endocrine studies of the sex offender who has a developmental disability to indicate if these results hold in this population. There are also extremely few studies of other endocrine conditions, such as diabetes or thyroid disorders, which can reduce emotional control, increase aggressiveness, and impair cognitive functioning in the average person (cf. Langevin & Bain, 1992). These disorders present one more disinhibiting factor that can contribute to sexually inappropriate acting out.

IATSO recommends a thorough physical examination of the sex offender, especially when physiological problems are suspected that may require specific treatment, e.g., brain damage, liver problems, or epilepsy. They further recommend that the medical/biological condition be treated first or at least in conjunction with other therapy directed at the sexually offensive behaviour. Thus, a collaboration of disciplines is needed for an ethically sound and thorough assessment of the sex offender who has a developmental disability.

Treatment Issues

Contemporary theorists are questioning whether any treatment works for sex offenders (Looman, Abracen, & Nicholaichuk, 2000; Marques, 1999; Marshall, 1993; Quinsey, Harris, Rice & Lalumiere, 1993). There has been a great optimism and naiveté over the past 40 years among sex offender treatment providers. In the 1960's and 1970's, behaviour therapy dominated and procedures such as assertion therapy and the potentially dangerous aversive conditioning, which is now banned in some locations, were used with the expectation that the sexually disordered male could be cured and his deviant behaviour forever eliminated. This optimism turned to cautious concern in the 1980's when relapse prevention therapy was introduced which did not promise a cure, but only to moderate behaviour and prevent deviant acting out. Marques (1999) notes that the question, "Does sex offender treatment work?" is too broad and needs to be addressed in terms of the specific groups treated and the program used. So too, sex offenders who have developmental disabilities should not be considered as one group. Offenders against adult females, for example, have a higher risk of recidivism than child sexual abusers or incest perpetrators (cf. Hanson & Bussiere, 1998). The confounding role of alcohol and drug abuse, antisocial personality and history, major mental illness, and the presence or absence of a sexual disorder, etc., should be taken into consideration along with the degree and nature of the developmental delay, as well as the individual's level of cognitive functioning and capacity to learn. Such a considered approach to treatment may find greater acceptability among decision makers who determine whether a sex offender who has a developmental disability will ever be in the community again.

Some current research suggests that lower intelligence scores are a predictor of both violent and sexual offense recidivism as well as treatment failure. It is difficult to evaluate the role of intelligence in recidivism and treatment outcome because too often men with lower IQs [i.e., below 80 on the Wechsler Adult Intelligence Scale (WAIS)] are excluded from studies (cf. Hall, 1988; Hanson, Steffy, & Gauthier, 1993; Quinsey, Rice, & Harris, 1995). Marques, Nelson, West, and Day (1994), raised the interesting question whether more intelligent (or more educated) offenders were better able to benefit from treatment, or the type of treatment offered; potentially reducing their risk of re-offense more so than in less intelligent subjects. Follow up results of their randomized group treatment study suggest IQ does play a role and may interact with treatment success, among other factors, albeit the effect size of IQ scores on recidivism is weak. Reddon (1996) noted that more intelligent individuals are better able to benefit from traditional therapy in general. He found in a sex offender population that higher verbal IQ was associated with greater treatment completion rate and with reduced recidivism. Verbal IQ and especially comprehension scores predicted recidivism. Reddon (1996) also noted that low WAIS-R IQ was a better predictor of recidivism than MMPI scale scores or the Buss-Durkee Hostility Inventory scales.

Tudiver et al. (1997) recommended that treatment methods for offenders who have a developmentally disability be based on those used to treat non-disabled offenders, but they should be tailored to address the learning needs and special issues facing individuals who have a developmental disability. They indicated that treatment time frames may need to be extended in order to meet the needs of individuals who have a developmental disability. Langevin and Pope (1993) reported that sex offenders with learning problems may have a negative attitude to the whole assessment process and to treatment, but this can be influenced by therapist intervention (cf. Langevin, Marentette, & Rosati, 1996). An important but unanswered question in the sex offender population is whether the lower IQ individual/learning disabled client is more likely to refuse treatment or to drop out of treatment if he starts (see also Marshall & Barbaree, 1988). Reddon's (1996) study offers support for this hypothesis. Nevertheless, there is wide variability in the level of functioning of the sex offender who has a developmental disability, which will have a significant bearing on both assessment and treatment prospects. Other factors which may be confounded with intelligence are institutional versus community setting as one may expect that higher functioning individuals are more likely to be placed in the community. Moreover, this group will have a greater opportunity to engage in conventional sexual outlets than individuals in institutions.

The role of IQ in treatability and treatment success is a weak one and it does not appear as a variable in the currently popular Violence Risk Appraisal Guide (VRAG) or Sex Offender Risk Appraisal Guide (SORAG) developed by Quinsey, Harris, Rice, and Cormier (1998), albeit treatment completion is considered a factor in reducing risk of recidivism (cf. Hanson & Bussiere, 1998). Nevertheless, attitudes about the sex offender who has a developmental disability may have a profound effect on assessment thoroughness and treatment planning.

If treatment is deemed appropriate for the sex offender who has a developmental disability, the question arises whether the same procedures used on sex offenders in general apply. Although some programs are broad-based, e.g., Haaven, Little, and Miller (1990); or may use relapse prevention therapy, the current treatment of choice; there appears to be a greater tendency in cases of the sex offender who has a developmental disability to resort to sex drive reducing medication such as medroxyprogestine acetate (Provera) (cf. Griffiths, Quinsey, & Hingsburger, 1989). These antiandrogen treatments have little acceptance among sex offenders generally and may have long term harmful side effects (Hucker, Langevin & Bain, 1988; Langevin, Wright, & Handy, 1988). Perhaps it is the frustration and inability of clinicians who have little training in treating individuals who have a developmental disability to communicate with them that leads to a chemical solution to the sexual problem. Perhaps it is the restrictive attitude toward any sexual expression in individuals who have a developmental disability that leads to a solution wherein sexual expression is suppressed (cf. Griffiths et al., 1989). The literature on sex drive reducing medication tends to provide single case reports in general and controlled studies are few in number. The cases tend to present "last resort treatment when everything else has failed." The long term effects of administering the antiandrogens to males is still unknown, although the list of side effects is daunting (cf. Mellela, Travin, & Cullen, 1989; Prentky, 1997). Some clinicians consider the alternatives to no medication worse than the consequences of taking the drugs.

However, it should be noted that it has never been conclusively demonstrated that sexual preference patterns, such as pedophilia, have been changed by sex drive reducing medication. Antiandrogens reduce libido and sexual thoughts and interest as long as the offender is taking the drug. Once the offender stops taking the drug, the original sexual preference invariably reasserts itself. In some cases, the antiandrogens appear to lose their effectiveness. The acceptability of Provera and other sex drive reducing agents remains a problem for sex offenders in general. Hucker et al. (1988) examined 100 consecutive cases of child sexual abusers and found only 41 admitted having a problem and only twenty were willing to engage in a three month course of Provera therapy with the 50% chance that Provera or a placebo would be administered. Eight more cases dropped out of treatment, leaving twelve who competed the three month procedure. One of the twelve faked taking the drug. Of course injections could have been used to insure compliance, but this would be no guarantee of cooperation with continued treatment. Some offenders "disappear" and others develop a number of side effects that leads to termination of treatment. Prentky (1997) has reviewed the issue of informed consent, noting that this is not usually a problem for individuals of average intelligence, although it is questionable whether an individual who is imprisoned can ever truly consent. Even if an offender advocate is present, can the sex offender who has a developmental disability appreciate the extent of the drugs effects and its potential harm? If antiandrogens are to be used, ability to consent must be evaluated in each case. Prentky (1997) argues that antiandrogen therapy should never be used on its own. Mellela et al. (1989) express concern over the growing legislation of antiandrogen treatment in the United States and suggest that there is a constitutional prohibition to involuntary use of this treatment. They argue however that voluntary drug treatment is promising, as long as the offender is not coerced.

Group therapy appears to be the dominant mode of treatment offered for sex offenders generally, although sex offenders prefer individual counselling to any other mode of treatment (Langevin et al., 1988). Group treatment is cost effective, but is it the optimal learning situation for the sex offender who has a developmental disability? It behooves professionals working with individuals who have a developmental disability to examine the full range of factors influencing their client's sexual behaviour and to develop a comprehensive treatment plan that has some chance of convincing administrators that an effective treatment is possible.

Griffiths et al. (1989) have noted the tendency to use aversive condition methods on individuals who have a developmental disability. Although these methods were more popular in the

1960's and 1970's, they continue to be used today in the form of olfactory aversion and the less noxious "covert sensitization". If a sexual disorder is present, aversive methods may only temporarily suppress deviant sexual desires which will return once treatment is terminated. Adaptation to a conventional or at least legal sexual relationship with a consenting adult has been recognized as a more suitable treatment aim but this may not be possible in every case (cf. Griffiths et al., 1989). Although there is a current emphasis on social skills training and sex education for the sex offender who has a developmental disability which may be especially valuable for those who do not have a sexual disorder, it is important to identify those who do suffer from a paraphilic sexual disorder. For example, some pedophilic or homosexual individuals have little or no arousal to adult females and may even find the contacts disgusting. Others may enjoy the contact with adult females and chances of successful treatment and adaptation to conventional heterosexual roles are more promising. Results of any study would be mediated by the level of functioning of the individual, degree of institutionalization, opportunities for conventional relations, level of social skills attained, and response to treatment (cf. Griffiths et al., 1989).

Assessing Risk

Historically, mental health practitioners have had enormous influence in deciding whether a person is a danger to the community and at risk for repeated offenses. Such decisions were traditionally based on clinical opinion. Contemporary theorists have turned to the actuarial method to assess risk (cf. Quinsey et al., 1998). Although these methods are still experimental and have limited research on their effectiveness, they are being used more frequently in court and in clinical risk assessment.

The best instruments now available are the Violence Risk Appraisal Guide (VRAG) and the Sex Offender Risk Appraisal Guide (SORAG). Professionals working with sex offenders who have developmental disabilities should therefore be aware of their utility and limitations. The VRAG and the SORAG, a development of the VRAG, appears to have been examined primarily at Penetanguishene (a maximum security mental health facility for individuals found "not criminally responsible" or "unfit to stand trial" by the courts) and has limited research elsewhere. However, the VRAG Manual was first published in 1998 and it is likely that more research studies on this promising instrument will appear in the near future.

Second, prediction of dangerousness and risk is not as reliable and accurate as clinicians and researchers would hope, even on the basis of actuarial methods. Hanson and Bussiere (1998) indicated that, in a meta-analysis of studies involving 23, 393 offenders, the best predictors were deviant sexual preferences, prior sexual offenses, marital status, and age. Offenders who failed to complete treatment were also at higher risk of recidivism. Unfortunately, the best combination of these and all other predictors only identified recidivism with limited accuracy. The VRAG predicted violent recidivism with 22% accuracy, but the SORAG predicted sexual offense recidivism with only 4% accuracy. Evidently much more research is needed.

Finally, there is a major problem of the validity of the measure of recidivism such as the VRAG and SORAG, which used only RCMP (Royal Canadian Mounted Police) federal prison records that they are far from complete. In a study by Langevin (1994) of over 2100 offenders seen between 1969 and 1994, the RCMP files only identified 56% of the cases. When the earliest files 1969 to 1974 were examined, only 25% of the cases were identified. Preliminary analysis of the ongoing study indicated that RCMP records tended to miss cases, wherein there was only provincial correctional time. It appears that multiple sources of data on recidivism are needed.

Conference Deliberations

The primary focus of the study group was their lack of training and resources available to assess and treat the sex offender who has a developmental disability. Concerns were expressed over what should be assessed and what treatment, if any, is appropriate. Do they have an obligation to provide treatment and is there a "right treatment" for offenders who have a developmental disability? What are the issues surrounding consent? What are the clients' rights? They wanted to know how to identify dangerous offenders who have a developmental disability and how to assess risk. How can an offender with a developmental disability and with a paraphilia be identified? In an atmosphere of uncertainty about the true nature of the population for whom they were responsible, they were also concerned about staff safety. Should a staff member legally charge a client who has a developmental disability who attacks them sexually or physically? They said they did not know what resources were available in the community to treat their clients who are also sex offenders.

Their concern reflects the findings of a survey done five years earlier by Tudiver et al. (1997) of a broad range of mental health, social services, and correctional agencies that deal with the sex offender who has a developmental disability. They concluded that services for this population were extremely limited. Agencies reported that they were faced with an increasing demand for services for this population, but they felt they could not meet the demand with their existing levels of knowledge, training, and resources. The consensus of the current consensus group was that little has changed. In part, the reluctance of authorities to provide training and resources may reflect a belief that sex offenders who have developmental disabilities are dangerous or untreatable. For political reasons and community safety, there may be a reluctance to permit treatment of individuals who have a developmental disability who may remain in an institution without criminal charges or trial or be detained indefinitely. The reluctance of administrators to train case workers in assessment and treatment methods may reflect the common attitude that nothing can be done for sex offenders who have a developmental disability or the false belief, noted by Griffiths et al. (1989), that individuals who have developmental disabilities should have no sexual expression, and, even if they are not deviant; "They should remain forever children."

Summary

State of the Art

Professionals working with the sex offender who has a developmental disability are encountering difficulties in terms of training and opportunities to provide appropriate assessments and treatment to their clients. A number of treatment programs tend to ignore sexual disorders that may appear in individuals who have a developmental disability. They address needs for socialization opportunities and institutional problems rather than address the need to select out specific individuals with developmental disabilities and possible sexual disorders who may present a danger to the community and/or have special treatment needs. Current reporting laws and legal matters are of special concern when dealing with the sex offender. Workers should turn to well established and recognized associations such as ATSA and IATSO for support on training and guidelines on assessment and treatment issues. A range of factors is important in the assessment of sex offenders who have developmental disabilities: sexual history and preference, substance abuse, mental illness and personality, history of crime and violence, neuropsychological functioning, and other biological factors that may influence sexual behaviour and cognitive functioning, especially endocrine disorders such as sex hormone abnormalities, diabetes, and thyroid dysfunction. It is especially important to have external sources of information on the sex offender in general who may omit for various reasons, important details of their history and on the sex offender who has a developmental disability who will not, or cannot, describe important historical items of information. It is further important to provide a complete assessment of the sex offender who has a developmental disability to examine biological variables that may play a significant role in his sexual misbehaviour. Neurological and endocrine factors may be especially significant to examine.

Intelligence has been considered a significant factor in treatability and treatment success. However, a number of factors are entwined with intelligence that may play an even greater role in treatment success and motivation. The role of IQ in treatment outcome is a weak one and lower IQ generally should not prevent treatment attempts. Although sex drive reducing medications appear as a first course of treatment of the sex offender who has a developmental disability, standard non-drug treatments have also been applied and may be effective. Contemporary theorists are debating the effectiveness of any treatment of sex offenders, but researchers' questions in the past may have been too broad. In treating the sex offender who has a developmental disability, specific groups such as offenders of adult females who are at greatest risk of recidivism versus child sexual abusers versus incest perpetrators who are a lower risk, should be considered separately. The individual's capacity to learn and cognitive strengths and weaknesses should be evaluated in terms of treatment goals and methods.

Finally, risk assessment has become more of a requirement in court and in clinical practice addressing violent offenders and sex offenders. These methods should be cautiously considered with sex offenders who have developmental disabilities as well. The willingness of administrators and government officials to introduce assessment and treatment procedures to the sex offender who has a developmental disability may be influenced by the comprehensiveness of assessment factors considered and the goals of treatment outlined.

Clinical Implications

Based on the information provided by the members of our conference group, many sex offenders who have developmental disabilities are not receiving appropriate assessment or treatment. Case managers lack the knowledge or skills to address the needs of these clients and to guarantee their own safety.

Agency Implications

Institutions for individuals who have a developmental disability should be aware of their responsibility to identify risk for sexual offense among their clientele who have developmental disabilities, as they may face lawsuits unless reasonable attempts have been made to protect the other residents and the community at large. It behooves institutions to provide suitable training in identifying and assessing the sex offenders among individuals who have a developmental disability who present a risk to the community and require special treatment. The agencies can turn to organizations such as ATSA and IATSO for individuals versed in the methods of assessing and treating sex offenders who may help to upgrade their staff training.

Final Consensus Statement

Much can be done for the sex offender who has a developmental disability. Some may be acting out of ignorance or lack of appropriate education, others present a risk due to paraphilic sexual disorders, and others due to criminality. Training resources are available to teach case workers the skills to asses, treat, and identify sexual disorders and other problems among sex offenders. Institutions need to take action to improve staff skills.

References

Association for the Treatment of Sexual Abusers (ATSA) (2001). *Practice standards and guidelines for members of the Association for the Treatment of Sexual Abusers.* Beaverton, OR: Author.

Bersoff, D. N., Glass, D. J., & Blain, N. (1994). Legal issues in the assessment and treatment of individuals with dual diagnoses. *Journal of Consulting and Clinical Psychology, 62 (1),* 55-62.

Coleman, E., Dwyer, S. M., Abel, G., Berner, W., Breiling, J., Hindman, J., Knopp, F. H., Langevin, R., & Pfaffline, F. (1995). The treatment of adult sex offenders: Standards of care. *Journal of Offender Rehabilitation, 23(3/4)*, 5-11.

Freund, K., McKnight, C. K., Langevin, R., & Cibiri, S. (1972). The female child as surrogate object. *Archives of Sexual Behavior, 12*, 119-133.

Freund, K., & Watson, R. (1991). Assessing the sensitivity and specificity of a phallometric test: An update of "Phallometric diagnosis of pedophilia." psychological assessment. *Journal of Consulting and Clinical Psychology, 3*, 254-260.

Griffiths, D., Quinsey, V. L., & Hingsburger, D. (1989). *Changing sexually inappropriate behaviour.* Baltimore, MD: Paul H. Brookes Publishing.

Haaven, J., Little, R., & Petre-Miller, D. (1990). *Treating intellectually disabled sex offenders: A model residential program.* Orwell, VT: Safer Society Press.

Hall, G. C. N. (1988). Criminal behavior as a function of clinical and actuarial variables in a sex offender population. *Journal of Consulting and Clinical Psychology, 55*, 773-775.

Hanson, R. K. & Bussiere (1998). Predicting relapse: A meta-analysis of sexual offender recidivism studies. *Journal of Consulting and Clinical Psychology, 66(2)*, 348-362).

Hanson, R. K., Steffy, R. A., & Gauthier, R. (1993). Long-term recidivism of child molesters. *Journal of Consulting and Clinical Psychology, 61*, 646-652.

Hucker, S., Langevin, R., & Bain, J. (1988). A double blind trial of Provera for pedophiles. *Annals of Sex Research, 1(2)*, 63-78.

Kuban, M., Barbaree, H. E., & Blanchard, R. (1999). A comparison of volume and circumference phallometry: Response magnitude and method agreement. *Archives of Sexual Behavior, 28(4)*, 345-359.

Lalumiere, M. L. & Quinsey, V. L. (1993). The sensitivity of phallometric measures with rapists. *Annals of Sex Research, 6(2),* 123-138.

Langevin, R. (1988). Defensiveness in sex offenders. in R. Rogers (Ed.) *Clinical assessment of malingering and deception* (pp. 269-290). New York: Guilford Press.

Langevin, R. (1992). Biological factors contributing to paraphilic behavior. *Psychiatric Annals, 22(6),* 315-319.

Langevin, R. (1994). *Report to the Solicitor General of Canada: A twenty-five year follow-up of sex offender recidivism.* Unpublished manuscript.

Langevin, R., & Bain, J. (1992). Diabetes in sex offenders. *Annals of Sex Research, 5,* 99-118.

Langevin, R., & Lang, R. A. (1990). Substance abuse among sex offenders. *Annals of Sex Research, 3(4),* 397-424.

Langevin, R., Marentette, D., & Rosati, B. (1996). Why therapy fails with some sex offenders: Learning difficulties examined empirically. *Journal of Offender Rehabilitation, 23,* 143-155.

Langevin, R. & Pope, S. (1993). Learning disabilities in sex offenders. *Annals of Sex Research, 6 (2),* 149-160.

Langevin, R., & Watson, R. (1996). Major factors in the assessment of paraphilics and sex offenders. *Journal of Offender Therapy, 23(3/4),* 39-70.

Langevin, R., Wright, P., & Handy, L. (1988). What treatment do sex offenders want? *Annals of Sex Research, 1,* 363-386.

Looman, J., Abracen, J., Nicholaichuk, T. P. (2000). Recidivism among treated sexual offenders and matched controls. *Journal of Interpersonal Violence, 15(3),* 279-290.

Marques, J. K. (1999) How to answer the question: "Does sex offender treatment work?" *Journal of Interpersonal Violence, 14(4),* 437-451.

Marques, J. K., Nelson, C., West, M. A., & Day, D. M.

(1994). The relationship between treatment goals and recidism among child molesters. *Behavior Research & Therapy, 32,* 577-588.

Marshall, W. L. (1993). The treatment of sex offenders: What does the outcome data tell us? A reply to Quinsey, Harris, Rice, & Lalumiere. *Journal of Interpersonal Violence, 8 (4),* 524-530.

Marshall, W. L. & Barbaree, H. W. (1988). The long-term evaluation of a behavioral treatment program for child molesters. *Behavior Research & Therapy, 26,* 499-511.

Mellela, J. T., Travin, S., & Cullen, K. (1989). Legal and ethical issues in the use of antiandrogens in treating sex offenders. *Bulletin of the American Academy of Psychiatry and Law, 17(2),* 223-232.

Prentky, R. A. (1997). Arousal reduction in sexual offenders: A review of antiandrogen intervention. *Sexual Abuse: A Journal of Research and Treatment, 9(4),* 335-348.

Quinsey, V. L., Harris, G. T., Rice, M. E., & Cormier, C. A. (1998). *Violent offenders: Appraising and managing risk.* Washington, D.C: American Psychological Association.

Quinsey, V. L., Harris, G. T., Rice, M. E., & Lalumiere, M, L. (1993). Assessing treatment efficacy in outcome studies of sex offenders. *Journal of Interpersonal Violence, 8(4),* 512-523.

Quinsey, V. L. & Lalumiere, M. L. (1996). *Assessment of sexual offenders against children: The APSAC study guide.* Newbury Park, CA: Sage Press.

Quinsey, V. L., Rice, M. E., & Harris, G. T. (1995). Actuarial prediction of sexual recidivism. *Journal of Interpersonal Violence, 10(1),* 85-105.

Rada, R. T. (1975). Alcoholism and forcible rape. *American Journal of Psychiatry, 132(4),* 444-446.

Reddon, J. R. (1996). Phoenix program for sex offender treatment: An evaluation update with recidivism data obtained in September, 1995. Submitted to Solicitor General of Canada.

Sinclair, C. (1998). Unique features of the Canadian Code of Ethics for Psychologists. *Canadian Psychology, 39(3),* 167-176.

Thompson-Cooper, I., Fugere, R., & Cormier, B. M. (1993). The child abuse reporting laws: An ethical dilemma for professionals. *Canadian Journal of Psychiatry, 38,* 557-562.

Tudiver, J., Broekstra, S., Josselyn, S., Barbaree, H. (1997). *Addressing the needs of the developmentally delayed sex offenders: A guide.* Toronto: Clarke Institute of Psychiatry.

Chapter 12

Sexual Offenses and the Legal System

Debbie Richards, Shelley L. Watson, and Randy Bleich

Introduction

Historically, reporting sexual abuse to the police when a victim has a developmental disability has been avoided more often than not. "Currently, many victims with disabilities are so severely disadvantaged in the criminal justice system that their right to personal security and equal protection of the law are almost certainly violated" (Sobsey & Mansell, 1992, p. 11). Crimes go unreported at exceedingly high rates when people with developmental disabilities are the victims. Wilson and Brewer (1992) found that 40% of crimes against people with mild and moderate mental retardation went unreported to the police and 71% of crimes against people with more severe mental retardation went unreported. Comparatively, Tharinger, Horton, and Millea (1990) estimate that only 3% of cases of sexual abuse involving people who have a developmental disability are reported to the police.

When an individual with a developmental disability commits a sexual offense, multiple factors contribute to a situation in which the crime often goes unreported. The offender is more likely to repeat the offense and continue to victimize (Sobsey, 1994). It has also been found that offending by people who have disabilities are likely to continue when treatment is denied. This is particularly true when the offender resides in an institution with continued access to potential victims (Sobsey, 1994).

Case Study

John is a 30 year old male who has a moderate developmental disability and has been living with his parents for the past year with support from a local agency. A goal of independent living has been established with ongoing community-based support. Historically, John had lived in various community residences for twenty years. He is bilingual but often has difficulty expressing himself in either language. John needs time and encouragement to express himself.

Bill is a 43 year old male who has a mild developmental disability and lives in an independent setting. He receives one hour of support per month from an adult protection service agency.

Sam is a 39 year old male who has a developmental disability. He lives in a support home affiliated with a local agency.

One day, John's mother called the agency requesting immediate help, explaining that her son had become violent in the absence of any apparent precipitant. When the support staff arrived, John was red faced, closed-fisted, and unintelligible. When asked what was upsetting him, he said that Bill had stolen his money on several occasions.

When asked if anything else took place, he described several incidents of sexual abuse and said that he feared Bill. John's mother said she was aware of these incidents which had occurred three weeks previously, but had instructed her son to try and forget what happened. However, she felt he was becoming more agitated each day, and attributed his current agitation to these assaults.

The support staff gave John the option of reporting the abuse to the police. With his consent, the police were contacted and two detectives interviewed John The police were frustrated during their attempts to elicit information from John. As a result, both detectives continually directed questions to the support staff and in turn, were redirected to John. At times, one of the officers was abrupt and loud in his questioning. After the interview, John clearly stated that he thought this detective did not believe him because "he yelled at me".

After the interview, the detectives stated that John was unable to give an "oath" or describe times or dates of the assaults. They indicated that no charges would be laid. However, they agreed to watch for Bill, the alleged perpetrator, returning to John's neighbourhood. They also stated that John would not be considered a credible witness by the court's standards due to the slowness of his speech, the lack of details given regarding the assaults, and the presence of a developmental disability.

Support staff accepted the role of providing appropriate supports for John to increase his awareness of any further situations that could potentially be dangerous or unsafe to him. This was done immediately. However, John never felt that justice had been served, nor did he feel safe from the perpetrator. John stated, "Bill should have had to go to jail".

Eight months later, Bill was charged with assaulting two children, aged nine and ten years and a male adult. The latter individual also had a developmental disability. Again, the police were hesitant in laying charges, since they were unsure if Bill understood his rights. Ultimately, he was charged.

With the commencement of court proceedings, both the defense and prosecution questioned whether Bill, in the event of a conviction, should receive a prison sentence. Both parties felt that Bill would be at risk of being victimized himself in a correctional facility. When convicted, Bill was sentenced to a two year probation period, the conditions stipulated the need for a full psychiatric assessment and treatment intervention plan.

Today, John lives in an independent setting with staff supports. He receives ongoing guidance and education in self-protection skills. There have been no subsequent disclosures of abuse from John to support staff or his family.

Bill lives in an independent setting with one hour of support per week, received from an adult protection service agency. He continues to be treated with medication from a court-appointed psychiatrist. Subsequent to his conviction, Bill was also identified as the perpetrator that sexually assaulted Sam. The alleged abuse had continued for a six month period. After support staff discussed options with Sam, he chose not to report the assaults to the police.

The agency felt an ethical dilemma as to whether they should overrule Sam's decision not to notify the police. The agency felt an ethical responsibility to report the incident to improve community safety, but this conflicted with their commitment to honour Sam's choices.

This situation remains an on-going issue for the police, the local service agency that assists individuals who have a developmental disability, and the mental health professionals treating the perpetrator.

This case study illustrates many of the issues that contribute to under reporting. Do human service agencies have an ethical responsibility to report all sexual offenses? Is there not an ethical responsibility to guarantee that victims are not revictimized? In examining these vital questions, no single correct answer emerges. Obstacles to reporting continue to be issues that need identification to ensure that appropriate action is taken, when indicated.

Literature Review

Several issues arise concerning the legal system and individuals who have a developmental disability. These include a lack of knowledge regarding developmental disability in the criminal justice system, a lack of understanding of the criminal justice system, a lack of reporting of abuse/assault to authorities, the belief that individuals who have developmental disabilities cannot testify competently, and the lack of treatment for victims and offenders who have developmental disabilities. The following literature review will address these issues.

Lack of Knowledge Regarding Developmental Disability

When individuals who have developmental disabilities inter-
face with the legal system, the system may fail due to a lack of
knowledge and expertise. Judges, lawyers, and police officers
receive little, if any, pre-service or in-service training regarding developmental disabilities (Schilit, 1979; Yuker, 1986).
Schilit (1979) found that 90.8% of law enforcement had not
received any training either formally or informally in the area
of developmental disabilities. Furthermore, only 31.5% of respondents had any professional contact with an individual who
had a developmental disability. Therefore, when law enforcement officers come into contact with an offender with a disability, they often do not know how to proceed (Schilit, 1979).

Yuker (1986) suggests that police officers possess little knowledge of people with disabilities, and that many officers harbour negative sentiments. This lack of knowledge regarding
offenders who have developmental disabilities often leads the
court to call upon psychiatrists, psychologists, and other human service professionals to guide it when working with people who have a disability. These consulting professionals are
influenced by their own attitudes, preconceptions, and misconceptions. Although the attitudes of these consultants are generally positive, they can sometimes communicate negative images of people who have disabilities (Sobsey, 1994).

Even when crimes against people who have developmental
disabilities are reported, law enforcement officials may demonstrate a reluctance to become involved (Sobsey, 1994). This
reluctance may be caused by a variety of reasons as cited by
Sobsey (1994):

1. The police may have negative attitudes or a lack of experience with people who have disabilities.
2. The police may believe that the prosecutor will reject the case because of the victim's disability.
3. The police may see the case as complex, making it likely to create a large demand on time and resources.

Sobsey, Wells, Pyper, and Reimer-Heck (1995) believe that crimes committed against individuals who have a developmental disability are sometimes given lower priority for investigation and prosecution, than crimes against other members of society. It has been shown that police are at times directed by senior administrators to stay out of the affairs of other government agencies, such as departments of mental health or disability (Sobsey, 1994).

All of these factors influence how the criminal justice system handles an offender who has a developmental disability. If criminal justice system personnel are not knowledgeable about developmental disabilities, the individual who has a developmental disability may be unduly charged, tried, and convicted of a crime of which the individual is not guilty (Schilit, 1979).

It has also been shown that lawyers are generally unaware of the rights of people with developmental disabilities, even when they are representing them as clients (Yuker, 1986). When charged with an offence, individuals who have intellectual disabilities are unlikely to be fully cognizant of the variety of criminal justice services at their disposal, or of how they may be accessed (Wilson & Brewer, 1992). They may have difficulty realizing that a particular event constitutes a crime. They may have difficulty expressing their lack of knowledge, or they may have difficulty instructing their lawyer. Individuals who have developmental disabilities may have only limited knowledge of their rights and responsibilities in this situation.

Lack of Understanding of the Criminal Justice System

Individuals who have developmental disabilities are over represented in offender prevalence rates (Murphy, Coleman, & Haynes, 1983). This may well be due to the cognitive impairment of individuals with disabilities, which makes them more likely to be caught than offenders without such impairments (Senn, 1989). The individual who has a developmental disability may also have difficulties with communication and comprehension (Ericson, Isaacs, & Perlman, 1999). For example, an individual may admit that he or she sexually assaulted someone, but may see no contradiction in describing the contact as accidental. Similarly, some individuals who have a disability may confuse their thoughts with their actions, and report sexual fantasies as if they actually occurred (Tudiver, Broekstra, Josselyn, & Barbaree, 1997).

Individuals who have a developmental disability may be more suggestible and predisposed to biased responding (Tudiver et al., 1997). The individual who has a developmental disability may be more likely to answer yes/no questions in the affirmative, even if the question posed does not make sense. The individual who has a developmental disability may also show increased compliance with persons in positions of authority in an attempt to please them (Tudiver et al., 1997). Therefore, these individuals may be vulnerable to undue influence during an investigative process.

In a study conducted by Brown and Courtless (1969), it was found that confessions or incriminating statements were obtained in two thirds of the cases when dealing with a suspected offender who had a developmental disability. In most cases, no psychological or psychiatric examination was conducted, nor was competency to stand trial discussed. In 88% of the cases, no appeal was filed. Santamour and West (1978) found that defendants who had a developmental disability plead guilty more often or confessed to the crime. There were fewer plea bargains or appealed convictions. These defendants were also granted probation and parole less frequently.

Impaired communication may also be a factor when a victim reports sexual assault. Individuals who have a developmental disability may be simply unable to report an occurrence of sexual abuse. In addition, when abuse is reported, it is often not investigated, generally because of the legal issues concerning the acceptability of the testimony of a person with a developmental disability (Sobsey, 1988).

Lack of Reporting Abuse/Assault to Authorities

Due to the increased vulnerability of the offender who has a developmental disability, service providers often avoid law enforcement notifications, except in cases of serious criminal conduct. In addition, because of the fear of adverse repercussions for service recipients and for their programs, service providers will often refrain from informing law enforcement of "minor" suspected or known criminal acts, including sexually assaultive behaviour (Ray, 1994).

To investigate additional factors contributing to the lack of reporting of sexual assault, Tudiver et al. (1997) conducted a survey of twenty seven human service agencies. These authors found that action was taken with respect to many serious sexual incidents. In almost half of the cases (44%), the incident was reported to the police and in 11.8% of the cases a report was made to a child welfare agency. Charges were laid in 34% of these reported incidents (Tudiver et al., 1997).

Reasons for not filing charges included the belief that the action was not considered a crime (35%), that the victim was too young to give evidence (5%), and the victim refused to give evidence (15%). It was also found that reports were not filed because parents did not wish to pursue charges (15%), the victim denied the incident, or there was not other evidence (10%) (Tudiver et al., 1997). There is also a reluctance on the part of many service providers to acknowledge the sexually abusive behaviour of persons with developmental disabilities as criminal (Tudiver et al., 1997).

Failure to report is also evident when dealing with victims of sexual assault who have a developmental disability. Victims and their advocates not reporting crimes is the most frequent reason that law enforcement agencies fail to lay charges. Sobsey and Doe (1991) reported that 65.9% of cases did not result in charges.

Agencies themselves are often directly responsible for conducting their own investigations of abuse (Sobsey, 1994). This process becomes a chief obstacle to effective criminal investigations of abuse in human services delivery systems.

Internal investigations often lead to the conclusion that the victim is unable to give an accurate account of the assault. Contributing to the victim's vulnerabilities are the assumptions that these individuals are unlikely to understand and report abuse and that they probably will not be believed if they do report (Senn, 1989).

An additional factor in the decision to not report a sexual assault appears to be that victims often fear the disruption of their current residential placements. Frequently, victims are directly intimidated by the abuser. In most cases, the victim knows the abuser in some capacity. 30% of offenders are family members (natural, step, or foster family), another 30% are friends or acquaintances of the victims, while 27% are specialized service providers (Sobsey, 1988). The interactions between the offender and victim are characterized by an inequity of power (Sobsey & Doe, 1991).

Individuals working within institutions where abuse has taken place often know more about the abuse that is occurring than they share with the general public (Sobsey, 1994). Staff members who have knowledge of sexual abuse do not usually report it to their supervisors. Staff are hesitant to report for a host of reasons. According to Stefan (1994), these reasons include fear of retaliation from colleagues or from administration, as well as believing that nothing will ever realistically come out of a report. Supervisors and administrators who are aware of the abuse may attempt to control the problem internally, but when they do, they avoid taking any action that could lead to public recognition. Even when authorities beyond the confines of an institution become aware of abuse, they often respond by referring the problem back to "institutional authorities" (Sobsey, 1994).

In a study conducted by Rindfleisch and Bean (1988), it was found that organizational support for reporting and affiliation with residential care have only minimal influence on willingness to report. Being an administrator and being a resident were more heavily weighted. Being a resident was positively related to willingness to report, while being an administrator was negatively related to this variable.

Administrators may be reluctant to inform police either because of fear of negative publicity, or repeated experiences of investigations, ending in yet another decision not to press charges (Stefan, 1994).

It has also been found that an abusive subculture often exists among staff in service provision for individuals who have a developmental disability (Sobsey, 1994). This subculture often predominates. Within such an abusive subculture, abuse is not viewed as either deviant or socially unacceptable. Daily abuse is viewed as normal and may become expected. Peer pressure may encourage abuse. Sobsey (1994) reports that in this looking-glass world, individuals who attempt to curtail the abuse or report the abusive behaviour become targets of social outrage and administrative retaliation.

People who commit abuse are implicitly or explicitly encouraged. The abusive subculture often intercepts any reports of abuse. Consequently, even when incidents clearly fit the criteria for mandatory reporting to outside agencies and law enforcements, studies suggest that 80-85% never reach the proper authorities (Levine–Powers, Mooney, & Nunno, 1990).

Belief that Individuals are Unable to Testify Competently

Individuals who have a developmental disability are often considered to be unreliable witnesses by service providers as well as by law enforcement agencies. This is a major stumbling block to charges being laid even after a report is filed. In a study by Sobsey and Varnahan (1991), it was reported that in 22% of cases, police declined to press charges, generally because the victim was viewed as an "incompetent witness".

Historically, people who have developmental disabilities have been regarded as unreliable witnesses, similar to young children, because of the belief that their memory systems are inherently defective. The acceptability of testimony by a person with a disability is often a legal concern; therefore, police investigations of assaults are often curtailed (Sobsey, 1988). The susceptibility to suggestibility and the lack of skills to report events accurately bias assessments of testamentary capacity (Perlman, Ericson, Esses, & Isaacs, 1994).

Because of the vulnerability of the individual who has a developmental disability to sexual abuse, it is important to determine whether and under what circumstances the individual can be considered to be a reliable witness. One must consider if they have the functional memory capacity to accurately and adequately report events. Proneness to suggestibility must be addressed. Certain question formats can be considered that might facilitate accurate reporting of particular incidents by individuals who have a developmental disability (Ericson et al., 1999; Isaacs, Ericson, & Perlman, 1994; Perlman et al., 1994).

It has been shown that individuals who have developmental disabilities vary greatly in their competence to report on events. It is the responsibility of mental health professionals to assist in the determination of specific witness capacities in individuals who have developmental disabilities.

Lack of Appropriate Treatment for Offenders

Access to treatment is another problem that arises for the individual who has a developmental disability. Abuse victims who have developmental disabilities are often denied access to treatment services. If they do access services, these services often fail to accommodate their individual needs (Sobsey et al., 1995). This is also true for the offender who has a developmental disability.

When the offender who has a developmental disability is charged with a sexual assault, treatment is often inaccessible even in institutional settings. In fact, offending may continue when offenders remain clustered in institutions with vulnerable people (Sobsey & Mansell, 1992). Offenders who do not receive treatment are likely to commit further offences. There is evidence that many adult sex offenders were victims of sexual abuse as children. Therefore, effective treatment of victims of child sexual abuse may not only help the victim, but also decrease the chance that some victims will later become offenders.

Murphy et al. (1983) reported that prisons and inpatient psychiatric facilities were most often used to confine offenders who had developmental disabilities. While these settings may be more likely to offer treatment than the institutions for non-offending individuals, there is no guarantee that the sex offender who has a developmental disability will be included in the treatment program. There is also evidence that offenders who have developmental disabilities in prison or in correctional programs are often victimized by other offenders (Murphy et al., 1983).

Police will often advocate for alternative treatment within a service agency for convicted offenders who have a developmental disability as opposed to traditional incarceration. The police are aware that these offenders are at greater risk of victimization in a penal system. Their vulnerability raises their attractiveness as victims. Lack of knowledge of rights and responsibilities may increase the impunity of the criminal who victimizes these individuals (Sobsey, 1994). Integrating individuals without specific safeguards who have a developmental disability with sex offenders who do not have disabilities may place these individuals at risk of victimization (Murphy et al., 1983; Tudiver et al., 1997). Sex offenders who have developmental disabilities have also been known to victimize "acutely psychotic patients" in inpatient facilities (Murphy et al., 1983). The literature reviewed suggests that the current system is not working. Sex offenders who have developmental disabilities are not receiving treatment to prevent further offending, may be continuing to abuse others sexually, and are being sexually abused while incarcerated (Senn, 1989).

Sobsey and Mansell (1992) state that offender treatment services should establish specific programs for offenders who have a developmental disability. Professionals who specialize in treating sex offenders often have limited experience with individuals who have a developmental disability. Likewise, professionals who specialize in developmental disabilities often lack training and knowledge regarding the treatment of sex offenders.

Conference Deliberations

During the group discussions concerning people who have developmental disabilities and the legal system, several areas were identified as primary concerns. These included the lack of an agreed protocol between agencies who serve individuals who have a developmental disability and the police, a lack of knowledge on the part of police officers when dealing with individuals who have a developmental disability, and an uneasiness on the part of service providers regarding how to report a sexual assault to the police.

The main area of concern was the relationship between the police and the community support network. Discussion revealed that police departments do not have working agreements or protocols with community support networks serving people who have disabilities. It is ironic that these same police departments have protocols for child abuse issues and adult sexual assault issues for individuals without disabilities.

Perhaps this lack of protocol is due to the lack of knowledge on the part of the police concerning individuals who have developmental disabilities. It is very difficult to find police officers who have an understanding and sensitivity to individuals who have special needs. There are few officers with specialized training in developmental disabilities, although there are officers who have received specialized training in dealing with other sexual assault victims. For example, child abuse investigators or adult sexual assault investigators are both trained in these perspective areas to perform their jobs. Police personnel present in the group argued that they do not deal with these investigations on a regular basis; therefore, it is difficult to have police investigators specially trained in the area of developmental disabilities.

Another area of concern was the need for improved rapport between agencies that serve individuals who have develop-

mental disabilities and law enforcement agencies. Many service providers have been disappointed with the interactions
that they have had with police in the past. They therefore do
not call upon the police when there is a sexual assault. Many
of the participants felt that police did not want to deal with offences committed by or against individuals who have a developmental disability. Participants agreed they often delayed or
denied reporting sexual crimes due to these past experiences.
They expressed the opinion that until there was significant improvement in the system, there were no actual benefits to reporting a sexual assault.

The lack of education police officers receive regarding the
topic of developmental disabilities was also an area of concern
for the group. Many questions were posed: How much do police officers know about individuals who have a developmental disability? Do they know the identifying characteristics of
a developmental disability? Do they have the ability to recognize the strengths and weaknesses of individuals with developmental disabilities? Are law enforcement officials aware of
how individuals who have a developmental disability interact
with others, how they function, how they think? Do they hold
stereotypes and misconceptions about individuals with developmental disabilities? Overall, the group felt that police are
not able to efficiently respond and deal with complaints by individuals who have a developmental disability because of their
lack of training in this area.

The group was informed that the Ontario Police College has
no training programs for educating police investigators to conduct investigations with persons who have developmental disabilities. The group felt police need to be aware of some of the
communication difficulties that these individuals may have.

Police officers need to receive training on how to communicate with individuals who have a developmental disability. They should receive assistance from individuals who work with these clients when conducting interviews. The group felt that police need to take ownership for their education and that police should also collaborate with local agencies to conduct joint training sessions.

The involvement of service providers in decisions surrounding the legal process was also discussed. Participants were unsure about issues regarding the timing of reporting incidents of sexual abuse to their agency or to the police. When discussing offending client behaviour, the fear of reprimand by their administrators for reporting was expressed. This fear was countered by the feeling of legal obligation to the community to report the offense. When talking about a client who is a victim of sexual assault, participants felt the need to protect their clients from the potentially painful emotional experience inherent in the reporting process.

Many issues arise regarding the preparation of clients for involvement in the legal system. Issues of suggestibility during interviews, confidentiality, appropriate documentation, and the potential for evidence to be contaminated were all discussed. Participants felt ill-prepared to participate in the legal process.

The conviction of offenders who have a developmental disability was another concern expressed by the group. Should offenders go to jail where they may be revictimized by other offenders? Alternatives to incarceration, such as diversion programs, were discussed.

The group articulated the difficulty in distinguishing if there has been a sexual assault or if the client has made a poor decision. They also acknowledged concern regarding issues of consent not being well addressed. The need for interviewers to be trained to effectively communicate with individuals with developmental disabilities was stressed.

Consensus of the Group

The group agreed there is a need to develop protocols and guidelines for use by the police and community support networks. The group felt that there has to be a consistent approach to sexual assault investigations. Education of investigators so that they are sensitive to the unique issues facing the individual who has a developmental disability was emphasized.

When dealing with a client who is a victim of sexual assault, there has to be more consultation with all persons involved to ensure that the victim's rights are protected. The fact that these individuals are presumed unlikely to understand and report abuse and that they will not be believed if they do report must be addressed (Senn, 1989). Police officers need to be more sensitive to the special needs of the victim who has a developmental disability and work with service agencies to ensure that the victim does not undergo any further harm.

If a person with a developmental disability is arrested and charged, there must be assurance that his/her rights are clearly explained and that the accused person understands his/her rights. Guidelines need to be set out for the reporting of offending behaviour by clients who have developmental disabilities. In order for this to happen, there is a need for the establishment of communication protocols between the police and agencies that work with individuals who have a developmental disability.

Summary

State of the Art

Sexually offending behaviour both by individuals who have a developmental disability and against individuals who have a developmental disability are community problems. Community mandates to address these problems fall under the jurisdiction of many different agencies and organizations, each with their own philosophy and mandate. There is often a lack of communication between agencies that support individuals who have developmental disabilities and police departments. The development of shared philosophies and improved communication could be the cornerstones of a successful working relationships between these agencies and police departments (Tudiver et al., 1997). Agency roles must also be co-ordinated so that there is a continuum of service and care for the individual who has a developmental disability who sexually offends, or is the victim of sexual assault. Formal guidelines would also ensure that law enforcement notifications are made consistently and fairly (Ray, 1994).

Clinical Implications

When dealing with a client who has sexually offended, law enforcement notification should be mandatory, regardless of the perceived harm or lack of harm to the victim. There should also be a requirement for law enforcement notification in cases of recurring criminal conduct where the offender's behaviour has not decreased, despite agency counselling, training, and support (Ray, 1994). If the incident is reported to the proper authorities, the legal system may serve as a means of holding the individual accountable for his/her behaviour and linking him/her with the appropriate intervention (Tudiver et al., 1997). The introduction of an offender with a developmental disability into the legal system may also enhance treatment participation and compliance. If the behaviour is not reported, then there are no consequences for the offender and the offensive behaviour could escalate (Tudiver et al., 1997).

It is imperative that police officers be aware of developmental disabilities and cognizant of the characteristics of individuals who have disabilities (Schilit, 1979; Yuker, 1986). Individuals with developmental disabilities may have difficulty with traditional communication methods. They may have a non-traditional form of communication. Police officials need to ask the victim or caregiver if there is an alternative method of communication required, such as Bliss symbols or Picture Communication Symbols. It has also been suggested that wallet-sized cards could be developed for law enforcement personnel that list important information on the recognition of individuals with a developmental delay (Tudiver et al., 1997). Strategies for effective communication should be included on these cards, as well as a phone number of an agency that can provide assistance in dealing with the individual involved.

Agency Implications

It is the responsibility of agency support staff to provide accurate details to the investigating police officers related to the special needs of the individual. This will facilitate an optimal interview with both victims and alleged offenders. Consideration should be given to providing the following information:

- The etiology of the individual's developmental disability
- Any accompanying disorders, such as epilepsy
- How the disability affects the individual's functioning
- What augmentative communication strategies are available
- Any medications the individual is using
- If the individual has had any sex education, and if so, what he/she has learned
- Have there been any previous experiences with this individual? (although the interview is specific to THIS incident)
- Any noted behavioural change within the individual
- Any emotional responses or previous coping strategies that could be facilitated to optimize the individual's participation in the interview

It is the responsibility of the police official to inform the detainee of his or her right to council. This includes the obligation to explain this right in a manner which the detainee can understand. Where, however, there is indication that the accused does not understand his or her right to counsel, police must take steps to facilitate that understanding. The police officer must possess effective communication strategies for dealing with individuals who have a developmental disability. As has been stated, there are a number of misconceptions about persons who have developmental disabilities that may contribute to whether or not a charge is laid. It is incumbent upon agencies supporting individuals with developmental disabilities to promote community education to counter these misconceptions.

What Should Be Done Now

Service providers should endeavour to ensure that community policing objectives incorporate procedures for assisting people who have a developmental disability (Wilson & Brewer, 1992). These objectives might include police undertaking some routine contact/checking designed to increase the likelihood that crimes will be reported. The following guidelines to reporting a sexual assault are an example of a protocol arising from a partnership between a local police department and agencies supporting individuals with developmental disabilities. The objective of these guidelines is to ensure a consistent community approach when an allegation of sexual abuse or assault is made involving an individual with a developmental disability. See Figure 1 for Guidelines and Practices to Reporting a Sexual Assault (Richards, Watson, & Bleich, 2000), a protocol in place in the Niagara Region, Ontario.

In order for protocols to be effective, special training should be provided to police personnel with regard to issues of disability. Sexual violence prevention and intervention should be a priority for law enforcement officials. In order to establish a more effective role in preventing and responding to such violence, police officials require specific training and resources to deal with this type of crime (Skoog & O'Sullivan, 1993).

Final Consensus Statement

Consensus achieved at the 1998 Sexuality: Ethical Dilemmas Conference articulated two major areas that need to be addressed with regard to sexual offenses and persons who have a developmental disability. While we can strive for abuse-free environments, we realize the immensity of this challenge, ac-

Figure 1

**Guidelines and Practices To Reporting a Sexual Assault
(for People who have a Developmental Disability)**

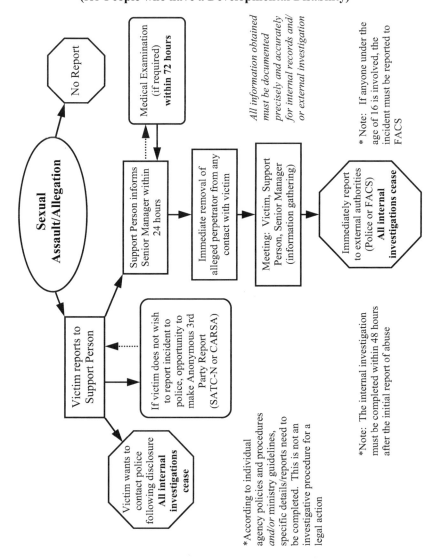

(Richards, Watson, & Bleich, 2000)

knowledging the fundamental dynamic of abuse, and its promotion by authoritarian structures that emphasize power and control within service agencies. However, through strategic planning and awareness, abuse can be significantly decreased, if we pursue the following two goals:

1. An increased educational standard established for law enforcement, the judicial system, agency employees, and individuals who have a developmental disability

2. A committed working relationship between the legal system and agencies supporting people who have a developmental disability

This belief is supported by Sobsey's (1994) statement, people with disabilities have often been systematically excluded from programs to prevent abuse from services that support victims. Even their basic right to personal security has often been denied through lack of access to the law enforcement and criminal justice systems that protect other members of society" (p. xiv). If an effort and commitment is made to promote education and partnerships within systems, positive change for people who have developmental disabilities is possible.

References

Brown, A. & Courtless, T. F. (1969). The mentally retarded offender. In R.C. Allen (Ed.), *Readings in law and psychiatry*. Baltimore, MA: Johns Hopkins University Press.

Ericson, K., Isaacs, B., & Perlman, N. (1999). Enhancing communication: The special case of interviewing victim-witnesses of sexual abuse. In I. Brown & M. Percy (Eds.),

Developmental disabilities in Ontario, (pp. 453-462). Toronto, ON: Front Port Publishing.

Isaacs, B., Ericson, K., & Perlman, N. B. (1994). Recall of the developmentally handicapped witness. *Canadian Journal of Human Sexuality, 3(1)*, 77-80.

Levine-Powers, J., Mooney, A., & Nunno, M. (1990). Institutional abuse: A review of the literature. *Journal of Child and Youth Care, 4(6)*, 81-95.

Murphy, W. D., Coleman, E. M., & Haynes, M. R. (1983). Treatment and evaluation issues with the mentally retarded sex offender. In J. G. Greer & I. R. Stuart (Eds.), *The sexual aggressor: Current perspectives in treatment* (pp. 22-41). New York, JY: Van Nostrand Reinhold Company.

Perlman, N., Ericson, K., Esses, V., & Isaacs, B. (1994). The developmentally handicapped witness: Competency as a function of interview strategy. *Law and Human Behaviour, 18*, 171-187.

Ray, N. K. (1994). Capitalizing on the safety net of incident reporting systems in community programs. In J. Sundram (Ed.), *Choice and responsibility: Legal and ethical dilemmas in services for persons with mental disabilities*, pp. 277-296. Albany, NY: New York State Commission on Quality of Care for the Mentally Disabled.

Richards, D., Watson, S, & Bleich, R. (2000). Guidelines and practices to reporting sexual assault (for people who have a developmental disability). *Journal on Developmental Disabilities, 7(1)*, 130-140.

Rindfleisch, N. & Bean, G. J. (1988). Willingness to report abuse and neglect in residential facilities. *Child Abuse & Neglect, 12*, 509-520.

Santamour, M. S, & West, B. (1978, October). The retarded offender and corrections. *Mental Retardation and the Law*, 25-37.

Senn, C. (1989). *Vulnerable: Sexual abuse and people with an intellectual handicap.* Downsview, ON: G. Allan Roeher Institute.

Schilit (1979). The mentally retarded offender and criminal justice personnel, *Exceptional Children, 46,* 16-22.

Skoog, D. M. & Sullivan, S. P. (1993). *Police training and family violence: A foundation for the future.* Ottawa, ON: Solicitor General of Canada and Canadian Association of Chiefs of Police.

Sobsey, D. (1988). Sexual offenses and disabled victims: Research and practical implications, *Vis-à-Vis, 6(4),* 1-2.

Sobsey, D. (1992). Sexual abuse in perspective and how to reduce the risks. *New Zealand Disabled, 5,* 20-23.

Sobsey, D. (1994). *Violence and abuse in the lives of people with disabilities: The end of silent acceptance?* Baltimore, MA: Paul H. Brookes Publishing Co.

Sobsey, D. & Doe, T. (1991). Patterns of sexual abuse and assault. *Sexuality and Disability, 9(3),* 243-259.

Sobsey, D. & Mansell, S. (1992). The prevention of sexual abuse of people with developmental disabilities. *Network, 2(3),* 8-17.

Sobsey, D. & Mansell, S. (1992). Teaching people with disabilities to be abused and exploited. *Active Treatment Solutions, 3(4),* 6-11.

Sobsey, D. & Varnhagen, C. (1991). Sexual abuse, assault, and exploitation of Canadians with disabilities. In C. Bagley & R. J. Thomlinson (Eds.), *Child sexual abuse: Critical perspectives on prevention, intervention, and treatment* (pp. 203-256). Toronto, ON: Wall and Emerson.

Sobsey, D., Wells, D., Pyper, D., & Reimer-Heck, B. (1995). *Violence and disability: An annotated bibliography.* Baltimore, MD: Paul H. Brookes Publishing.

Stefan, S. (1994). "Dancing in the sky without a parachute":

Sex and love in institutional settings. In J. Sundram (Ed.), *Choice and responsibility: Legal and ethical dilemmas in services for persons with mental disabilities*, pp.219-244. Albany, NY: New York State Commission on Quality of Care for the Mentally Disabled.

Tharinger, D., Burrows Horton, C., & Millea, S. (1993). Sexual abuse and exploitation of children and adults with mental retardation and other handicaps. In M. Nagler (Ed.), *Perspectives on disability* (2nd edition), pp. 235-246. Palo Alton, CA: Health Markets Research.

Tudiver, J., Broekstra, S., Josselyn, S., & Barbaree, H. (1997). *Addressing the needs of developmentally delayed sex offenders: A guide*. Health Canada.

Wilson, C. & Brewer, N. (1992). The incidence of criminal victimization of individuals with an intellectual disability. *Australian Psychologist, 2,* 114-117.

Yuker, H. E. (1986). Disability and the law: Attitudes of police, lawyers, and mental health professionals. *Rehabilitation Psychology, 31(1),* 13-25.

Chapter 13

Summary of Ethical Issues

Gordon DuVal

Introduction

The twelve chapters in this volume canvas the diverse and challenging range of ethical problems arising in the sexuality of persons with developmental disabilities. Although practitioners and caregivers seek clear norms and standards to assist with the resolution of these dilemmas, a determination of ethically appropriate choices necessarily involves the balancing of disparate and often conflicting values. At the heart of ethical issues regarding sexuality and persons with developmental disabilities, two important values, or clusters of values, are in tension. Watson, Venema, Molloy, and Reich characterize these values in Chapter 1.

Persons with developmental disabilities have the right to develop and engage in caring and intimate relationships, which may have sexual expression. As a number of the authors point out, these relationships are natural and intrinsic to personhood, dignity and positive conceptions of the self. We all share the need for affection and intimacy, and persons with developmental disabilities are no different. To deny such opportunities is a violation and treats them as less than full persons.

Persons with developmental disabilities are also entitled to privacy and to have personal information treated confidentially, as an expression of this respect, in the same way as we treat others without such disabilities. Persons with developmental disabilities should be given information relevant to the choices they may reasonably make. Such persons are often poorly informed about sexuality and socially acceptable sexual expression. They are often misinformed or poorly informed about their right to sexual expression, to choose their own partners, to be free of coercion, exploitation, and abuse, about their rights and obligations in the agency supervised setting, and about the impact of their disability on sexual functioning.

While these principles and values are essential to the just treatment of persons with developmental disabilities, it is important to note also that there are a number of problems and dangers surrounding their sexual activity. Clinicians and caregivers rightly see such persons as sometimes requiring assistance and protection by reason of their disability. Risks attending sexual activity include unwanted pregnancy, sexually transmitted disease, and sexual coercion, exploitation, and abuse. For a variety of reasons, persons with developmental disabilities are at increased risk of being harmed in these ways and often need help and education to reduce or avoid such harm. In the agency supervised setting, caregivers and staff have a fiduciary obligation to take reasonable steps, and have reasonable procedures in place, to protect individuals in their care.

Ethical dilemmas in this context often arise when these two principles, respect for self-determination and protection of vulnerable persons, come into conflict. Neither value is inherently more important and the particular context and narrative of the situation is always essential to determining a proper balance between these values. Nevertheless, there are other ethical considerations that can be helpful in striking that balance.

Persons with developmental disabilities are presumptively entitled to make and act on their own choices when they have the appropriate decisional capacity to do so. Assessments of capacity raise challenging questions, and will be addressed more fully later. However, such determinations must be made in the context of the particular choice to be made. That is, a person may be incapable of making particular kinds of decisions, in particular situations, but may be capable of making other choices, or the same choice in other circumstances or at other times.

Restrictions on the self-determination of an individual must be reasonable and aimed at avoiding significant harms or risks of harm. Such limitations of freedom must be the least possible, consistent with achieving the valid protective purposes for which they are imposed. Limitations on freedom of choice must be made on the basis of protection of the person or others from harm, and not on enforcing caregivers' or family's values. Sexual expression by such persons can inspire strong emotions and often makes others uncomfortable. Respect for persons includes accepting difference. While caregivers and families have an important obligation to advocate for and assist persons with developmental disabilities, they must be wary of infantilizing them or creating dependence in doing so.

Overview of Subsequent Chapters

In Chapters 2 and 3, Owen, Griffiths, Lindenbaum, and Arbus-Nevestuk address sexual policies in agencies supporting persons with developmental disabilities. The authors argue that agencies should develop clear policies with respect to sexuality, noting that problems will inevitably arise. It is preferable to have policies available to address these problems in a way that expresses the values of the institution. A sexuality policy permits staff to address problems in a coherent way and allows for consistent treatment of clients and staff when difficulties arise. It should be developed and approved with the input of clients, families, and other stakeholder groups to reflect the broad range of needs and perspectives.

Such policies have a number of purposes:

- To clarify the agency culture and values and give context and background to particular policies and practices.
- To supply decision models and guidelines that staff can apply in particular circumstances while at the same time allowing flexibility to adapt to unusual situations.
- To provide clear sanctions for policy violation.
- To train staff to apply the policy in keeping with agency values, ethical and legal standards, and with an awareness of the issues of counter transference.
- To encourage a frank discussion of ethical boundaries and to encourage staff to come forward to seek help and guidance in case of uncertainty.

The authors argue that policies should not to be overly restrictive of sexual activity. They should not, for example, prohibit all sexual behaviour but focus instead on education and protection from abuse and exploitation. They should give consistent direction, delineate agency responsibilities clearly and provide guidelines to assist staff in handling difficult situations. Policies should establish procedures for dealing with inappropriate or criminal sexual behaviour, since persons with developmental disabilities may be vulnerable both to victimization and also to developing sexually offending behaviour.

Policies should make provision for access to medical services including birth control, information about and treatment for sexually transmitted disease, pregnancy, and sexual issues relating to the individual's disability, including sexual dysfunction and the effects of medications on sexual activity. Prevention of sexual abuse is a key component of a sexuality policy. This includes educating potentially vulnerable clients about the nature of abuse, their rights with respect to physical contact and sexual activity, the practices of abusers, and strategies for avoiding or reducing the incidence of sexual abuse.

A policy should provide standards for consent to sexual activity. Valid consent requires adequate information, decision-making capacity and a voluntary choice. There should be an understanding of simple anatomy, avoiding pregnancy and sexually transmitted disease, the right to say no for any reason, and the social and emotional consequences of engaging in sexual activity. Although decision-making capacity should be presumed, valid consent requires that the person understand and appreciate this and other information relevant to a decision to engage in sexual activity.

Finally, consent must be voluntary and not take place in the context of a coercive relationship. Consent to have sex with a caregiver or staff member can never be voluntary.

There should also be education about healthy boundaries with caregivers, both to promote a healthy therapeutic relationship and to reduce abuse. Caregivers should be vigilant to the power dynamics of the staff-client relationship, including the potential for coercion or intimidation. The therapeutic alliance requires a relationship of trust. Such trust however, cannot be confused with an expectation of unquestioned compliance to authority. Clients should be encouraged to speak freely about their feelings toward abuse and any concerns about the appropriateness of staff behaviour.

Agency sexuality policy should be premised on an understanding of the dynamic and psychology of the abusing caregiver; physical, emotional, and psychological indications for the existence of abuse; standards for investigating suspected abuse, and appropriate involvement and interactions with police. The policy should provide opportunities for client education about relationship development and should encourage a range of positive relationships. There should be adequate resources for training staff to implement the policy, which should be applied consistently by all staff and throughout the agency.

In Chapter 4, Sheehan examines the crucial issue of consent to sexual relations. She focuses on the balance between individual freedom and privacy, and protecting potentially vulnerable persons from abuse and possible psychological and physical harms. In analyzing requirements for consent to sexual activity, both criminal and health-care perspectives are examined.

Sexual contact without consent is a crime. The criminal standard of valid consent is high, such that most persons with developmental disabilities would not be capable of consenting. This is particularly true of young persons, except where the age difference between the parties is small. In this regard, the law focuses on a presumed lack of maturity and judgment in young people and the potential for coercive exercise of authority or persuasion. A position of trust or authority precludes valid consent by minor children.

What should be the standard of valid consent by persons with a developmental disability who are of adult years but have the mental age and maturity of a minor? According to Sheehan, valid consent requires "... informed and voluntary consent by a person of social maturity who appreciates the moral context of the activity and is free of coercive influence" (p. 145). Consent must be based on knowledge of significant relevant factors including an understanding and appreciation of the nature of sexual activity, its emotional and psychological consequences and social context.

Sheehan argues that the capacity to consent to sexual activity involves the following:

• The ability to appreciate the nature of sexual activity, the risks involved, and ways of reducing those risks,
• An understanding that the person may refuse at any time, and
• Appreciation that there are physical risks (such as pregnancy and sexually transmitted diseases) as well as emotional risks, including rejection, guilt, and embarrassment.

Capacity to consent to sexual activity is context-dependent. A person with a developmental disability may be incapable of engaging in certain activities, with some persons, under some circumstances, but capable in others. Decision-making capacity can change over time. So, a person may be incapable of making a particular choice at one time, but capable at another.

Accordingly, there is a need for individual clinical evaluation of capacity that relates to the particular circumstances of the choice. For the protection of others, it is important also to identify and assess persons who would not be capable of appreciating the language and behaviour of non-consent by another.

Assessments of capacity should be on-going and should acknowledge the contextual and dynamic nature of decision-making capacity. Once such determination is made, caregivers should take steps to protect those who are not capable of consenting, but respect the privacy and dignity of those who are capable, whether or not they have a developmental disability.

In Chapter 5, Watson, Griffiths, Richards, and Dykstra address the particular needs of persons with developmental disabilities for sexuality education "... to enable their successful transition from childhood into adulthood and...be able to enjoy the rights and responsibilities as a member of adult society." (p. 175) Such education is often neglected for persons with developmental disabilities. However, it is vital for a number of reasons:

- Persons with developmental disabilities often have gaps in their knowledge and experience about sexual issues and little opportunity to discuss and learn about sexual matters.
- Persons with developmental disabilities have been shown to have many misconceptions about sexuality that not only confuse, but also create risks for them.
- Deinstitutionalization has resulted in large numbers of persons with developmental disabilities living in the community with increased opportunities for developing sexual relationships, arguably with less direct support and guidance.
- There is an increasing awareness of sexual exploitation and abuse against this population.
- The increasing prevalence of HIV/AIDS renders the need

for information on these topics particularly acute.
- There is increasing interest expressed by persons with developmental disabilities themselves for such education.

The authors identify an exhaustive list of topics that should be taught to persons with developmental disabilities. These include: medical and physiological information about birth control, pregnancy, sexually transmitted disease, and other consequences of sexual behaviour, including parenthood; relationship skills and sociosexual training, including self-esteem, sexual lifestyles, social and emotional aspects of sexuality and attitudes about sex; appropriate limits to sexual expression including consent and "good touching/bad touching"; methods of protection from abuse and common tactics of exploitative persons; and ways that the person's particular disability may impact his or her sexuality.

The authors argue for the development of guidelines for teaching sexuality to persons with developmental disabilities. They encourage that teaching be incorporated into the every day living environment and employ primarily non-didactic techniques. Training should be non-judgmental and should avoid value-laden words and expressions. In training, as in treatment, educators should seek to build trust with clients and ensure confidentiality of clients' responses and input.

With respect to sex education, three particular ethical problems are raised. First, the authors acknowledge the lack of evidence of effectiveness of sex education and training for persons with developmental disabilities, yet they strongly encourage its use. Studies demonstrating effectiveness are inconclusive and some studies have suffered from significant methodological flaws. Clearly, more research is needed to demonstrate both the effectiveness of educational techniques themselves and the effectiveness of education for individual clients. Second, there is a worry that very comprehensive education sends a mixed message to clients, families and other caregivers. While agency staff is encouraged to foster independence in other areas, they may be strongly paternalistic and directive in sexuality education. Clearly, the focus should be on supporting and providing resources to persons with developmental disabilities and not simply protecting them or imposing agency values on their sexual lives. Third, it is difficult for educators to avoid imposing their own values in sex education, in view of the sensitive nature of the subject matter and the strong feelings and beliefs that the topic inspires in everyone, including educators.

In Chapter 6, King and Richards trace the history and canvas the ethical issues involved in sterilization and birth control for persons with developmental disabilities. The right of individuals to control their own procreation must be balanced against the welfare of their prospective children. Because of the far-reaching effects and irreversibility of sterilization, and the sensitive context of the situation, the issue is one that must be approached carefully. If a person is capable of making a decision with respect to sterilization and birth control, others should not make such a decision. There should be no presumption of incapacity to make these decisions. Even assuming the presence of decision-making capacity, education and counselling is necessary to ensure that the decision is voluntary. Requirements for information and voluntariness are high, due to the serious and irreversible nature of these decisions. Competent persons with developmental disabilities should be provided accurate information in a clear and understandable way. A client considering sterilization should be aware of other options for contraception and should be encouraged to select the least restrictive method of birth control, while permitting the greatest freedom of social activity. In general, the least permanent method of birth control is preferable if consistent with other goals.

In Chapter 7, Feldman describes the significant impediments and supports to successful parenting faced by persons with developmental disabilities. The purpose is to guide determinations of the suitability of parents or potential parents. While full inclusion of people with developmental disabilities includes sexual expression, there is less public endorsement for parenting by these individuals. A personal interest in having and raising children can conflict with the best interests of potential children.

The author identifies a number of impediments to successful parenting by persons with developmental disabilities:

- Parents with developmental disabilities are disproportionately involved in child protection cases, although this may be to some extent the result of subtle discrimination, rather than a fair assessment of risk to the child. In such cases, the concern is more often neglect than abuse.
- Parents with developmental disabilities are almost always poor, poorly educated, and un- or under-employed. These factors create family stresses that may negatively impact on children. In addition, low IQ may interfere with effective parenting, and result in parents adopting a "cloak of competence" that interferes with obtaining services and supports that would otherwise be available.
- Parents with developmental disabilities may themselves be especially vulnerable to financial or sexual exploitation, with negative repercussions for children. Further, they often have co-occurring medical or mental health problems,

including high rates of depression, which may result in dysfunctional parent-child interactions and other problems. Parents with developmental disabilities often suffer social isolation and a lack of needed supports. They may also lack insight into the kinds of services and supports they require. Children of parents with developmental disabilities are at increased risk for developmental problems. These factors, together with society's enduring stigmatization of this population, cause significant parental stress that may interfere with adequate parenting.

Services that are compassionate, appropriate, and effective can greatly enhance the quality of life of parents with developmental disabilities and their children, and attenuate the impediments they face. A majority of parents with developmental disabilities can learn child-care skills with proper support. Further research is needed to determine the effectiveness of interventions and support aimed at parents with developmental disabilities. Some agencies are working toward finding resources and supports for parents with developmental disabilities and there is a trend in court decisions favouring keeping natural families together.

The author makes a number of recommendations. Among them:

- In making decisions about their suitability as parents, persons with developmental disabilities should be judged on the same criteria as those without disabilities
- Assessments of parental capacity should take account of relevant impediments and supports
- Education should be considered as an initial alternative to terminating parental rights

- Consideration should be given to specialized foster arrangements, whereby parents may keep the child but receive assistance in giving care. "[T]he biological parents can sometimes be taught to carry out some child-care activities with guidance and supervision provided as needed by the foster parents." (p. 281)

In Chapter 8, Cox-Lindenbaum and Watson explore the ethical issues surrounding sexual assault against persons with developmental disabilities. Such individuals are more vulnerable to abuse than those without disability. To some extent, this increased abuse is related to negative social attitudes toward persons with developmental disabilities and their sexuality.

Power inequities are important factors in abuse by caregivers, who comprise roughly one-half of perpetrators of abuse. Indeed, the perpetrator is known to the victim or to their caregivers in 96% of cases. Perpetrators who exploit the caregiving relationship typically do so many times before being apprehended. Often, the agency response is to blame the victim or ignore indications of abuse by staff.

The victim's insufficient knowledge of appropriate physical and sexual behaviour, poor judgment, and over-compliance to the authority of caregivers or others also contributes to victimization. Society's de-sexualized image of persons with developmental disabilities often results in a failure to recognize the possibility of abuse. Society's subtle devaluation of these persons contributes to abuse against them.

Dependence on caregivers may render persons with developmental disabilities more trusting, compliant, and passive, and may create a fear of losing ties to caregivers. Impairments in communication may create greater vulnerability since persons with developmental disabilities often lack the ability to protest effectively, or report incidents of abuse. Even when abuse is reported, they may be seen as less credible in criminal justice proceedings. Social isolation and institutionalization may result in increased vulnerability to abuse.

While training potential victims to avoid or resist abuse is a standard approach, it must be supplemented by steps to reduce abusive situations encountered by persons with developmental disabilities. Within agencies, proactive preventive programs can reduce vulnerability. An example is implementation of stricter staff screening and hiring procedures. In addressing these problems, there must be vigilance to identify cues that abuse may be occurring.

Treatment programs for offenders are also important, since treatment can reduce the incidence of future abuse. Understanding abuse is particularly important because without adequate treatment a significant proportion of victims will themselves become abusers. When abuse occurs, charges should be laid and convictions obtained wherever possible.

In Chapter 9, Goldman and Morrison address the sources of and responses to inappropriate sexual behaviour by persons with developmental disabilities. Sexual misbehaviours are over represented in this population. A number of factors may play a role in increased sex offences by persons with developmental disabilities. These include: a history of being abused, ignorance about appropriate sexual or physical behaviours, segregation by gender, absence of sex education, and impaired mental abilities and adaptive skills.

Some apparently sexually deviant behaviour is in fact "counterfeit deviance," defined as "... behaviours that appear deviant upon initial observation that can be attributed to factors other than deviant arousal upon closer analysis" (Hingsburger, Griffiths, & Quinsey, cited on p. 8). A lack of privacy may result in persons with developmental disabilities carrying out sexual activities in non-public places. If sex is prohibited by agency policy, any such activity may be characterized as illicit. However, consensual sex should not generally be characterized as inappropriate or deviant. There is a need for education of parents and staff members to understand the individual client as an adult with normal sexual urges and needs. Sexual expression is not inherently wrong or inappropriate for a person with developmental disability.

Predatory sexual behaviour by persons with developmental disabilities arises from a number of factors. While such offenders often require close supervision to protect the community, they should be confined in the least restrictive setting in which they can safely reside, and should be offered treatment. An offender should be comprehensively assessed, including screening for the presence of alcohol, drugs, mental illness, and environmental conditions, to determine appropriate treatment approaches.

Prompt reporting of truly aberrant sexual behaviour helps reduce predatory activity and facilitates getting help for both victim and offender. More research is required to determine effective education and intervention to reduce sexual misbehaviour. Education is needed to help caregivers and others distinguish counterfeit deviance from true sexual predation. Criminal justice officials should have information to help them understand that persons with developmental disabilities who engage in sexual misbehaviour are not all predators requiring incarceration, although some may need treatment and possibly restricted confinement. Residential settings should be designed and operated in ways that promote sexual health and discourage inappropriate behaviours.

In Chapter 10, Fedoroff, Fedoroff and Peever discuss ethical issues in consent to treatment by sexual offenders with developmental disabilities. Even for offenders convicted and given a sentence conditional upon seeking treatment, neither the agency nor the treatment team is obliged to offer treatment, and the accused maintains the right to refuse treatment. The team must decide whether he or she meets the criteria for involuntary commitment under local laws, typically if the accused poses a danger to self or others by reason of mental illness. Although a person is involuntarily detained, the treatment team is not entitled to administer medications without valid consent. Under a conditional sentence, the accused may still elect to refuse treatment. If he or she is incompetent, consent must be obtained from a legally authorized substitute decision-maker. Other normal obligations with respect to treatment apply. Consent must be voluntary, capable, and informed. So, the person must be told the risks and benefits of treatment as well as the availability and effectiveness of alternative treatment, including no treatment.

At a court-ordered assessment, the accused must be made aware that the agency is obliged to report any relevant clinical information to the court. For purposes of treatment however, the level of disclosure to the court or others is a matter to be negotiated with the accused, who has the right to know and control what will be done with the information obtained.

There are certain exceptions however, since the treatment team has an obligation to report otherwise confidential information for a variety of purposes, primarily to protect the safety of others. For example, under child protection laws, clinicians are obliged to report known and suspected sexual offences against identifiable minors. In addition, contemplated dangerous or criminal behaviours may have to be reported under certain circumstances. The reporting obligations of the treatment team should be disclosed at the outset, so there is no subsequent confusion.

Relations with family members can be complex, particularly with regard to clinical information about the client. In dealing with families, the treatment team must not engage in or encourage deceptive behaviour. Limits on the release of clinical information imposed by a competent client/patient must be respected, even when it is parents that request it. While the team must safeguard confidential information, except to the extent required by law, there is no prohibition against the team gathering information, from parents or others, to assist in the effective treatment of the patient/client. Indeed, in planning care, it is important to involve trusted individuals, including family members in care.

In Chapter 11, Langevin and Curnoe argue that when persons with developmental disabilities are charged with or convicted of a sexual offence, they should be treated much like any other offender. Special treatment may result in violation of the person's civil liberties. However, there are a number of difficulties surrounding the assessment and treatment of persons with developmental disabilities involved, or alleged to be involved, in sexual offences.

A comprehensive assessment of sexual offenders, or alleged sexual offenders, should include all pertinent factors relating to the person, including sexual history and preference, substance abuse, mental illness and personality, history of crime and violence, neuropsychological functioning, and other biological factors that may influence sexual behaviour and cognition. However, tools for such assessments are at best variably effective in this population.

Under child welfare laws, a person who reveals thoughts of sexually or physically abusing an identifiable child must be reported, compromising confidentiality and harming the therapeutic relationship. While clients should be advised of this reporting obligation in advance, persons with developmental disabilities may be particularly unguarded in making such disclosures, and criminal charges may result.

Many therapists are hesitant to engage in treatment, especially with a client judged to be dangerous or difficult to treat. They may fear an allegation that they have failed to treat the person properly and face the threat of lawsuit by a future victim if their client re-offends.

The therapist owes a number of loyalties, primarily to the client and the legal system, but also to the public, to his or her own institution, and others. These obligations will often come into conflict and managing such dual agency or multiple agency situations can be ethically challenging.

Mental health practitioners have traditionally been relied upon to make assessments or predictions about a sexual offender's danger to the community. Such assessments have serious limitations, although some predictors have been shown to be at least somewhat reliable. These include deviant sexual preferences, prior sexual offences, marital status, age, and failure to complete a previous course of treatment.

There is some reluctance on the part of agencies to offer treatment to sexual offenders with developmental disabilities or to train therapists in the techniques of assessment and treatment. This may be due to the belief that there are no effective treatments for these offenders. However, this population is in need of treatment both for their own sake and for public safety. While more research is needed to develop and test a variety of potential treatments, some effective treatments exist and ought to be used.

In Chapter 12, Richards, Watson, and Bleich survey ethical issues involved when persons with developmental disabilities become the victim or the perpetrator of a sexual offence. They urge that incidents of abuse by or against persons with developmental disabilities be reported in the same way as such offences involving non-disabled persons. The failure to report raises particular problems because those who victimize persons with developmental disabilities are likely to repeat the offence if not apprehended and persons with developmental disabilities who abuse are likely to continue to victimize others so long as they remain untreated.

There are a number of reasons for the low rate of reporting of crimes against persons with developmental disabilities:

- Police officers and court officials typically possess little knowledge of persons with developmental disabilities and may harbour negative sentiments towards them. This can result in allegations of abuse being discounted and such reports thereby discouraged.

- It may be determined that the victim is too young, or is otherwise unable to give reliable evidence in court, often arising from a belief that the memories of persons with developmental disabilities are inherently defective, or that they are prone to suggestibility.
- The victim may fear disruption in their current residential placement, or feels intimidated by the abuser and wishes not to draw attention to the abuse.
- Staff members may be hesitant to report abuse either in fear of retaliation by colleagues or administrators, or because they believe no action will be taken.
- Administrators of agencies may fear lawsuit or adverse publicity if a report is made.
- Caregivers may seek to protect victims from the potentially painful emotional experiences inherent in reporting and prosecuting incidents of abuse.

The reasons for under-reporting of crimes alleged to be perpetrated by persons with developmental disabilities are less clear. However, the authors speculate that there is some hesitation to characterize sexually abusive behaviour by such persons as criminal. Responsible persons may also believe that such persons would anyway be found unfit to stand trial or not criminally responsible by reason of mental disorder. If so, prosecution of offenders may seem pointless if offenders will simply be re-institutionalized for treatment in a similar setting.

Once in the system, persons with developmental disabilities charged with or suspected of committing sexual offences face a number of particular problems. Because of their impairments, some individuals may confuse their thoughts with their actions and report sexual fantasies as if they actually occurred.

In addition, they may be more suggestible and compliant to authority than others accused. Persons with developmental disabilities will tend to confess to crimes more readily. There are fewer plea bargains and appeals of conviction when such persons are accused. Interestingly, persons with developmental disabilities are also granted probation and parole less frequently. Often, such offenders do not have access to treatment for the offending behaviour. If so, they are more likely to commit similar offences in future. Offenders with developmental disabilities in the prison system are particularly vulnerable and at greater risk of being physically or sexually abused than others.

The authors make a number of recommendations. Primarily, notwithstanding these problems, suspected sexual offences should always be reported. Police and others in the criminal justice system must be sensitive to the special needs of victims with developmental disabilities to ensure that the criminal justice process does not further victimize them. Introduction of the developmentally disabled offender to the criminal justice system serves to enforce accountability for the misbehaviour and may enhance treatment participation and compliance. If the person with developmental disability is arrested and charged, he or she must be assured that legal rights are explained and will be respected, and that the particular problems and vulnerabilities arising from their disability are sensitively addressed.

Summary

This volume opened with the story of Jason, a kind-hearted, soft-spoken, 27-year-old man with a moderate degree of developmental disability. The question was asked, how do we deal fairly and sensitively with Jason's need for sexual connection and intimacy while acknowledging his particular vulnerabilities? Consistent with his own safety and that of others, surely we owe Jason the same freedoms and opportunities enjoyed by others in society. To the extent Jason is capable of exercising reasonable judgement, he should be permitted, indeed encouraged, to do so. While his impairments may sometimes necessitate imposing restrictions, these must always be reasonably related to the prevention of significant harms and no greater than required for such protection.

Jason is entitled to live in an environment that is as safe from abuse and exploitation as possible, and to education to help him avoid being abused. If he does become a victim of abuse, he is entitled to the same treatment as other victims, including counselling and support. If Jason should himself engage in abusive behaviour, he should be confined as necessary to deter future abuse, but also treated to ensure that such an offence is not repeated.

Jason's impairments impose an obligation to help and support in exercising liberty and accessing as many opportunities as possible. This means providing Jason with assistance and education to understand the ways of intimate relationships and ensure that he and intimate others are safe in their sexual expression. It also requires an acknowledgment that for Jason, sexual activity may not be simply a physical act, but is almost certainly an expression of his care for, and desire for intimacy with another human being.

References

Hingsburger, D., Griffiths, D., & Quinsey, V. (1991). Detecting counterfeit deviance: Differentiating sexual deviance from sexual inappropriateness.   *The Habilitative Mental Healthcare Newsletter, 9*, 51-54.

Appendix A

Contributors

Kimberly Arbus-Nevestuk, M.A.

Kim is completing a Doctorate in Clinical Psychology at the Chicago School of Professional Psychology. Kim has worked with children and adolescents who have a dual diagnosis. She currently works with children who have psychiatric disorders in Chicago, Illinois.

Randy Bleich

Randy is a Staff Sergeant for the Niagara Regional Police in Ontario, Canada, with extensive experience in child abuse and sexual assault. Randy's special interest in working with agencies and develop protocols and standards has been a positive step within the legal system for individuals who have developmental disabilities.

Eli Coleman, Ph.D.

Eli is the founding and current editor of the Journal of Psychology of Human Sexuality, is one of the past presidents of the Society for the Scientific Study of Sex (SSSS), and is the current President of the World Congress of Sexology. Dr. Coleman is the Director of the Program in Human Sexuality, Department of Family Practice and Community Health, University of Minnesota Medical School in Minneapolis, Minnesota. He is the author of numerous articles on the topics of sexuality.

Diane Cox-Lindenbaum, A.C.S.W., M.S.W.

Diane is a psychotherapist and clinical consultant specializing in training and abuse focused treatment for children, adolescents and adults with developmental disabilities and their families. Diane founded the first Mental Health Clinic in New York State specifically for persons with developmental disabilities. She is an original NADD board member and is currently on the Executive board of NADD. She is a Diplomat in Forensic Counselling.

Suzanne Curnoe, B.A.

Suzanne is on staff with Juniper Associates in Toronto, Ontario. She is presently involved in a twenty five year follow-up study of sex offender recidivism. Suzanne has an extensive background in working with families and children.

Gordon DuVal, S.J.D.

Gordon is a Lawyer and Bioethicist at the University of Toronto Joint Centre for Bioethics and the Centre for Addiction and Mental Health. Dr. DuVal has a Master's degree in moral philosophy and a doctorate in law and bioethics. He has been a Fellow at the University of Chicago MacLean Center for Clinical Medical Ethics and at the National Institutes of Health Department of Clinical Bioethics.

Len Dykstra, M.S.W.

Len currently wears several hats, including Psychotherapist in private practice, Education Co-ordinator serving individuals who have brain injuries, and mutual support groups in multidisciplinary structures for individuals who have developmental disabilities. His affiliation with the Habilitative Mental Health Resource Network brings another dimension to his knowledge.

Beverley Fedoroff, R.P.N., B.S.

Beverley is a Forensic Psychiatric Nurse with experience in the assessment and management of individuals with mental illness or developmental disability who are before the courts.

Paul Fedoroff, M.D., F.R.C.P (C)

Paul is Co-Director of the Sexual Behaviours Clinic, Forensic Program, at the Royal Ottawa Hospital in Ottawa, Ontario. He is also the Associate Professor of Psychiatry at the University of Ottawa. His involvement with individuals who have developmental disabilities has been widespread. This has included research and a treatment program for people who have developmental disabilities, over the past several years in Ontario, Canada.

Maurice Feldman, Ph.D.

Maurice is renowned for his primary research in the area of parenting skills for parents who have developmental disabilities. Maurice is a Behavioural Therapist and is affiliated with Queen's University and Ongwanada Hospital in Kingston, Ontario.

Marc Goldman, M.S.

Marc has diversified experience in the field of developmental disabilities and mental illness. He has designed and supervised treatment programs for individuals with challenging sexual behaviour. Marc has spoken internationally on topics surrounding treatment designs and forensic psychology. Marc is also a Board member for the NADD Board of Directors.

Dorothy M. Griffiths, Ph.D.

Dorothy is a Professor at Brock University in St. Catharines, Ontario. She is known for her extensive writing and lecturing on developmental disabilities and behaviours that challenge the system, in particular sexuality.

Robert King, M.D., F.R.C.P. (C)

Bob is currently a Consulting Psychiatrist with the Developmental Disabilities Program of the North Bay Psychiatric Hospital in North Bay, Ontario. He lectures in the area of developmental disabilities and mental health issues, and is the recipient of the 1998 Robert D. Sovner Memorial Essay Award.

Ron Langevin, Ph.D.

Ron is an Associate Professor at the University of Toronto and is in private practice. He has been involved in research, assessment, and treatment of sexual and violent offenders for over 30 years. He has a special interest in the biological and psychological factors in sexual behaviours.

Louis Lindenbaum, Ed.D.

Lou has a doctorate in counselling psychology and is a licensed Psychologist in the states of New York and Connecticut. Louis Lindenbaum is an original NADD board member and is currently holding the position of President. He is also the Associate Executive Director of the Resource Centre for Developmental Disabilities in New York and speaks internationally on people who have developmental disabilities.

William Molloy, M.D., F.R.C.P (C)

Willie is the Director of the Memory Clinic and the Geriatric Research Group at the Hamilton Health Sciences Corporation, as well as Associate Professor of Medicine and Director of Research in the Division of Geriatric Medicine at McMaster University in Hamilton, Ontario.

Orson Morrison, M.A.

Orson is a doctoral student of clinical psychology at the Chicago School of Professional Psychology in Chicago, Illinois. Orson is committed to a variety of research interests particularly those relating to cross-cultural and multi-cultural issues in mental health treatment.

Frances Owen, Ph.D.

Fran is an Associate Professor at Brock University in St. Catharines, Ontario. Fran is a registered psychologist in Ontario and Quebec and the former Director of Niagara Region Behaviour Management. She has worked as a psychologist in schools and community service agencies. Her research interests are currently involving systems and sexual abuse with individuals who have developmental disabilities.

Cheryl Peever

Cheryl is in the school of Social Work at the University of Toronto. Together, with Dr. Paul Fedoroff she has conducted research on the assessment and management of sexual disorders.

Meg Reich, R.N.

Meg is a Registered Nurse and is presently managing the Windsor Essex Geriatric Assessment/Consultation Program in Windsor, Ontario. She has a varied clinical background, including emergency, surgical, long-term care, and public health.

Debbie Richards

Debbie is the Senior Resource Advisor for the Welland District Association for Community Living in Welland, Ontario. She has specialized expertise and interest in the area of sexuality and developmental disability. She has spoken to various groups on issues relating to sex education, sexual abuse prevention, along with training the trainer models which have included conferences, workshops, and educational settings.

Stacey Sheehan, L.L.B.

Stacey is the Designated Child Abuse Specialist for the judicial district of Niagara North in St. Catharines, Ontario. Prosecuting offenses of sexual assault, child sexual assault, and physician/patient sexual assault has led to a unique perspective on the start and subtle issues surrounding consent for sexual interaction. She is a well respected prosecutor who has supported individuals who have developmental disabilities.

Thomas Venema, M.S.W.

Thomas is a Psychotherapist in a well established private practice in St. Catharines, Ontario, with specialized training in cognitive therapy and sexual abuse. He serves as consultant to several agencies that serve individuals with developmental disabilities.

Shelley L. Watson, M.Ed.

Shelley's primary research interests are in the field of sexuality and developmental disability, as well as dual diagnosis. She has been involved in research and projects that include assessment, sexual abuse prevention and social/sexual education. Shelley is currently a doctoral student of Educational Psychology at the University of Alberta.

Appendix B

Consensus Group Leaders and Assistants

Human Rights
Group Leader: Thomas Venema
Assistant: Leslie Monger

Sexual Policies and Procedures
Group Leaders: Dorothy Griffiths & Frances Owen
Assistant: Kimberly Arbus

Treatment Issues for Sexual Offending Behaviour
Group Leader: Ron Langevin
Assistant: Amanda Oosterveer

Sexual Abuse
Group Leader: Diane Cox- Lindenbaum
Assistant: Juli Goldhawk

Sexual Policies and Procedures
Group Leaders: Frances Owen & Dorothy Griffiths
Assistant: Orson Morrison

Sex Education
Group Leader: Michael Barrett
Assistant: Melanie McClury

Masturbation
Group Leader: Keith Anderson
Assistant: Julie Koudys

Parents Who Have Developmental Disabilities Group
Leader: Maurice Feldman
Assistant: Kathy Tweedy

Sexually Transmitted Diseases
Group Leader: Susan Ludwig
Assistant: Melanie McClury

Sexual Relationships
Group Leader: Louis Lindenbaum
Assistant: Melanie Dawn

Spirituality, Sexuality, and Developmental Disabilities
Group Leader: Barry Hollowell
Assistant: Beverley Moran

Consent for Sexual Interaction
Group Leader: Stacey Sheehan
Assistant: Amanda Oosterveer

Inappropriate Sexual Behaviour
Group Leader: Marc Goldman
Assistant: Orson Morrison

Birth Control and Sterilization
Group Leader: John Martin Ellison
Assistant: Julie Koudys

Personal Responsibility and Sexuality
Group Leader: Len Dykstra
Assistant: Kathy Tweedy

Sexual Offenses and the Legal System
Group Leader: Patricia Clements
Assistant: Shelley Watson

Human Rights
Group Leaders: Sharon Bural & Meg Reich
Assistant: Rose Scott

Gender Identity and Sexual Orientation
Group Leader: Eli Coleman
Assistant: Kimberly Arbus

Consent to Treatment
Group Leader: Paul Fedoroff
Assistant: Beverley Moran

Guardianship
Group Leader: Patti Bregman
Assistant: Ingrid Zastrow

Appendix C

Conference Participants

JoAnne Aarts
Melissa Abrahams
Gina Aiello
Keith Anderson
Kim Arbus
Lisa Arthur
Phyllis Baines
Shari Ball
Ann Barrett
Michael Barrett
Joyce Bax
Elsie Belanger
Sue Benko
Sue Bessems
Jillaine Bieda
Carolyn Bielby
Sharol Bilodeau
Randy Bleich
Diana Boot
James Borysko
Heather Bozik
Patti Bregman
Cathy Bruce

Sharon Bural
Kathryn Burton
Lori Button
Sandy Calvert
Cindy Carl
Debra Cassidy
Jean Paul Caza
Karen Chartier
Theresa Chubak
Liz Clarke
Patricia Clements
Eli Coleman
Cindy Connors
Suzanne Coomber
Lynn Costabile
Diane Cox-Lindenbaum
Nancy Jo Cressy
Lesley Cross
Suzanne Curnoe
Melanie Dawn
Michelle Della Ventura
Patricia Deprima
Mark Dickie

Teresa Donaldson
Maria Douglas
Len Dykstra
Erinne Edwards
John Martin Ellison
Kristine Ericson
Wendy Faragalli
Paul Fedoroff
Maurice Feldman
Neil Flindall
Kevin Forrest
Tom Francey
Thom Gall
Jean Gilmour
Juli Goldhawk
Marc Goldman
Jeff Goss
Cathie Green
Nelly Green
Dorothy Griffiths
Robert Grimes
Dianne Grummett
Lois Hanes
Lani Harris
Barbara Hawke
Cathy Higham
Lesley Hiscoe
Bill Hlywka
Barry Hollowell
Cathy Huson
Donna Janzen
Paul Keary
Carol Ann Keighan

Beth Kent
Sandy Kish
Roslyn Kocot
Julie Koudys
Tracey Krysa
Paul Kyte
LeeAnne Lamarche
Diana Landwehr
Ron Langevin
Andy Lapointe
Carol Lawley
John Lee
Tracy Lehman
Debbe Liddycoat
Louis Lindenbaum
Sue Lindsay
Alexander Livingstone
Susan Ludwig
Cosmo Mannella
Whilhelmine Mason
Dwayne McClentic
Melanie McClury
Lana McKague
Diane McLean
Lynette Meecham
David Middleton
Linda Middleton
Ken Miles
Helen Millar
Leslie Monger
Durene Monz
Michael Moore
Beverley Moran